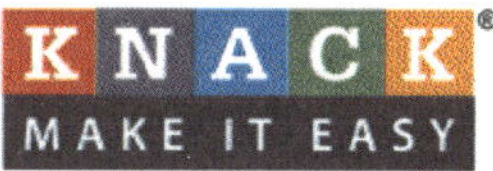

DIABETES
COOKBOOK

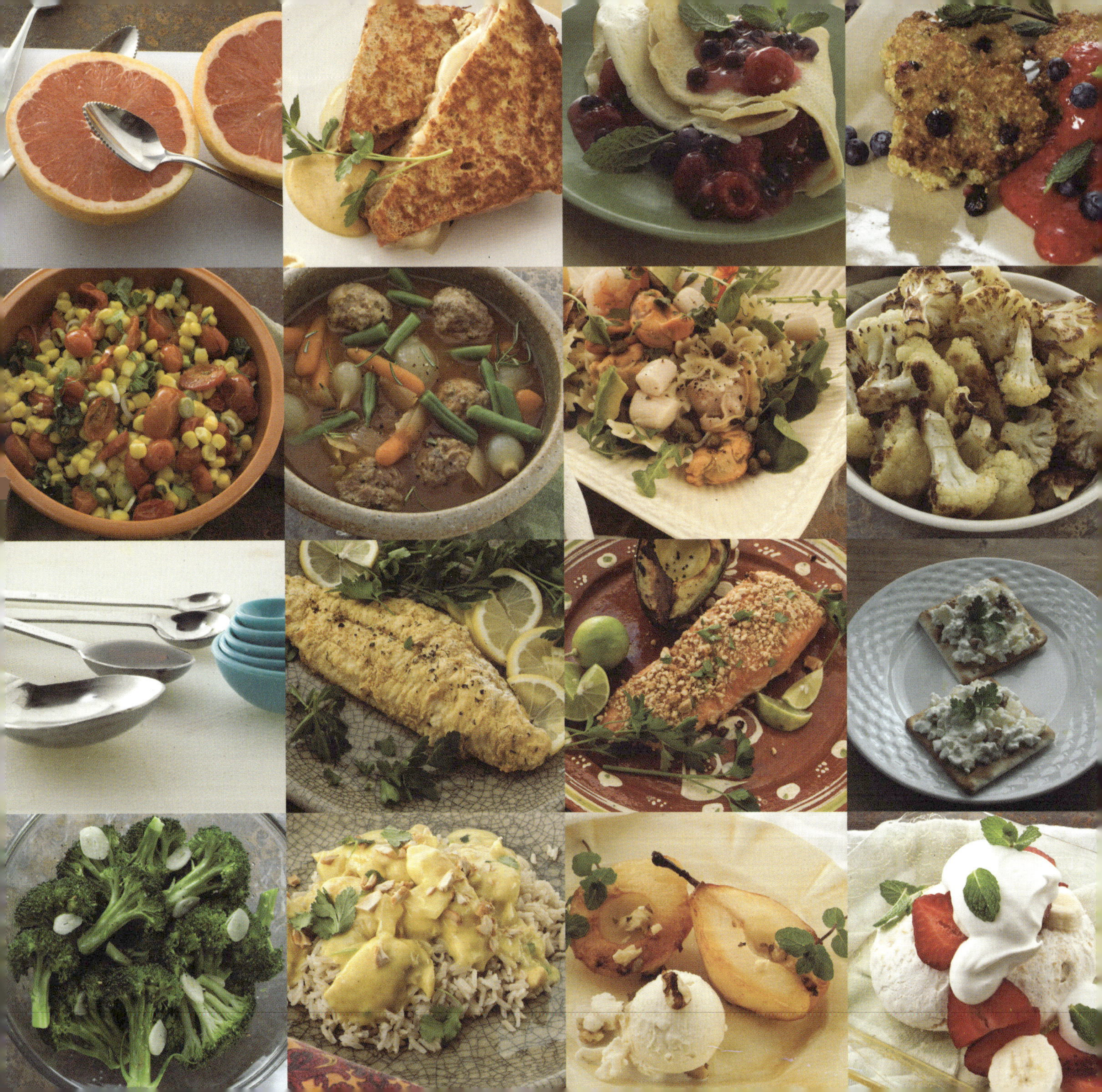

KNACK®

DIABETES
COOKBOOK

A step-by-step guide to delicious, healthy meals

NANCY MAAR

Technical Review by Nancy Held, M.S., R.D., C.D.E.
Nutritional Information by Jean Kostak, M.S., R.D., C.D.E.

Photographs by Viktor Budnik

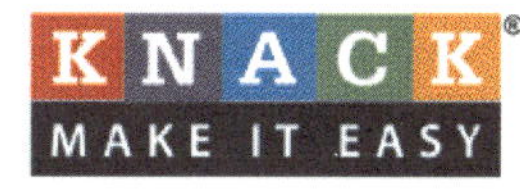

Guilford, Connecticut
An imprint of The Globe Pequot Press

Editor in Chief: Maureen Graney
Editor: Katie Benoit
Text Design: Paul Beatrice
Layout: Maggie Peterson
Cover photos by Viktor Budnik except back cover, far left: © Monkey Business | Dreamstime.com; front cover, far left: © Rorydaniel | Dreamstime.com

All interior photos by Viktor Budnik with the exception of p. 16 (left): jirkaejc/shutterstock; p. 18 (left): © Gsermek | Dreamstime.com; p. 18 (right): Kerry Garvey/shutterstock; p. 19 (left): Shutterstock; p. 19 (right): © Vladmax | Dreamstime.com; p. 22 (right): Jo Williams; p. 29 (left): © Alamy; p. 34 (left): © Monkeybusiness | Dreamstime. com; p. 34 (right): © Dreamstime.com; p. 35 (left): © Josefbosak Dreamstime.com; p. 35 (right): © Jjphotos | Dreamstime.com; p. 93 (right): © Ever Dreamstime.com; p. 97 (left): © Rorydaniel | Dreamstime.com p. 101 (right): sjeacle/shutterstock; p. 137 (left): Milos Luzanin/shutterstock; p. 155 (right) Jane Rix/shutterstock; p. 183 (left): Jo Williams; p. 190: Jo Williams.

CIP DATA: A catalogue record for this book is available from the British Library.

ISBN 978-0-7627-5925-5

Globe Pequot Press International
Footprint Handbooks
6 Riverside Court
Lower Bristol Road
Bath
BA2 3DZ
UK
T+44(0)1225 469141
F+44(0)1225 469461

The following manufacturers/names appearing in Knack Diabetes Cookbook are trademarks:
Colman's
Pyrex
Splenda
Tabasco

The information in this book is true and complete to the best of our knowledge. All recommendations are made without guarantee on the part of the author or The Globe Pequot Press. The author and The Globe Pequot Press disclaim any liability in connection with the use of this information.

Printed in India by Replika Press Pvt Ltd

About the author

Nancy Maar has written five previous cookbooks, including *The Everything Sugar-Free Cookbook*, *The Glycemic Index Cookbook*, and *The Gluten-Free Cookbook*. A resident of Norwalk, Connecticut, she writes restaurant profiles for *Norwalk Plus* and *Stamford Plus* magazines.

CONTENTS

INTRODUCTION

Healthy Cooking: An Introduction

Healthy cooking is not about depriving yourself of the foods you love, but rather about adopting a health-conscious lifestyle that allows you to cook the foods you love and crave, but with fresh, healthier ingredients and a greater understanding of your fundamental nutritional needs. Healthy cooking is a lifestyle decision, and one that can be made with relative ease by following some of the quick tips provided throughout this book, including buying fresh foods locally, occasionally using salt and sugar substitutes, and being mindful of what you are eating.

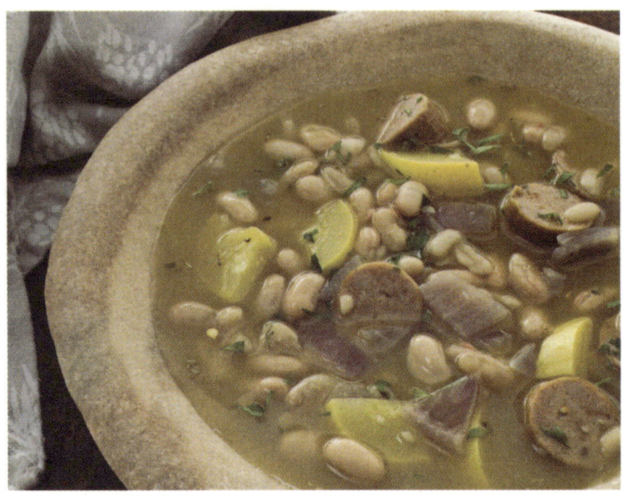

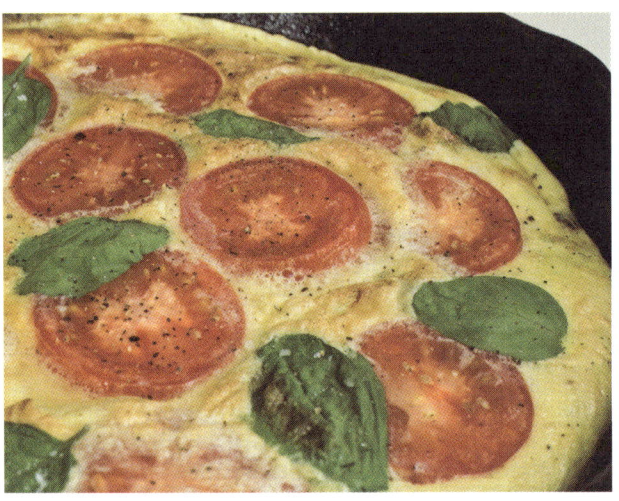

The *Knack Diabetes Cookbook* provides you with healthy, balanced, mouth-watering recipes for every meal of the day, whether it's savoury stuffed French toast for breakfast, a warm lentil salad for lunch or a Mediterranean rice and seafood dish for a hearty dinner. Being healthy does not mean compromising on taste; in fact, by using fresh ingredients, taste is often enhanced.

For someone with diabetes, the most important thing to consider is downsizing portions. You can eat a wide variety of foods and still maintain good blood sugar control by eating lots of fresh fruit and vegetables, whole grains, lean meat, fish and poultry. 'All in moderation' is a good motto to follow when planning your meals for the week.

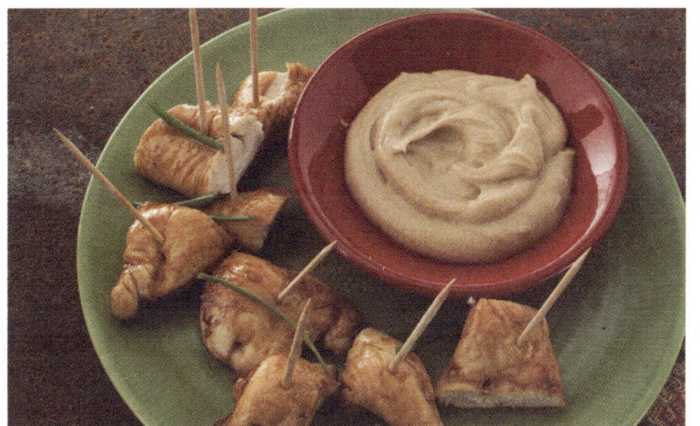

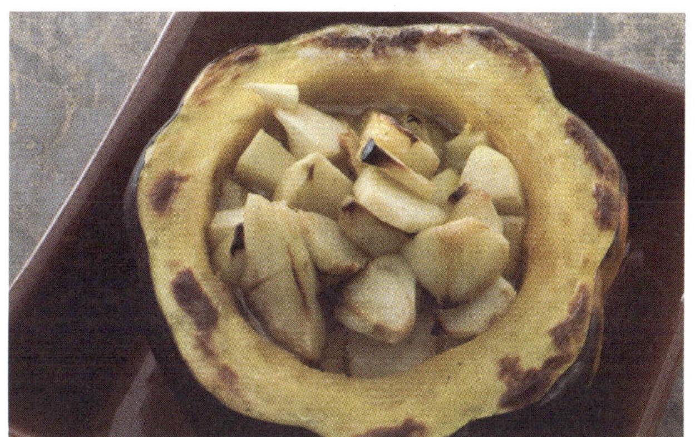

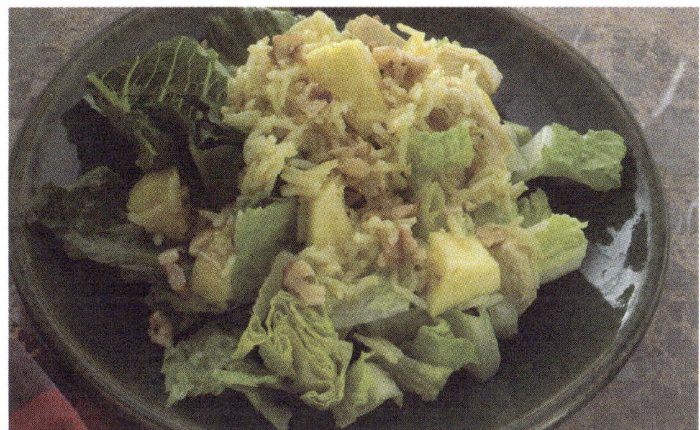

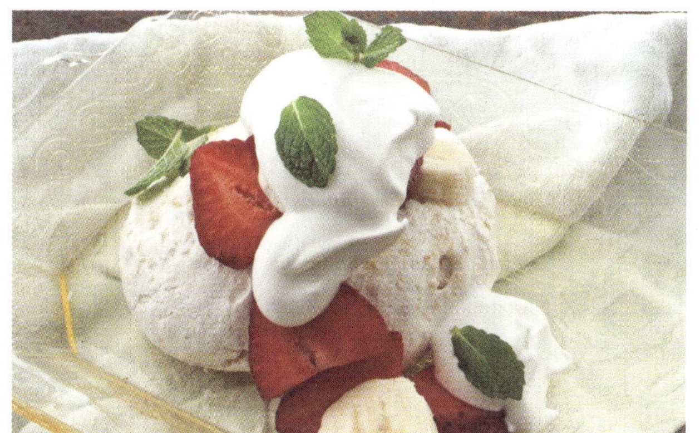

This cookbook also helps you stock your kitchen and store cupboard, providing information on the essential equipment and food items you need to create balanced, delicious meals for yourself and the ones you love. Included are wonderful recipes for homemade ketchup, mustard, vinaigrette and other dressings and sauces, which are perfect for finishing touches on a grilled vegetable salad or a pistachio and pepper steak.

In a short time, you'll find you can indulge your cravings and feed your family – and yourself – with healthy meals that are good for both the soul and the body. So please flip through these pages and be inspired.

Healthy Eating: A Diabetes Educator's Perspective

What does healthy eating mean for someone with diabetes? It is essentially the same as for anyone without diabetes but with attention to specific issues. Healthy eating is the first priority for people with diabetes. This means a diet with high-quality carbohydrates and fibre, low in saturated fat and calorically appropriate to lose or maintain weight. Controlling carbohydrate intake and monitoring blood sugar can go a long way to achieving glucose control.

Carbohydrate is the nutrient that affects blood sugar the most, compared to other dietary components. Foods that contain carbohydrates are potatoes, bread, cereals, pasta and

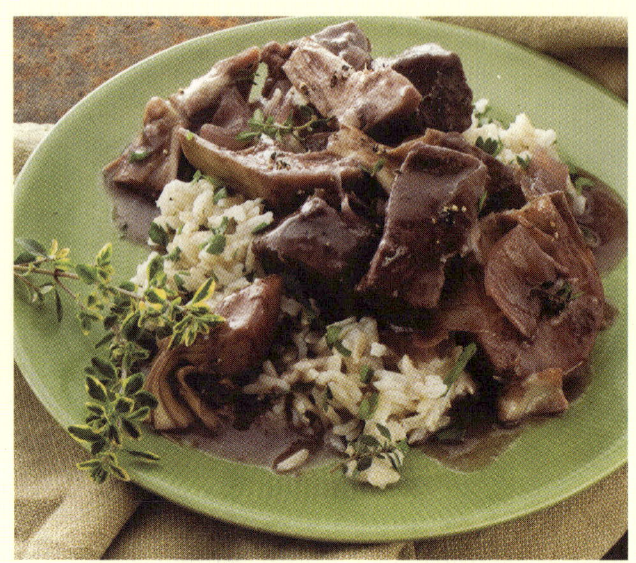

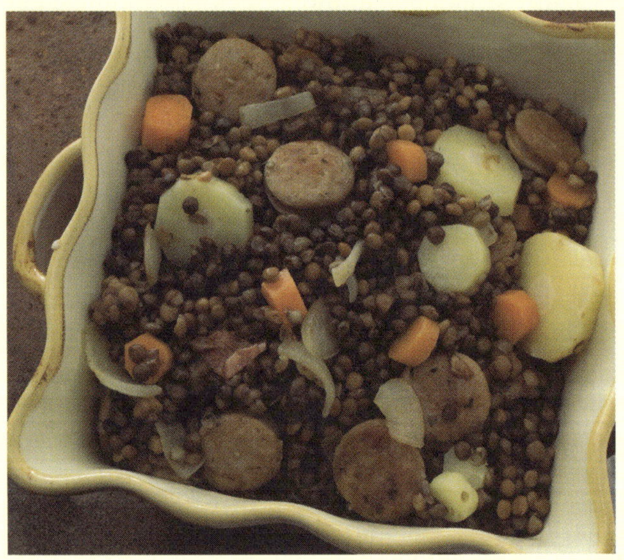

starchy vegetables such as peas and sweetcorn. Milk, yogurt and fruit also contain carbs. Vegetables have them but in small amounts. Fibre is a carbohydrate but affects the blood sugar less than starch and sugar. Monitoring blood sugars with a home blood glucose meter is critical to effective diabetes self-management. Observing how food, activity and other factors affect blood sugar assists in making changes.

Carbohydrate counting is a helpful tool in controlling blood sugar and can also help reduce caloric intake. In basic carb counting, one learns how much carbohydrate is in each food and the amount to eat for meals and snacks. Those on rapid-acting insulin can adjust the insulin depending on the amount of carbohydrate they have eaten. People with diabetes will be given guidelines by their dietician. For those who count carbs, I suggest that there may be 30 to 60 grams of carbohydrate in a meal and 15 to 30 grams in a snack. Of course, the grams in each meal depend on the overall amount in the meal plan and the caloric level desired.

The glycaemic index (GI) is a ranking of foods based on their effect on blood sugar levels. It is a measure of how quickly carbohydrate-containing foods raise the blood sugar. There are many factors that affect the GI, but generally foods that are less processed and have more fibre, such as vegetables, fruits, beans, whole grains, cereals and breads, produce a slower rise in blood sugar.

Since heart disease is one of the potential complications of diabetes, dietary factors that have an impact on

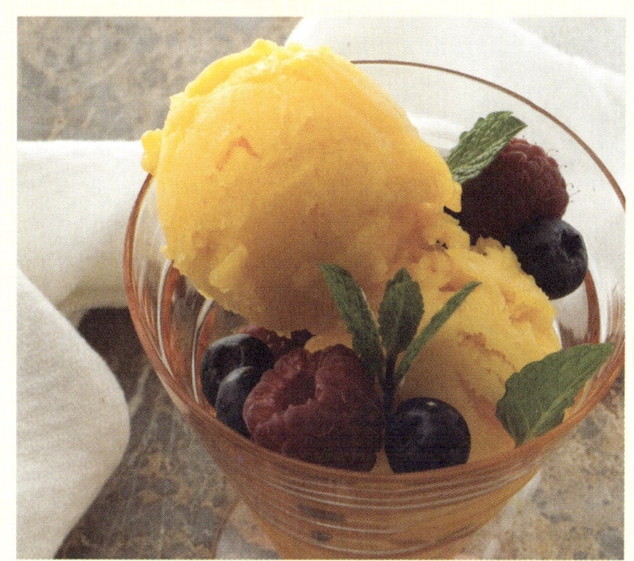

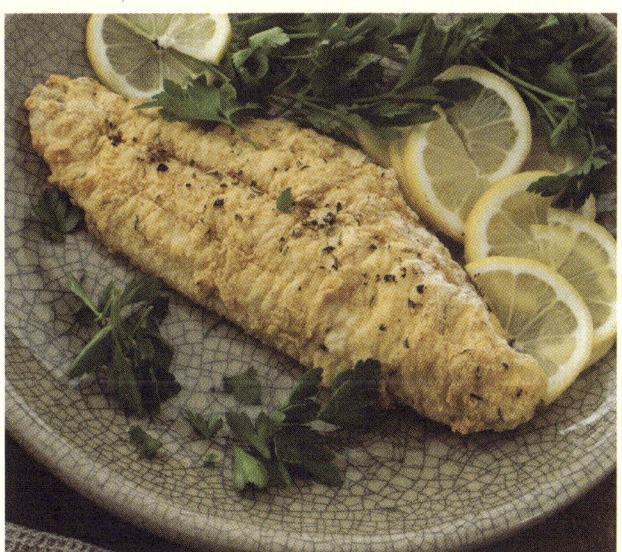

cardiovascular disease should be modified. Saturated and trans fats have the most adverse effect on blood fat levels. These include animal fats, as in high-fat meats and whole-milk dairy products such as butter and cream. The fats to choose are omega-3 fats (healthy fats found in foods such as salmon and other oily fish, walnuts and linseed) and mono-unsaturated fats (found in foods such as olive and canola oil, avocado, nuts and olives).

The key to successful diabetes control is learning how to self-manage – paying attention to blood sugar, making reasonable changes in food or lifestyle, and eating healthily to prevent or minimize diabetes complications.

Nancy Held, M.S., R.D., C.D.E.

FOODS FOR HEALTHY LIVING

Essential foods include fruit, vegetables, proteins and olive oil

To achieve a healthy diet, every kitchen should be stocked with a supply of healthy food: fruit, vegetables, proteins, olive oil and whole grains. It should exclude 'bad carbs' and fats. Bad carbohydrates are the foods that contain processed sugars and bleached flour. Butter, cream, whole milk and ice cream should be replaced by olive oil, skimmed milk and sugar-free sorbet.

The fruit in your diet may include any fresh, frozen, dried or canned fruit. If canned, it must be packed in water, not syrup. Vegetables include dried grains, beans and pulses as well as leafy and root vegetables. Green and yellow vegetables may be fresh, frozen or canned. Proteins include cheese, meat, fish, eggs, dairy, beans and pulses. Olive oil works well with vegetables. In addition, the human body

Fresh, Dried and Canned Fruit

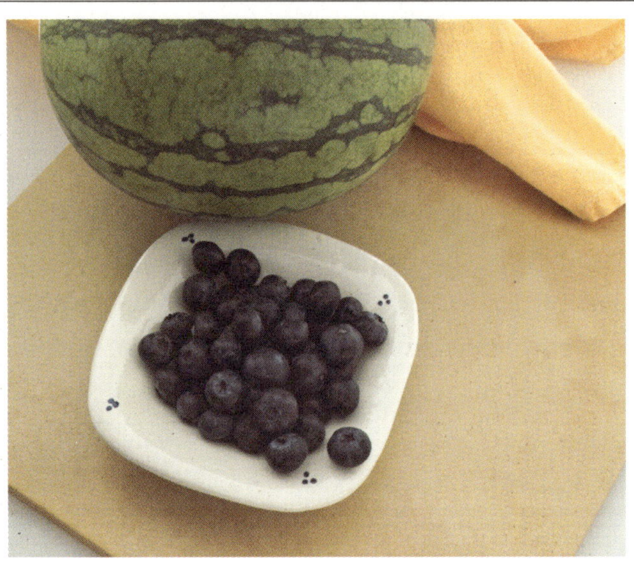

- Fresh fruit is the best to use in recipes and, when locally grown, will have spent the least amount of time in a refrigerator or on a train or lorry.

- Be exceptionally careful of canned fruits – even when they are packed in light syrup, they'll be loaded with sugar.

- Some frozen fruits are also packed in sugar.

- Dried fruits concentrate the natural sugars. However, the fibre helps to overcome the sugar content.

Vegetables and Grains

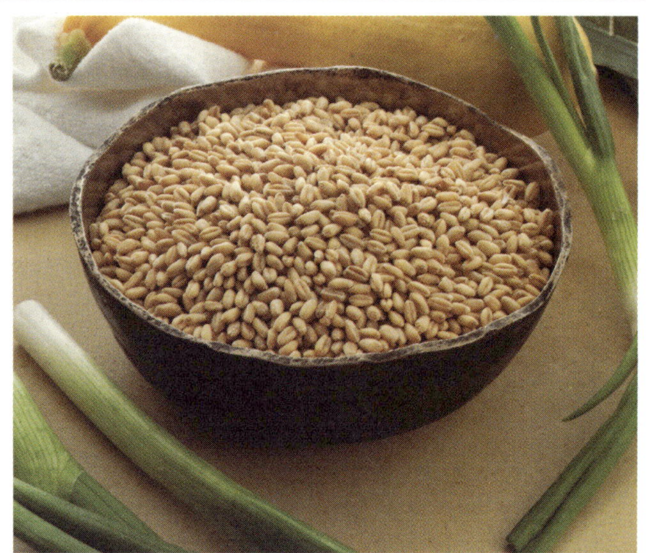

- Be careful of white, processed flour in breads and cereals. Always look for whole-grain breads, pastas and cereals.

- Yellow vegetables are important. Carrots, yellow courgettes and parsnips are good examples.

- Tubers, including potatoes, and root vegetables such as beetroot, parsnips and carrots, though sweet, are part of a healthy diet.

- Fill up on low-calorie 'good carb' like spinach, broccoli and cabbage for health.

needs some healthy carbs. Good carbs are less processed ones, as in whole grains, fibrous fruits and vegetables.

A healthy kitchen should also limit fats and not so healthy carbs. The carbs to avoid are the white ones, including processed flour, white sugar and any products made with them. Fats should be minimized in most cases, since they are so calorically dense. Even though certain oils actually heighten your good cholesterol, all fats and oils contain the same amount of calories. For example, one tablespoon of butter contains the same number of calories as one tablespoon of oil.

It's a good idea to freeze as much fresh summer fruit as possible to use in winter recipes. A peach pie in February, made from fruit that you've blanched, cut up and packed with lemon juice, can literally bring summer to the table even though it may be freezing outside.

Protein

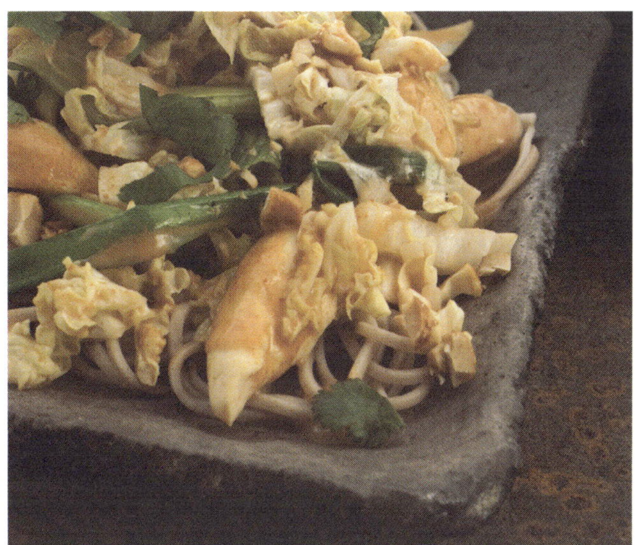

- Protein is a building block of strength and health. There are many forms of protein, from vegetable sources, such as beans and pulses, to low-fat milk, yogurt and cheese.

- Lean meats, such as chicken, turkey, veal and lamb, are good sources of protein. Just be sure to cut off all of the fat from the meat before cooking.

- Fish is an excellent source of lean protein.

- Some grains, such as quinoa, have a significant amount of protein.

Oil

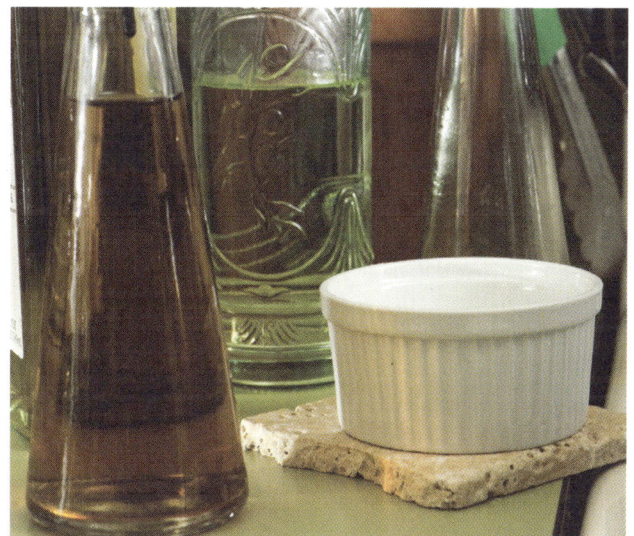

- When you must use fat, choose olive oil, canola oil and the oils from peanuts and various vegetables.

- Hydrogenated fats should be avoided. They stick to the arteries like glue.

- The process of hydrogenation makes oils solidify, so these fats will look and act more like butter, a saturated fat.

- Fats and oils from animals are very bad for arteries. Fried foods should be avoided, as should fatty meats, such as bacon, ham, sausages and some cold meats.

STOCKING YOUR STORE CUPBOARD

Have your favourite basics stored conveniently, and keep them well-organized for easy, speedy food preparation

Keep a basic range of food items to hand in your store cupboard. The shelves should be sensibly organized so you can easily find ingredients when cooking or see when you have run out of anything.

All foods that are not perishable can be kept in the cupboard. Sugar and flour need to be put in airtight containers to prevent them from attracting insect pests or going mouldy if it's damp. Dry items, such as pasta and rice in airtight containers, canned goods, and items in bottles can all go on the store cupboard shelves. Build up a collection of glass jars and biscuit tins in various sizes to hold biscuits, rice, pasta, beans and flour.

Baking Supplies

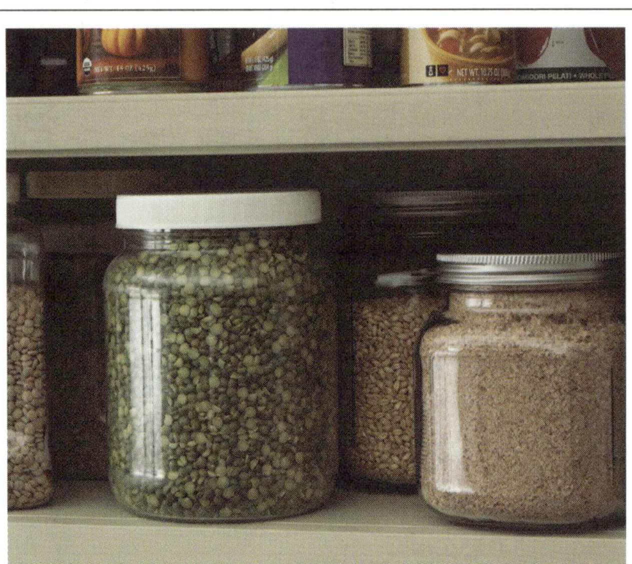

- Shelf organization is handy for keeping everything you need for one kitchen task together. If there is room to keep baking tins, pie dishes, baking sheets and muffin tins together, then do so.

- Keep flour, sugar, salt, bicarbonate of soda and baking powder in clearly labelled containers. Keep bottles of vanilla extract and other flavourings on hand, too.

- Keep your extra cake and scone mixes (if you use them) in this area.

- Rice, pasta and soup mixes should all be kept in the kitchen store cupboard.

Spices

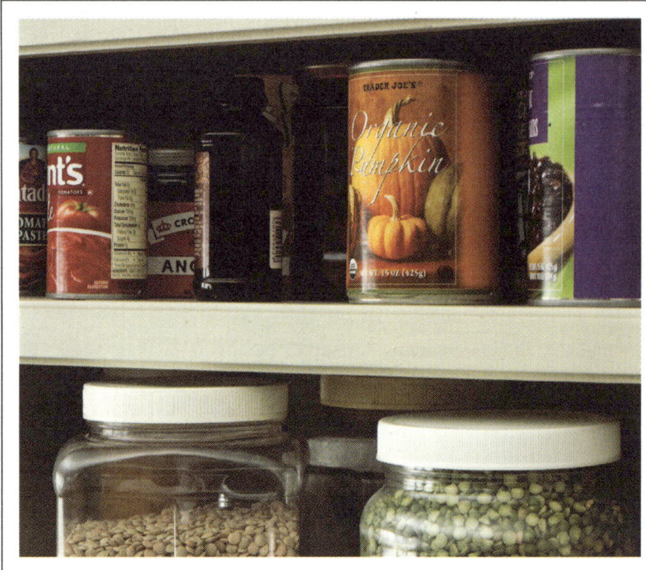

- Keep the flavourings and spices that go with your baking supplies on a shelf near them. These include vanilla and almond extract, cinnamon, nutmeg, whole cloves and ground cloves.

- Honey, maple syrup and salt substitute should be stored here as well.

- Keep packets of shelled nuts with the baking supplies.

Assemble all your baking supplies in one area. Include containers of flour, sugar, baking powder, large boxes of salt or salt substitute and bottles of vanilla and other flavourings.

Put dry pasta in another area, with canned tomatoes and tomato purée. Condiments that do not need refrigeration can also be stored in the cupboard, such as bottles of ketchup, Worcestershire sauce, hot sauce and so on. Herbs should be closer to the workspace, typically next to the stove.

Packets of ground coffee and tea, and jars of instant coffee can be stored on the shelves.

Canned Goods

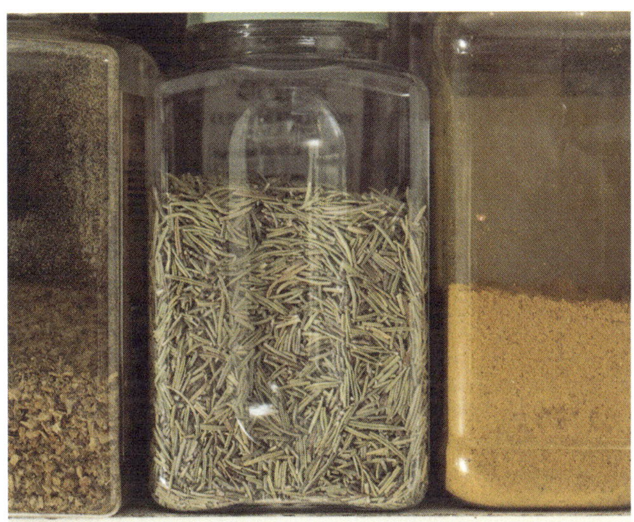

- Place all your dried fruits and nuts in airtight containers or resealable plastic bags.

- Keep canned fruits and fruit juices together, arranging the smaller tins at the front and the tall ones at the back so you can see what you have.

- Keep any canned vegetables together.

- Canned soup and dried beans and pulses for soup-making can all be put together.

Extra Containers

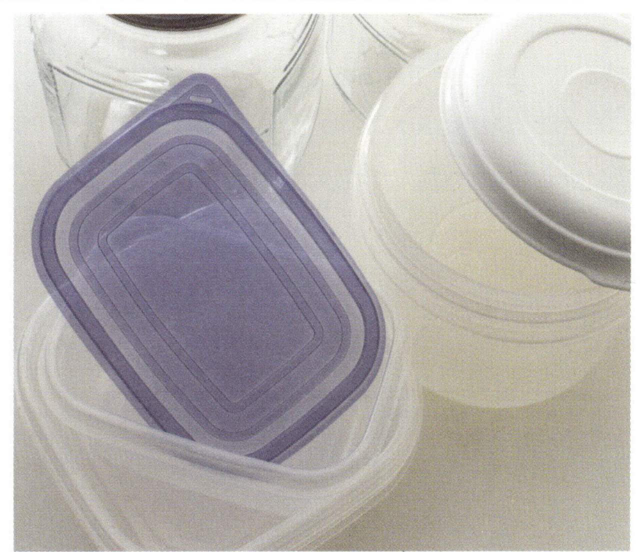

- It's good to have plenty of plastic containers of various sizes on hand.

- You will also need tins for open packets of biscuits and crackers.

- Kilner jars are good for holding open packets of tea and coffee.

THE REFRIGERATOR

Before electric refrigerators were invented, a few fortunate people had ice boxes stocked with natural ice, some of it shipped huge distances from Arctic regions, which was delivered by horse-drawn cart daily during the summer and every few days in winter. Housekeepers would put a sign for ice in the window, and the man with the cart would deliver it to the kitchen door. Thankfully, electric refrigerators came along in the 1920s, though many homes in Britain did not have one until the 1970s. What a blessing! With refrigerators, food stays fresher longer. Even so, when stocking your fridge, remember that local foods bought daily are the freshest.

A well-organized fridge is vital for any cook; it allows for items to be found more quickly and minimizes the chances that foods will go bad while sitting hidden in the back of the

Foods That Last One Day

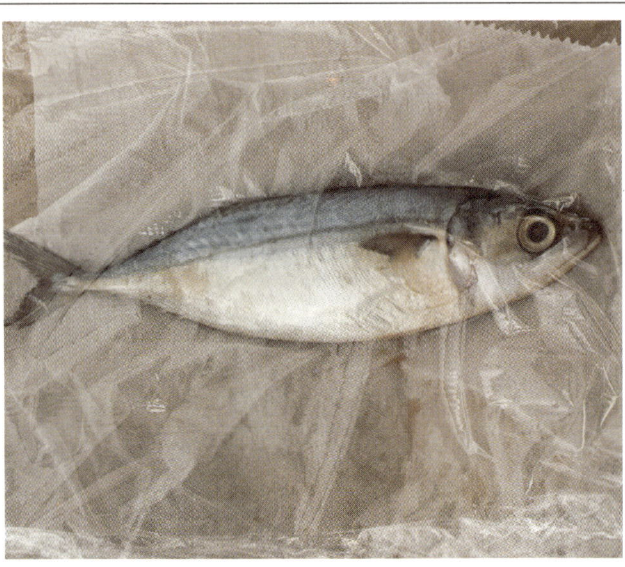

- Fresh fish (buy it the same day or the day before you plan to use it). Fresh or defrosted prawns, scallops, crab and lobster meat.

- Completely defrosted minced meat and chicken.

- Freshly picked ripe berries and cut up fruit (these will last overnight).

Foods That Last up to One Week

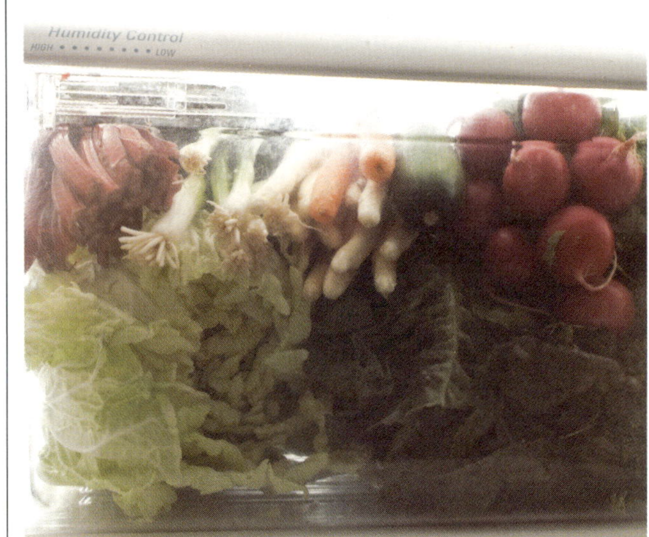

- The way vegetables are packaged dictates their fridge life. Some plastic bags keep soft vegetables fresh for up to a week.

- Fruits and vegetables that have been in the refrigerator for too long get limp, mouldy or gooey at the edges.

- Homemade soups and stews are good for a week. Soft fruit may last for a week if not ripe.

- All unpackaged foods should be labelled with the date you bought or made them. Bring older things to the front and use them as soon as you can.

fridge. Foods should be organized with like foods (all vegetables in crisper drawers, for example) and used in good time. All packaged food is labelled with expiration dates. Remember to check these regularly to make sure that you're using fresh foods. Foods that are past their best can make you and your family sick if they are eaten.

Keeping a running shopping list will also ensure that you never run out of a key ingredient just when you need it most. When you discover that you're running low on something, add it to your list for the next time you go shopping.

Keep your fridge clean: Wash it out every 2–3 months with a solution of washing-up liquid, white vinegar and 1 teaspoon of bicarbonate of soda to deodorize it. Remove the vegetable drawer; wash it thoroughly to clean away any mould. If there is mould in your refrigerator, you breathe the spores every time you open the door. If mould gets into your sinuses or lungs, it can make you very sick. Even a small refrigerator can harbour dangerous mould.

Foods That Last for One Month

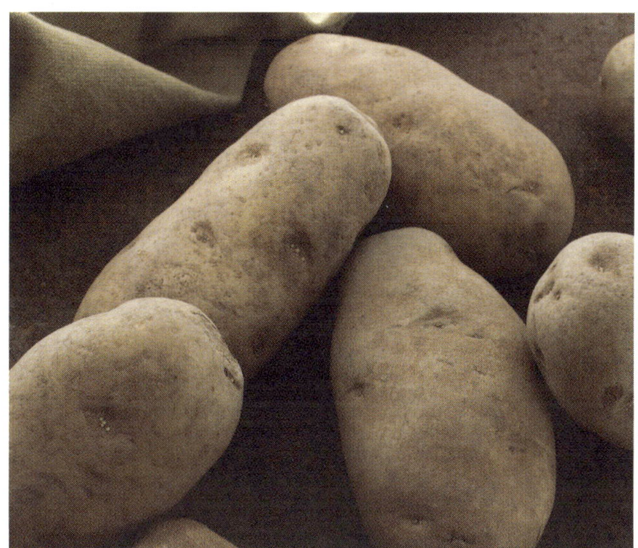

- Foods that last for one month include root vegetables, soups, stock and other well-packed and well-sealed items.

- Always look at the 'sell-by' dates on any packaged foods you buy that you plan to keep for a while.

- If you buy onions in a plastic bag, take them out of the bag; these bags are often moist inside and will contribute to spoilage.

- Check your refrigerator regularly for 'science projects' – things that have been pushed to the back and forgotten.

Keep Track of Foods

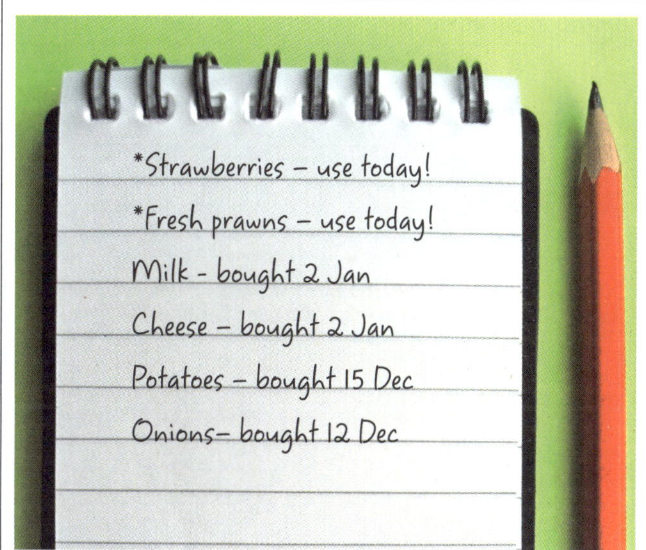

- List foods as you buy them.

- Star foods to be used right away.

- Cross off foods as you use them to add to next shopping list.

- Plan meals in advance to use up ingredients already in your refrigerator.

THE FREEZER

The freezer might be the greatest food storage tool since canning

Your freezer is a great place to store foods that you intend to use in the longer term.

Frozen items do not last forever; however, if you use a vacuum packer to freeze them, you'll find that they will last months longer than if you simply wrap them in plastic. The vacuum packer is especially good for individual servings of meat and fish, for example.

Liquids such as soups and stews, frozen fruits and tomatoes, should be stored in plastic containers with airtight lids. Chicken, beef and vegetable stocks are handy for soups, stews and sauces when frozen in 500-ml and 1-litre containers.

Freeze items such as peeled and grated fresh ginger by the tablespoonful in small bags. Lime and/or lemon juice can be frozen in ice cube trays and then stored in plastic bags.

Freezing Herbs

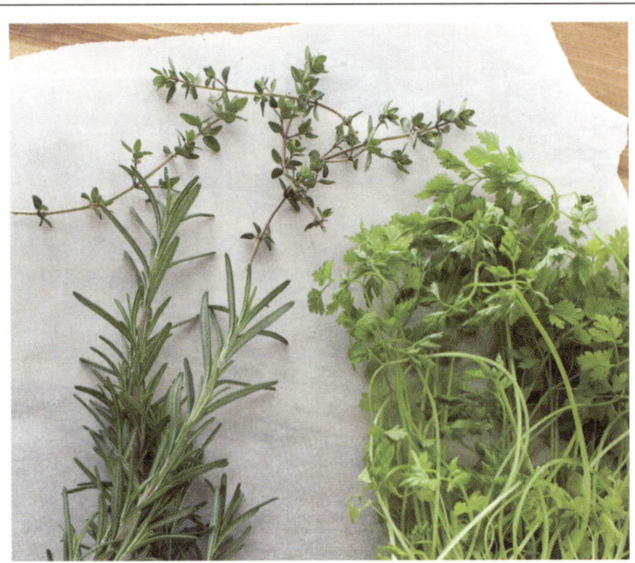

- To freeze fresh herbs, first rinse and dry them.

- When they are dry, line a baking sheet with baking parchment.

- Lay the herbs on the parchment and place in the freezer for 1 hour.

- Label plastic bags with the names of the herbs you are freezing. Place the herbs in the bags and keep frozen.

Freezing Berries

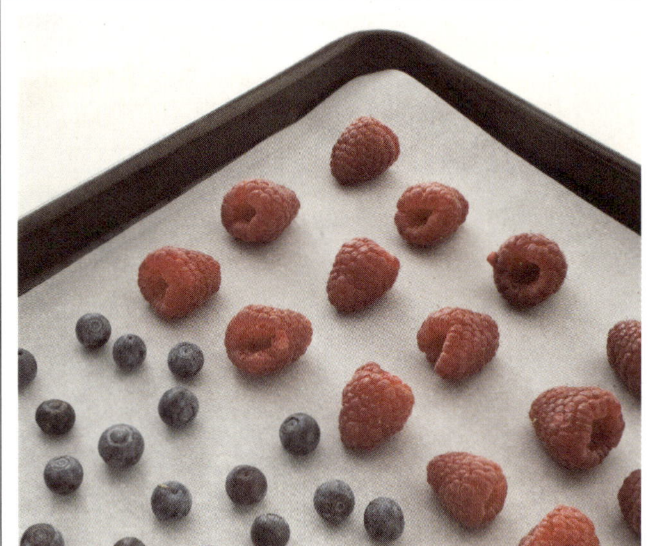

- Wash and dry ripe berries, leaving them whole; remove stems after washing or the juice will run out.

- Place a piece of baking parchment or aluminium foil on a baking sheet.

- Spread the berries on the sheet so they are not touching. Place in the freezer for at least 1 hour and no more than 3 hours.

- Put the frozen berries in plastic bags and return to the freezer for future use.

As with your refrigerator, organize like food items together so that they're easy to pull out and use. Also, label all foods with the date of freezing so that you know in which order you should use them.

There's nothing less appetizing than a piece of meat or fish that's been in the freezer for too long. Freezer burn is a drying out process that means it's too late to use the item as intended. In the case of steak or a roasting joint of meat, you might be able to stew it instead.

Freezing Tomatoes

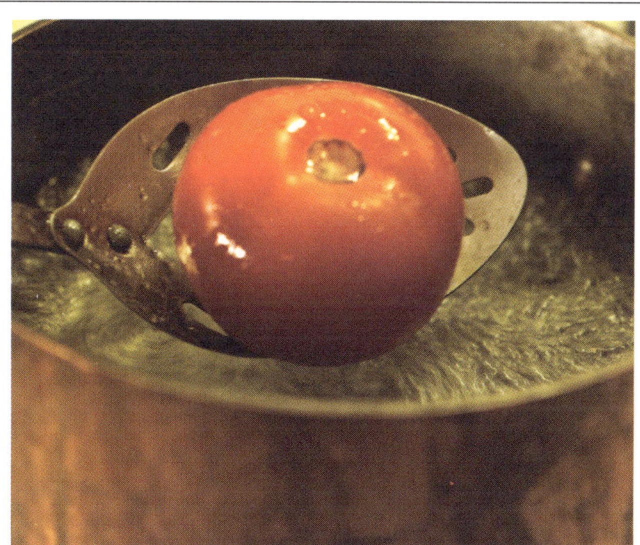

- Freeze tomatoes for soup, sauces or stews.

- Bring a saucepan of water to the boil. Place a colander in your sink.

- Blanch tomatoes by adding them to the boiling water a few at a time for 1–2 minutes, until skins split and are loosened. Place the tomatoes in the colander.

- Let them cool, then pull off skins. Cut tomatoes in quarters and place in plastic containers with about 1 teaspoon lemon juice as a preservative. Cool completely before freezing.

Freezing Peaches

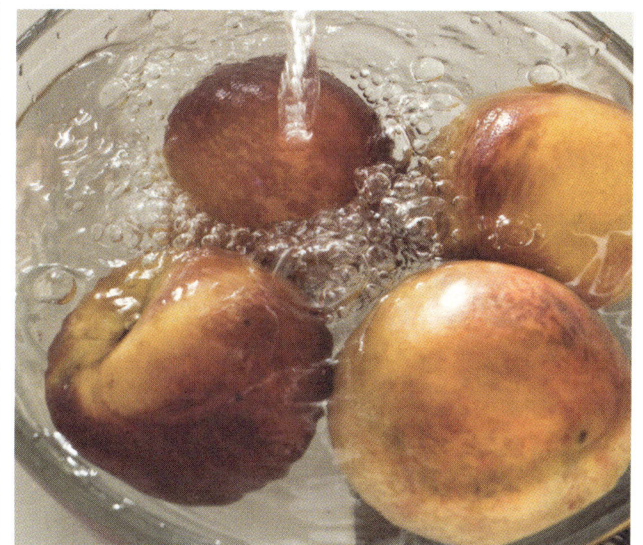

- Ensure that you'll have fresh pies, tarts and flans all winter.

- Bring a saucepan of water to the boil. Place a colander in the sink.

- Place a few peaches at a time in the boiling water for 1–2 minutes.

- Lift out peaches and place in the colander to drain and cool. When cool enough to handle, slip skins off and cut fruit in halves, removing the stones.

- Place halved peaches in a freezer container. Sprinkle each layer of fruit with fresh lemon juice. Cover; freeze.

FRESH FOODS

Chefs and good cooks agree: the fresher the food, the better

Fresh foods are always a good option when cooking a delicious meal. Fresh foods taste more vibrant than frozen options, and if they are grown locally cooking them supports the community.

Proper storage of fresh foods in your kitchen is paramount for ensuring the quality of the food. Place items you want to ripen, such as avocados and melons, on a sunny windowsill.

Conversely, if you want these items to ripen slowly, place them in a cool, dark area of your kitchen or in the refrigerator.

Most fresh foods need to be refrigerated. Even 'winter' vegetables keep longer when refrigerated. Salad greens are the most delicate. Cabbage, endive, chicory, kale, spinach, spring greens and mustard greens should never be left out at room temperature.

Using Fresh Fruit

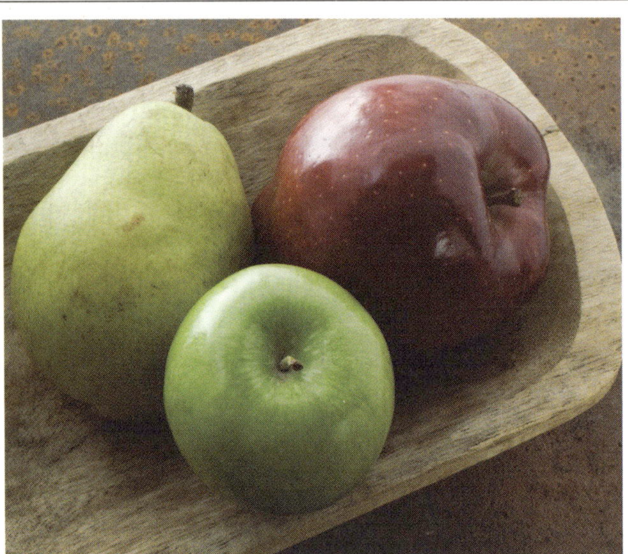

- Pears and apples do not have to be refrigerated if they are going to be used promptly. If you have a cool larder, place pears, apples and bananas there.

- Do not refrigerate bananas.

- Always wash fruit before eating or cooking it to remove any pesticides or germs.

- Don't wash fruit until just before you are ready to eat it. The moisture will hasten the rotting process.

Colourful, Nutritious Meals

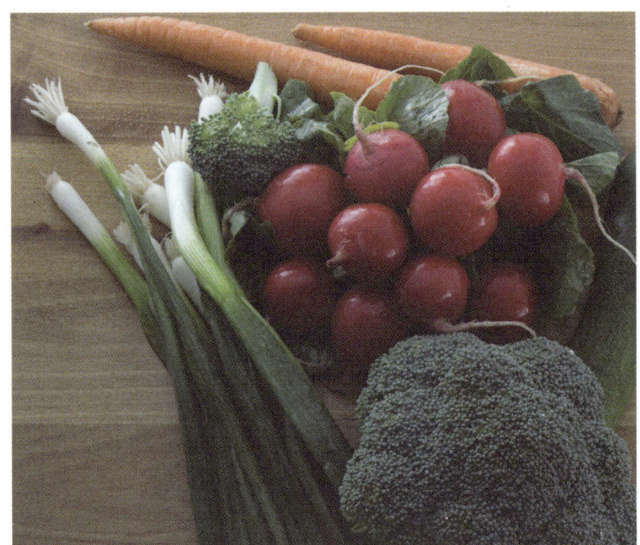

- Use as much colour as you can find in the produce section of your market. Get greens (lettuce), reds (tomatoes), and yellows (peppers, carrots) into your meals.

- Peppers are excellent garnishes, while baby spinach goes happily into soups, stews and omelettes.

- Buy greens in the supermarket or at the farmers' market, or use what's flourishing in your garden. Go seasonal for fresh. Always look for the darker greens, as they have more nutrition.

- You can also buy frozen vegetables. Nutrition quality is not lost in freezing.

Make sure vegetables are dry before you store them, as moisture rots green vegetables very quickly. Always dry fruit and especially salad greens before storing. Use a salad spinner or a clean tea cloth.

Always smell fish and seafood before you buy it. Make sure fish has shiny scales and bright eyes. Fresh seafood and fish should ideally be bought on the day you plan to cook it. Meat can usually be stored for a few days in the fridge, but check the expiration date when you buy it.

Add Greenery to Salads

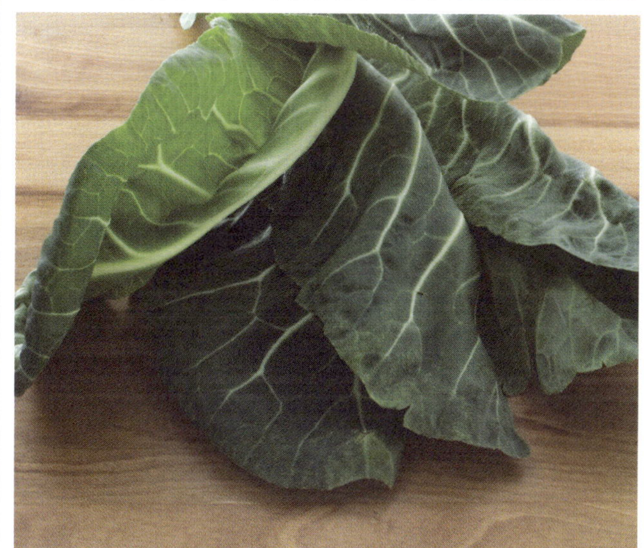

- When making salads, add darker greens to iceberg lettuce or Chinese cabbage. Greens come in all sizes, from small and bitter, such as rocket and watercress, to large and sweet, like romaine and iceberg lettuce.

- Rinse leaves before use and dry in a salad spinner.

- Before using heads of lettuce, remove outside leaves. Slice lengthwise and then crosswise. Add shredded watercress or rocket for extra nutrition.

- Wrap all salad leaves in paper towels before storing in plastic bags.

Preparing Fresh, Aromatic Vegetables

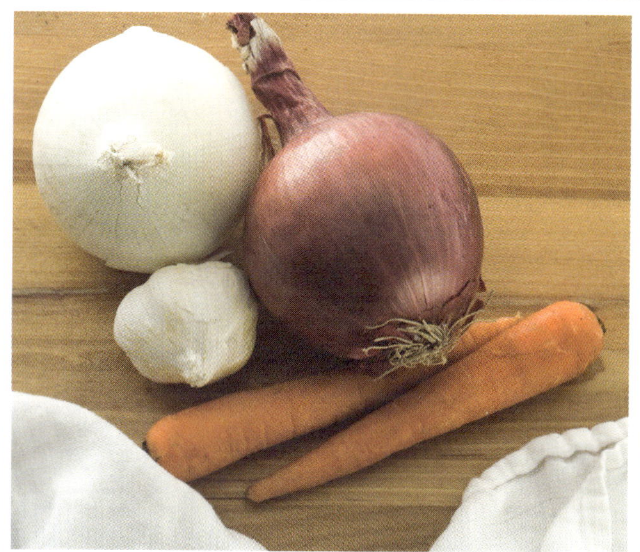

- Aromatic vegetables include carrots, parsnips, celery, onions, garlic and turnips. They add flavour, fibre and minerals to your recipe repertoire.

- Prepare garlic by breaking it into cloves. Slam cloves with the side of a cleaver, which separates them and makes them easy to peel. Place in a plastic bag in the fridge for quick access, or slice and freeze.

- Cut off and discard ends of onions; peel and chop. Place in freezer. Peel and slice carrots and parsnips; store in the fridge. Potatoes should be peeled at the last minute.

FLAVOURINGS

Every kitchen should have a variety of flavourings, from oils and vinegars to herbs, spices and extracts

When thinking about the kinds of flavourings to add to your recipes, start with the basics: sea salt or salt substitute, black peppercorns and red chilli flakes, or ground red pepper (cayenne) and pepper sauce.

You will also need herbs. All herbs begin as green leaves. You may grow your own or buy herbs fresh, dry them yourself or buy dried herbs in jars. Basic herbs include basil, oregano (the darling of the pizza parlour), thyme (think of turkey stuffing), dill for fish and seafood, and sage for all sorts of soups and stews. There are dozens of others.

Spices include twigs, roots (such as ginger), seeds (mustard, fennel, anise, coriander, celery seed and dill seed), and

Acidic Dressings

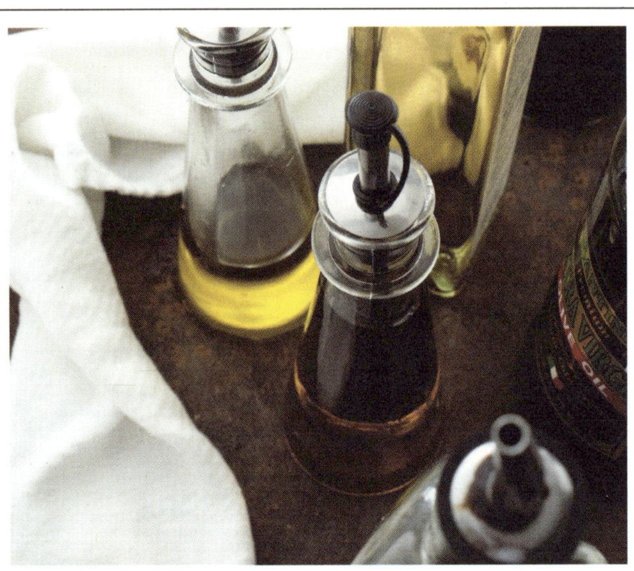

- Every salad needs an acid for flavouring, to counterbalance oil and bring out the flavours of greens.

- Basic dressing is made of one part vinegar and three parts oil. Vinegar can be based on red or white wine or sherry, and flavoured with raspberry and herbs such as basil and tarragon. Lemon or lime juice can be added or substitute for vinegar.

- Orange juice is a nice cooking liquid.

- Most mixed dressings are blends of mayonnaise and citrus or vinegar.

Oils

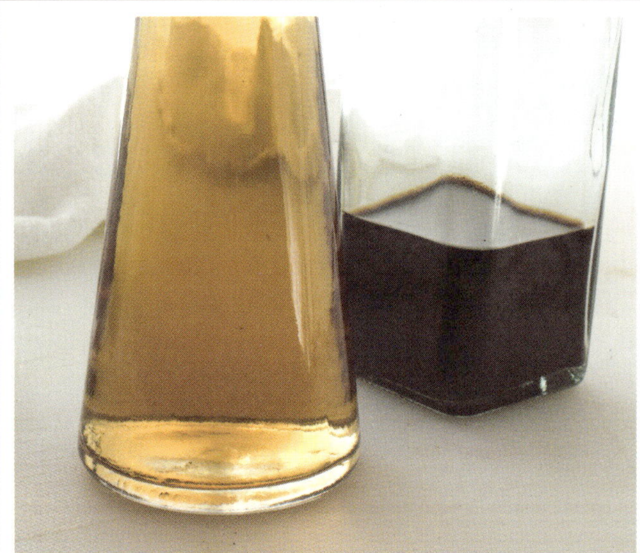

- Oil is a crucial ingredient in almost all dressings, marinades, soups, stews and sauces. Extra virgin oil comes from the first pressing. Virgin olive oil (the second pressing) and plain olive oil (the third) are often mixed with other oils.

- Once you've added vinegar, spices and herbs, only an educated palate can tell the difference between pure olive oil and blends.

- Salads, grilled or sautéed chicken, duck or seafood will be dry without oil in some form, whether it's olive, canola, groundnut, flavoured or mayonnaise.

dried berries (cumin, pepper, juniper berries, nutmeg, cloves and allspice).

Other important flavours come from extracts, such as vanilla, lemon and almond. Sauces, such as soy, Tabasco and Worcestershire, are combinations of spices and a carrier. Many flavoured oils are also useful in the kitchen. Oils include the basics, canola and olive oil, as well as sesame seed, walnut oil and truffle oil, for starters.

Wines also make excellent flavourings. Red and white wines that are good enough to drink are good in small amounts.

Sherry and Marsala have strong flavours and should also be used sparingly.

A well-stocked kitchen will have the basic flavourings ready and available. When stocking your kitchen each week, remember to check your herbs, spices and extracts for any necessary refills. Chances are, you'll be using these ingredients a lot in your dishes.

Bottled Flavourings

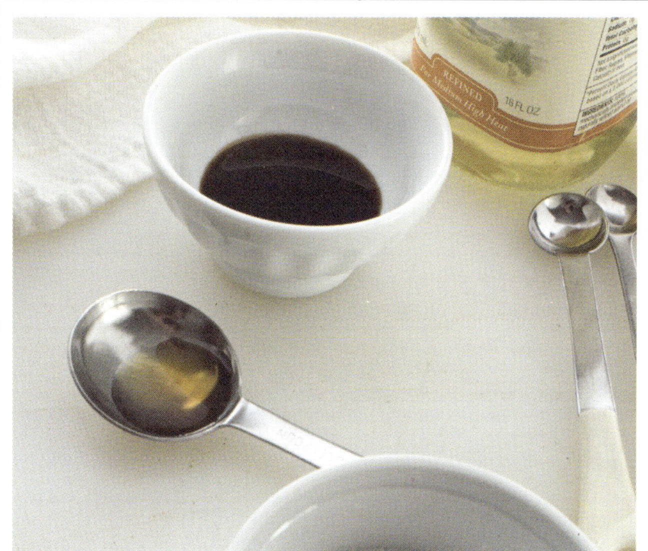

- When setting up your kitchen, you'll find that there are many goodies to add to basic oils, vinegars and spices.

- Worcestershire sauce and low-sodium soy sauce are invaluable as soup and stew flavourings. They don't require refrigeration.

- Always refrigerate opened barbecue sauces, ketchup and chilli sauce; pickles, roasted peppers and artichokes; olives, ground coffee and mayonnaise.

- Don't refrigerate extracts or unopened jams or jellies.

Sugar Substitutes

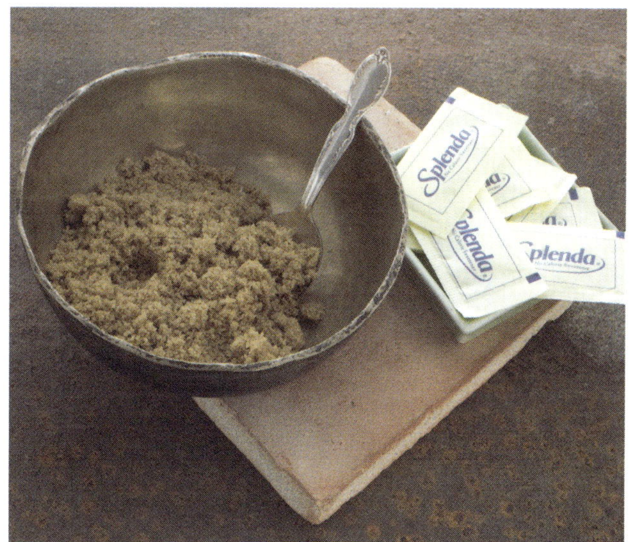

- Store sugar and sugar substitutes in airtight containers. They absorb humidity and the steam from boiling, grilling and poaching.

- Sugar substitute is important for baking, and in chilli sauce and barbecue sauce.

- Sugar substitutes labelled 'for baking' have some real sugar in them. But without the real sugar, the baked product will be dry, with a coarse texture.

SMALL TOOLS

These kitchen implements are essential for preparing delicious and nutritious recipes

There are four small tools that you should always have on hand in your kitchen: a lemon/lime reamer, a wire whisk, a box grater and a small spatula. Many of the recipes in this book use fresh lemon or lime juice. Lemon/lime reamers are generally made of wood and are fluted to twist out all the juice and pulp.

Wire whisks come in many sizes, from tiny to huge. Get a medium-size whisk, which is useful for beating eggs, whipping cream, whipping egg whites and generally mixing things up.

A box grater is essential if you don't have a food processor. And for many recipes, the box grater works just as well. Use it for cheese, carrots and other ingredients.

Lemon Reamer

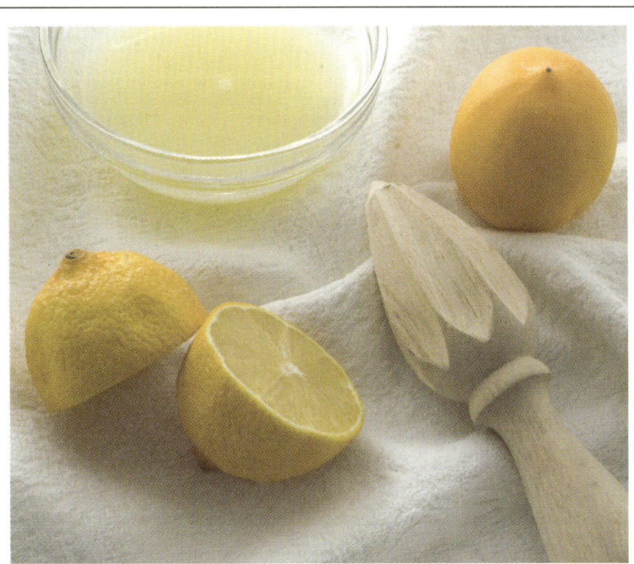

- With a lemon reamer, you can control quantities of liquid, from a few drops to half the lemon (or lime).

- Lemon juice is essential to flavour fish and prevent fruit from discolouring. It also keeps the colours true in vegetables.

- Lemon juice is used in sauces, braises and dressings.

- Lemon wedges are used as garnishes, for squeezing over fish and other foods.

- Lemon 'cures' foods, cooking the food in its acidity.

Wire Whisk

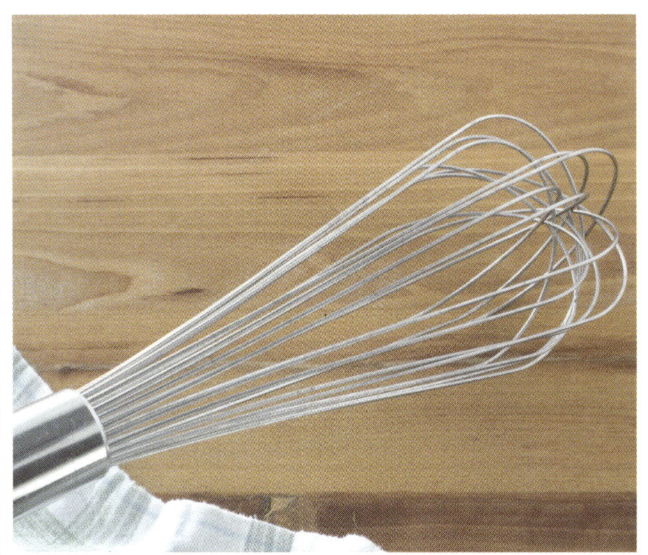

- The wire whisk is useful for beating eggs. It's also fine for whisking egg whites into a mass of peaks and for whipping cream.

- The whisk is also useful for getting lumps out of sauces.

- When making pan gravy, use the whisk to break up the brown bits on the bottom of the pan while adding hot liquid. This requires a good whisk.

- The whisk is also good for making salad dressings, blending the oil and acid thoroughly.

A small spatula is also essential. Not just for turning food as you cook it, but for peeping under pancakes and other foods to see if they are done.

Some other small tools are also great to have on hand. A garlic press pushes a peeled clove of garlic through tiny holes – the smaller the garlic is cut, the stronger it will be. For making garlic bread, the garlic press produces very small, juicy fragments. This is also a good way to add garlic to salad dressings. A citrus zester/canelle knife, which removes thin strips of lemon, lime or orange peel or larger strips of peel, is excellent for adding twists and making garnishes for many dishes. Keep it with your lemon reamer. A mandoline is handy for making paper-thin slices of cheese, onions, potatoes or other vegetables. Be careful to get the type of mandoline with a holder. If you have to hold the food while you move it across the blade, you may easily slice the tips of your fingers.

Box Grater

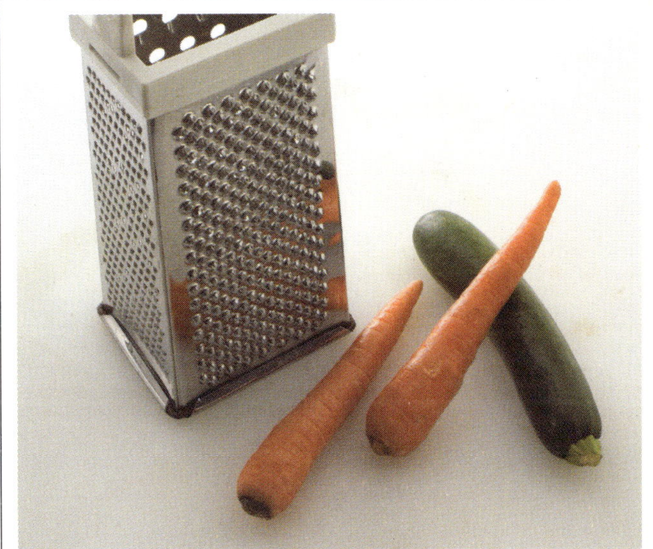

- Box graters may be old-fashioned, but they are very useful. Each side has a function. One wide side grates; the other wide side slices; one small side scrapes and the other is a minigrater.

- Grating is done on one side. It is easier to control than a food processor.

- Scraping is done on the other side of the box. Use the rasp to zest a lemon or lime quickly.

- The slicing side is fine for various types of vegetables, such as cucumbers.

Plastic Spatula

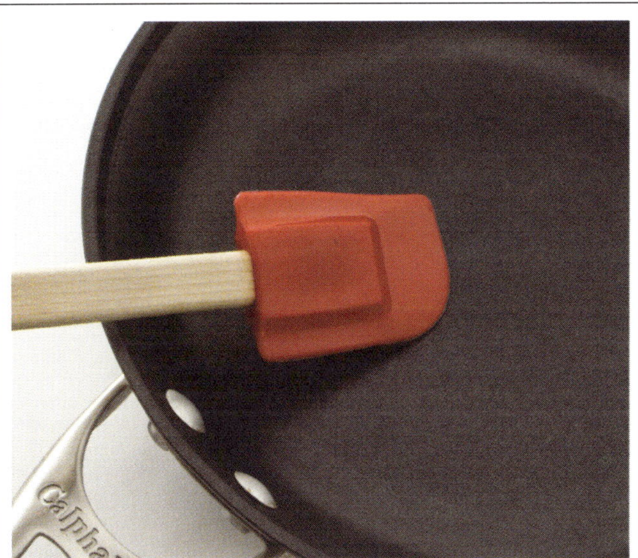

- A small spatula is useful for turning pancakes and omelettes.

- It's also good for checking under an omelette to see if it's browning nicely.

- A small spatula can be used for scraping up brown bits on the bottom of a pan.

- Plastic spatulas are more versatile than metal ones, as metal spatulas cannot be used in nonstick pans.

SMALL, SHARP CUTTING TOOLS

Cooks need easy access to knives, peelers, kitchen scissors and grapefruit spoons

When it comes to cutting and preparing food, a seasoned chef will turn time and again to certain kitchen essentials. A set of really good, sharp knives, from a short paring knife to a serrated bread knife to a cleaver, is important, because cooks need different knives to cut, slice and chop. Blunt knives are dangerous, as they slip off the food and into fingers. Many good knives are sold in sets with a knife sharpener, which is a worthwhile investment.

A really good knife is worth the gold you spend on it. Cheap knives do not sharpen properly. They will tear, even bruise the food rather than cutting through it. Good quality stainless steel knives are excellent, but old-fashioned carbon steel

Knife Set

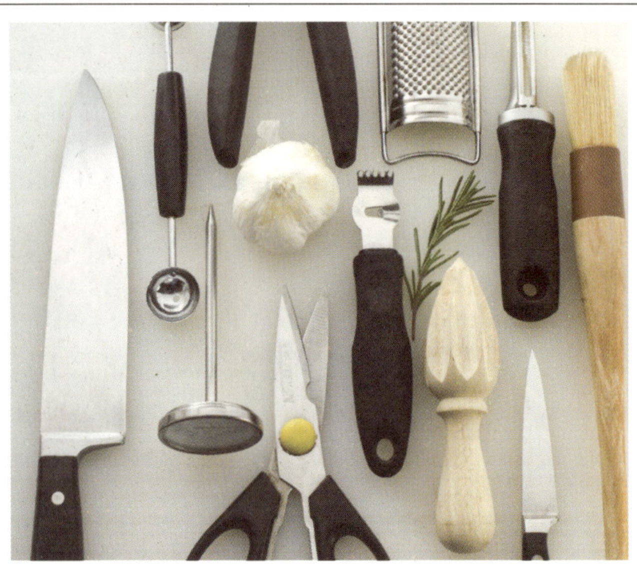

- A knife set has knives for various purposes. A paring knife is used to cut the hulls from strawberries, pare off the skins of small vegetables and remove stems.

- A serrated knife is for slicing bread and cakes. It acts like a saw and does not crush the bread or cake.

- A chef's knife, with its slightly curved blade, is excellent for carving meat and poultry.

- A cleaver is important for chopping and dicing vegetables and other foods.

Vegetable Peelers

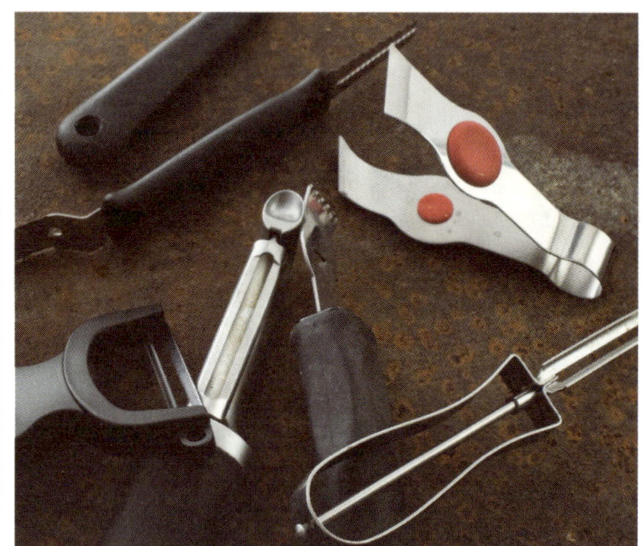

- When you find a style of vegetable peeler you are comfortable with, buy a couple – then if you are preparing a big meal, you can get others to help peel. Throw out blunt ones.

- Peeling techniques vary, and for left-handed cooks, the crossbow style is best for agility. Get the sharpest stainless-steel peeler you can find.

- Adjust your stroke speed and length depending on the food you are peeling. Some work best with small strokes, while bigger foods, such as large aubergines, work well with long strokes.

knives are also good: they aren't pretty, as they turn dark grey and can rust, but they are easily sharpened to a razor's edge.

Peelers come in two designs, the 'crossbow' and the 'up and down'. Either works well if the peeler is sharp. Use peelers for potatoes and other vegetables. Every kitchen needs scissors, both heavy poultry shears for cutting up a chicken, and smaller ones for opening plastic bags, cutting string, etc.

Perhaps the most surprising tool here is the grapefruit spoon: its pointed tip is good for removing grapefruit and orange sections, but also has many other uses.

Knives must be kept sharp with either a sharpening stone or a butcher's steel. Simply hone your knife with a few strokes on each side every time you use it, always moving in the same direction. Store the knife so that it isn't rattling against other knives and utensils, which could chip or dull the blade. Serrated knives and steak knives do not need to be sharpened.

Kitchen Scissors

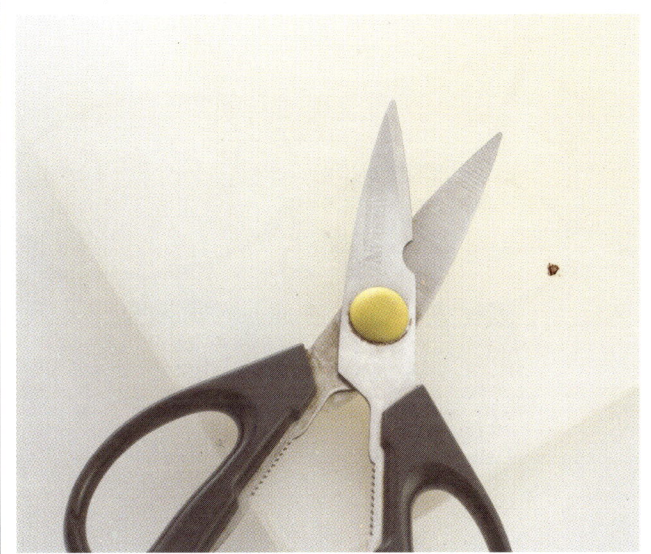

- Scissors are essential for a variety of jobs. Little jobs include cutting string and opening plastic packets.

- Big jobs include cutting up chickens and various cuts of meat, which is easier to do this way and more accurate than sawing away with a knife.

- Large poultry shears are excellent for cutting the wing tips off turkeys, ducks, and chickens for the stockpot.

- You also may find them more convenient and easier to wield than a knife for cutting up racks of baby ribs.

Grapefruit Spoon

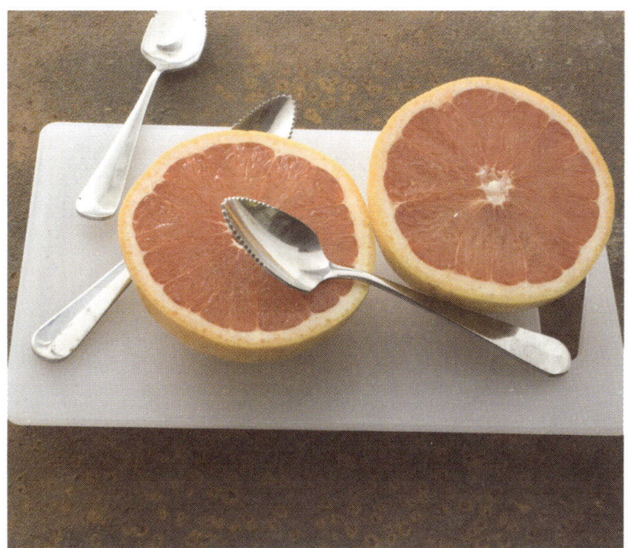

- The grapefruit spoon is as delicate as a surgical tool when used with a little practice and skill.

- It was originally designed for segmenting grapefruit for eating. Its genius is in the spoon's slender tip. This works around stones, seeds and skins.

- When making baked potato skins, cut the raw potato in half and scoop out the pulp with the grapefruit spoon.

- Use the spoon to scoop out avocado stones, melon pips and the cores from apples and pears.

MEASURING TOOLS

Measuring tools come in handy when following recipes, while when baking accurate weighing makes all the difference

When you are adding stock to your stew, a few millilitres more or less doesn't make much difference. When you are baking a cake, however, a few grams more or less flour, baking powder or sugar can mean success or failure.

There are two kinds of measures: dry and liquid. Scales are essential if you do a lot of baking, as it's important to weigh ingredients accurately. These days you can buy digital scales that speak the weight of your ingredients and even calculate your calorie intake, but traditional balance scales are accurate and easy to use.

Liquid measuring jugs are almost always made of glass, so you can see the quantities printed on the sides of the jugs.

Weighing Scales

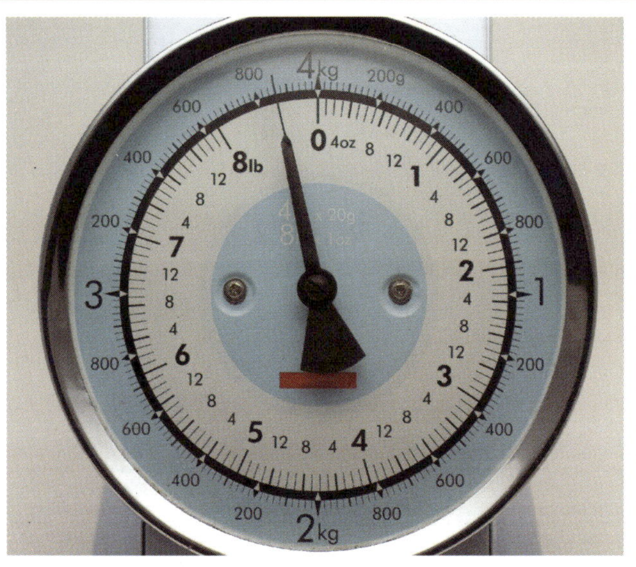

- Scales, whether manual or digital, measure ingredients accurately and can help to control portion sizes.

- When baking, measuring ingredients by weight is the most accurate way and will give you the best results.

- High-tech scales can have the nutritional content of the food you are weighing programmed into them. You can add up to 1,000 foods to the programmes in these dietary computer scales. You can also record food intake and keep track of total calories.

Liquid Measuring Jugs

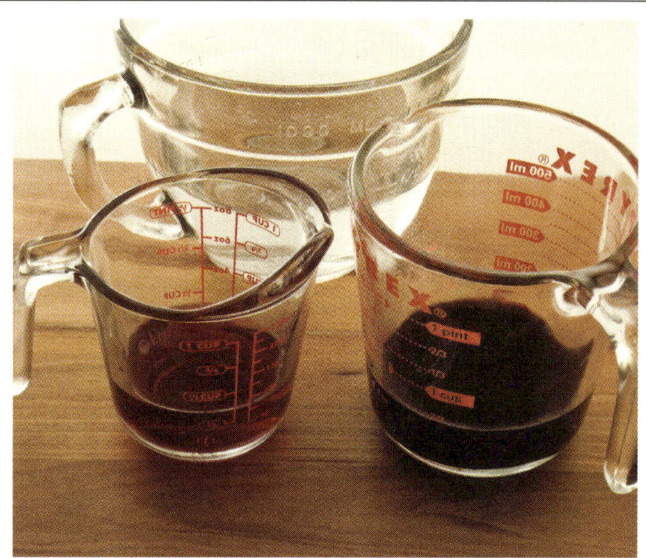

- When cooking, you need to know the quantities of the liquid measurements in terms of volume.

- Grams, cubic centimetres, and litres are marked on the side of the measuring jug.

- Pints and fluid ounces are usually marked on the other side of the jug, for recipes given in imperial units.

- You can use measuring jugs for mixing ingredients too.

They are available in various sizes, marked in both metric and imperial units.

A set of measuring spoons, from $1/8$ teaspoon to 1 tablespoon, works for both dry and liquid measures. For people on theraputic diets, these are a fairly accurate way to measure small quantities of food.

There is one caveat: although measuring spoons are based on using teaspoons and tablespoons, it is best not to use ordinary teaspoons and tablespoons for measuring. This is because the size of the spoons is not standardized, and the bowls are shallower than those of measuring spoons. You are more likely to spill your vanilla extract when using a teaspoon from your cutlery set than with a measuring spoon. Also, with a set of measuring spoons, the ½ teaspoon and $1/4$ teaspoon sizes are included, too. An $1/8$ teaspoon is equal to a pinch or a dash. So especially when baking but even as a general cooking rule, use dry and liquid measures to be exact.

Measuring Spoons

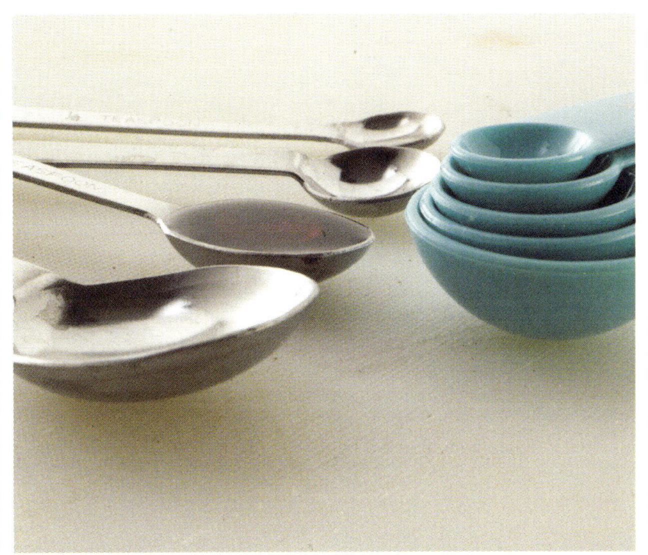

- Plastic measuring spoons are kept together by a plastic ring. The metal spoons are kept nested by a metal ring.

- Many cooks detach them for easy use; if you use just one while it's still attached, you end up having to clean them all.

- If you detach them, it's easy to misplace parts of the set. So detach and then store them in a ziplock bag.

- Measuring spoons will give you a more accurate measurement than your cutlery spoons, due to the depth of the spoon.

Old-Time Measuring

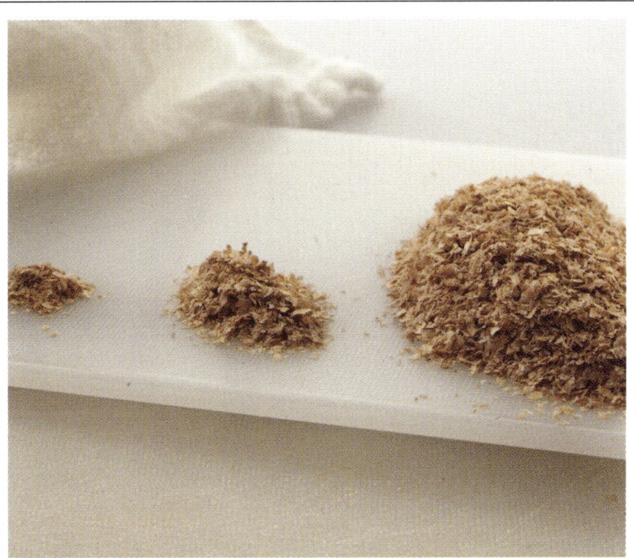

- If you come across an old family cookbook and want to translate, here's a guide:

- The old silver or stainless teaspoon or tablespoon is equivalent to the measuring spoon.

- A pinch is equal to $1/8$ teaspoonful. A dash is equivalent to a $1/2$ teaspoon.

- A handful is equal to about 120 ml.

LESS USED BUT NECESSARY TOOLS

While you may not use these items on a daily basis, always keep your kitchen stocked with them

Many of the gadgets you see in gourmet cooking stores are not absolutely necessary, but they are fun. When looking for kitchen gadgets, think about the foods you like to eat every day. Are you big on salad or spinach? In that case, you will probably need both a colander and a salad spinner in your kitchen. Sieves and colanders are necessary for rinsing and draining fruit and vegetables. If you rarely blanch and freeze tomatoes yourself, on the other hand, you probably don't need a food mill if you have a food processor.

Some gadgets can be used for multiple purposes. Fine sieves, for example, are used to separate out small foods, but they can double as sifters for flour and icing sugar. You'll find

Sieves and Colanders

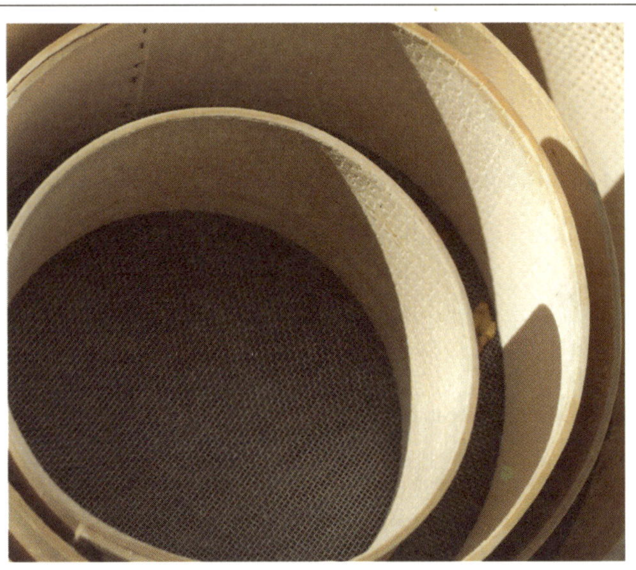

- Beside rinsing and cleaning food, a fine sieve can be used for making a purée. By pushing berries or tomatoes through, seeds and lumps are removed.

- A fine sieve can also be used in place of a flour sifter when baking.

- A large colander is excellent for washing spinach and lettuce. It's easy to put the colander in a large bowl of cold water and swish lettuce around to remove the dirt.

- When you remove the colander from the water, you should have clean leaves.

Salad Spinners

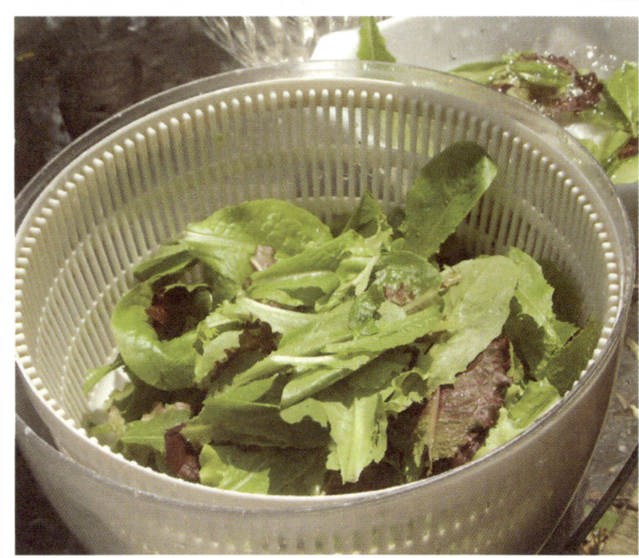

- These clever inventions use centrifugal force to spin water off the leaves.

- After you wash your greens, spin them as dry as possible. Drain off the water in the bottom of the container and spin the leaves again for good measure.

- If you are storing the leaves, wrap them in paper towels and then place them in a plastic bag.

- Salad leaves will stay crisp in the refrigerator for up to 4 days.

that sifters are most important for baking. You can also use a salad spinner as a colander for large, leafy vegetables.

Depending on your needs, you will determine what is necessary and what isn't. Many chefs will agree, however, that the following tools, while perhaps not used often, are still a great addition to your gadget collection.

When organizing your kitchen, remember to keep these tools tucked away in an easy-to-reach location for occasional use.

MAKE IT EASY

If you run out of shelf space, try this: use pegboard with holes in it for hooks to hang your gadgets. Arrange your least-used mills, colanders and sieves where they are out of the way. Check out your local kitchen or hardware shop for various other forms of accessible storage.

Sifters

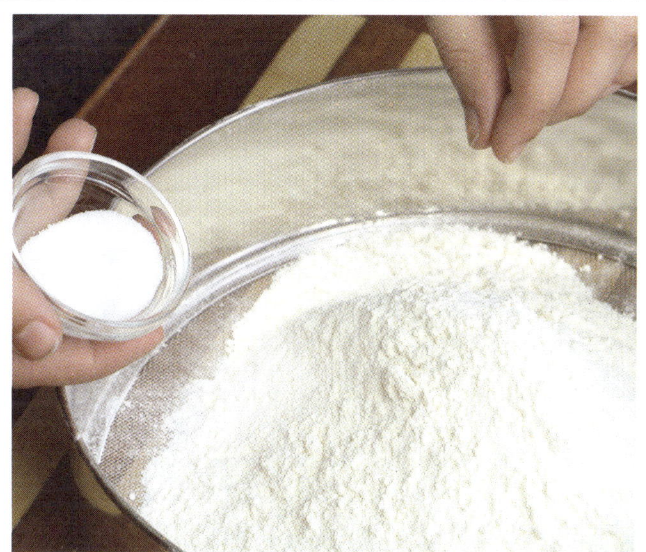

- Cooks who do a lot of baking need sifters. Since many recipes call for up to 350 g flour, a sifter that will hold that amount is about all a home baker needs.

- Sifting is more important when making cakes than it is when making pies, as it's essential to incorporate lots of air in the mixture as well as eliminating lumps.

- You'll also need to sift icing sugar for icings and cake mixtures, and for dusting the tops of pies and cakes.

Food Mills

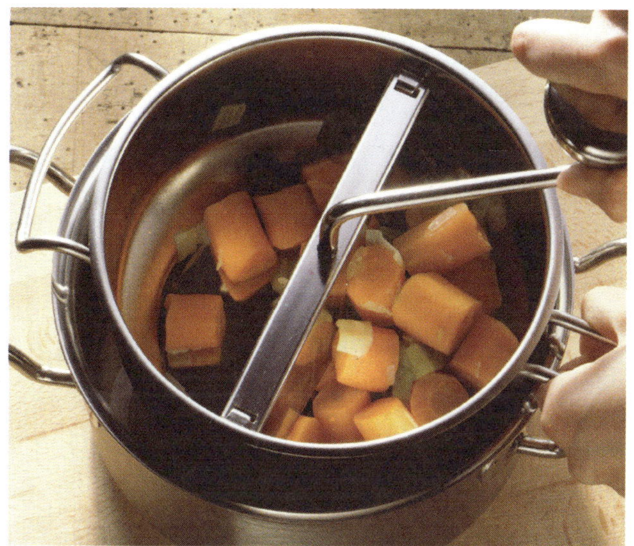

- Food mills are available in both electric and hand-crank models. Often known as moulis, they have been in use by cooks for years.

- Food mills separate the skin and seeds from the pulp of tomatoes and berries.

- Mills can be found in very large sizes for cooks who are canning large amounts of tomatoes or for cooks who make jams and jellies.

- Mills preceded the food processor, which purées food but does not remove the seeds, instead simply grinding them up with the skins and flesh.

SMALL APPLIANCES

These gadgets are important and handy to have around the kitchen

While not every appliance is needed for a gourmet kitchen, every kitchen does need a food processor, a blender and, ideally, two electric mixers – one hand-held for small jobs and a large, stand mixer for making cakes and whipped egg whites (for use in soufflés, for example).

Food processors are equipped with blades that have different uses. The basic grinding blade also chops, minces and purées. It works well with carrots, onions and nuts. It is an alternative to a blender for puréeing soups and smoothing out sauces. While the basic blade works from the base up, the grating blade works from the top down. It grates potatoes, carrots and cheese, among other things. The slicing blade works well on vegetables such as carrots and cucumbers, for salad. It also slices potatoes very efficiently. The food

Immersion Blender

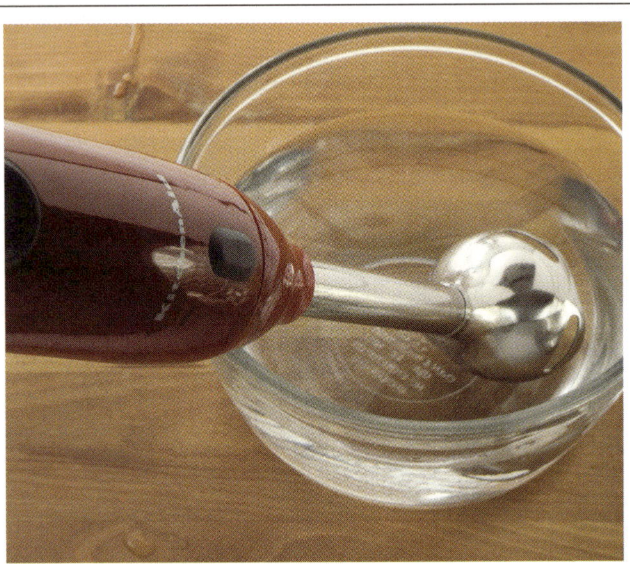

- Immersion blenders are good for mixing foods together, especially smoothies and sauces.

- There are disadvantages: some blenders can slop food or liquids over the side of the bowl; some are difficult to clean. It is best to experiment with various sized bowls and varying levels of liquids, starting with water.

- To clean, immerse the blender in hot, soapy water. Turn on the motor and run it until the blades are clean. Rinse the blender under hot running water first, then immerse it in cold water.

Food Processor Blades

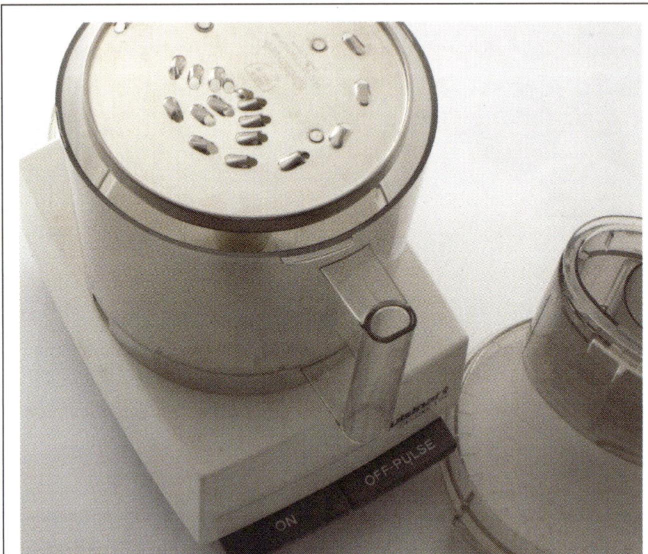

- The food processor chops, minces and purées, but not as finely as does the blender. Use this gadget to chop onions and garlic for soups or to chop vegetables for stews.

- The grinding blade chops when you pulse it. You can fine- or coarse-chop nuts, vegetables and fruits by starting and stopping (pulsing) your processor. The longer the machine is on, the finer the chop will be.

- Use the slicing blade for thin slices of celery, cucumber, or potatoes.

processor can do most of what a blender does, but blenders are not as versatile as food processors.

Blenders are, however, important, especially for making smoothies, fruit sauces and salad dressings. Some blenders are equipped with an additional small goblet, which is great for making small quantities of salad dressing.

Hand-held and electric stand mixers are useful for beating eggs and making meringues, cake mixes and pancake batter.

Hand-Held Electric Mixer

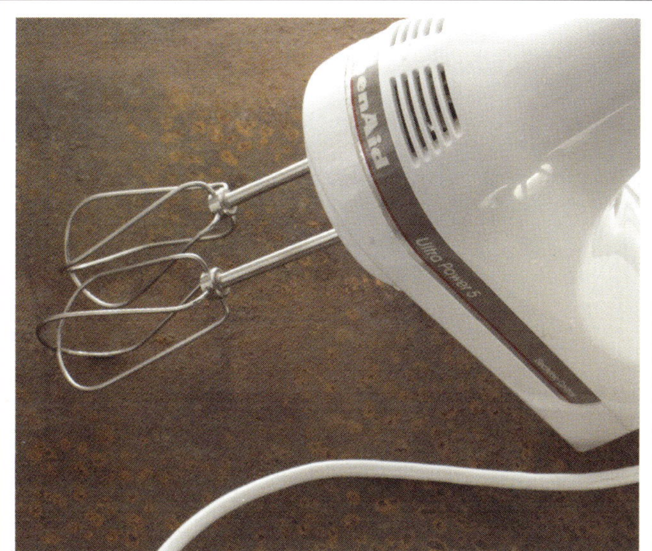

- A hand-held electric mixer can be used for a variety of mixing tasks. Use it to mash potatoes for a very good consistency.

- The hand-held electric mixer also works well for beating eggs for the World-Class Scrambled Eggs recipe.

- Use this mixer to beat eggs for omelettes. The Egg White Omelette recipe will be puffier if you use the mixer to whip up the whites.

- You can also use the mixer for whisking cake mixtures.

Electric Stand Mixer

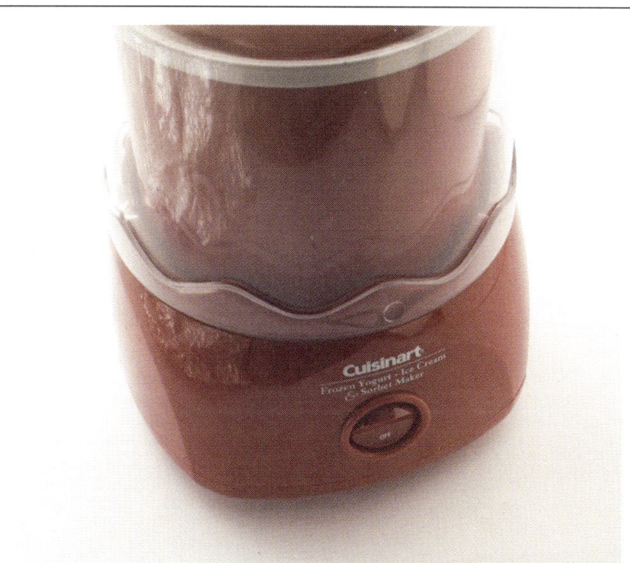

- The electric stand mixer is most useful when you are cooking for a crowd and making dishes by the litre rather than in small quantities.

- The electric stand mixer also frees you up to do something else while the mixer does the work.

- Large mixers are equipped with dough hooks, which enable you to make bread dough with them.

MID-SIZE APPLIANCES

These kitchen items will help expedite many dishes and save you time in the kitchen

Every chef can appreciate the help of some time-saving appliances in his or her arsenal of tricks. The microwave, breadmaker and slow cooker are three items a modern-day cook need not live without. Even a luxury item like the ice cream/sorbet maker will help make things easier for the gourmet cook.

A microwave helps with faster preparation. When you want green beans, asparagus or Brussels sprouts, heat them in the microwave and they're ready in 90 seconds. Carrots, parsnips and winter squash soften up quickly in the microwave.

An automatic breadmaker is great for fresh, homemade bread every morning, and it will also mix pizza dough. An ice cream/sorbet maker is excellent for homemade desserts,

Microwave

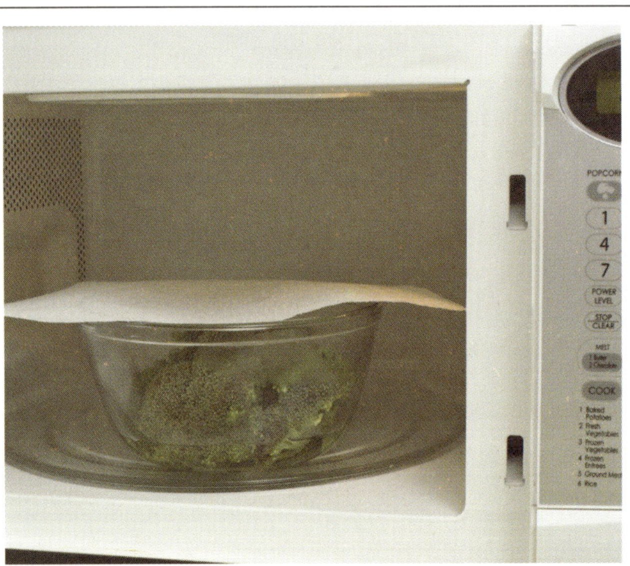

- Of all the things you can do with a microwave, cooking vegetables is prime.

- Try this: trim an artichoke, cutting off bottom and outside leaves. Put it in a glass bowl with 2 tablespoons of water and 1 teaspoon of lemon juice. It will be ready in 4 minutes.

- Always cover food with freezer paper, greaseproof paper or paper towels.

- Never cover food with cling film, as the plastic releases harmful chemicals, considered carcinogens, that leach into your food.

Automatic Breadmaker

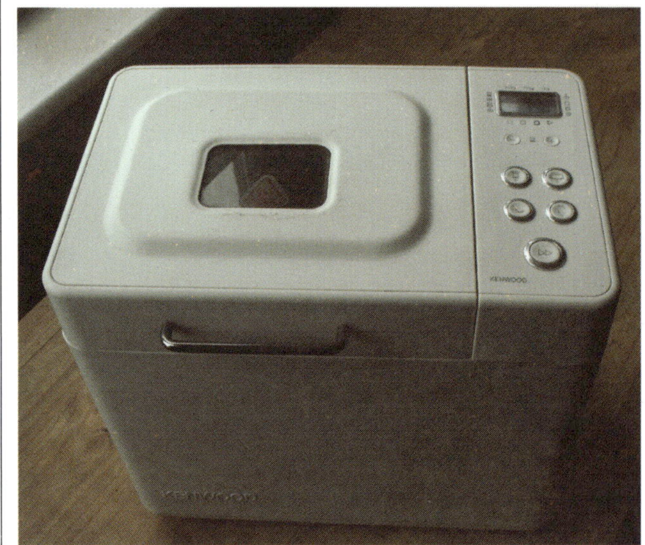

- A programmable automatic breadmaker allows you to enjoy fresh-baked bread every day.

- The ingredients are measured into the pan and once the programme is set the machine mixes and kneads the dough, waits for it to prove and then bakes it.

- Breadmakers use instant yeast, which is activated only when it comes in contact with the liquid in the recipe.

- Modern breadmakers can also be set to prepare dough without baking (for pizzas), and to add ingredients such as fruit and nuts.

allowing you to control their sugar content – a big help for people who have strict dietary needs.

Slow cookers are a household favourite, and there are many different types, sizes and brands available. Slow cookers make dinners easy for the working chef, who sometimes may not always have the most time in the world to prepare a five-star meal. Slow cookers take care of your stocks and simmer your hearty soups and stews.

Ice Cream Maker

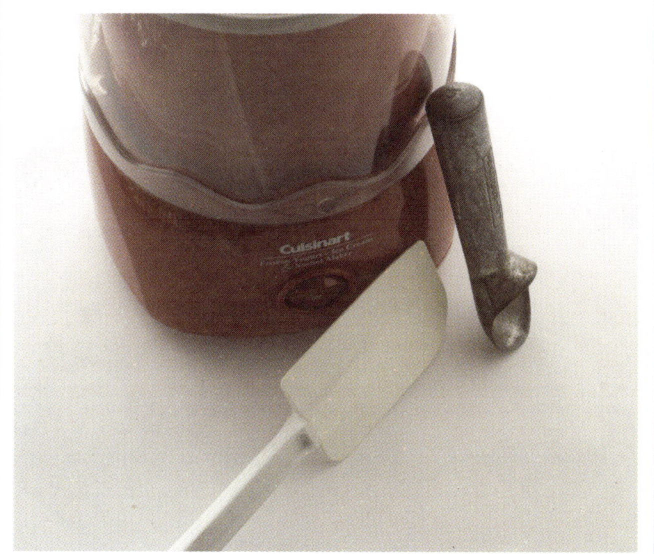

- When using an ice cream maker, be sure to follow the directions exactly and never overfill the bowl.

- If you do, the appliance will overflow as the ice cream is churned.

- Make sure that all ingredients are very cold before you add them.

- Set aside toppings such as fruit, nuts and raisins to eat with your ice cream, sorbet or frozen yogurt.

Slow Cooker

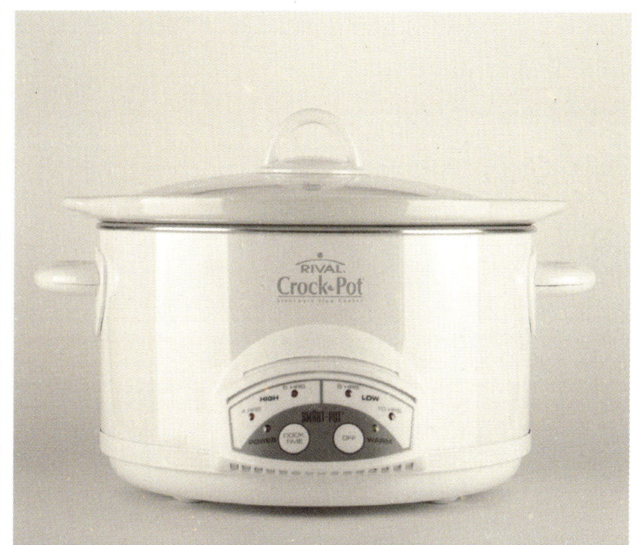

- Slow cookers are made from heavy ceramic ware. These thick pots are excellent heat carriers.

- Beside soups and stews, there are plenty of recipes that are easy and good in the slow cooker.

- Make your pot roasts in the slow cooker, for example.

- Keep an eye on the slow cooker the first time or two that you use it so that you will know if it over- or under-heats.

SAUTÉING

The sauté technique is used for vegetables, meat and fish

The art of sautéing is a versatile skill that every good cook should learn. A sauté pan is made of tin-lined copper, heavy stainless steel, enamelled metal or good-quality nonstick material. It is reasonably deep, to allow a sauce to be made after browning meat and other ingredients. It can be substituted for a wok when stir-frying but is not as conveniently designed for the purpose.

Aromatic vegetables are sautéed prior to using them in soups, stews and braises. Meats such as fillet steak and veal escalopes are also sautéed or pan-fried, keeping them low in fat. The same is true of delicately fleshed fish, such as fillet of sole or flounder.

Even when you use a nonstick pan, it's wise to add a little olive oil. The first part of the sauté is to sear the food. This

Preparing to Sauté

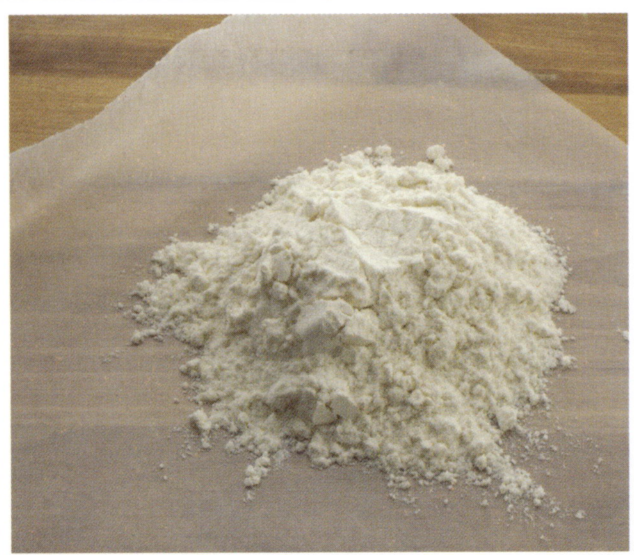

- First, sprinkle a piece of greaseproof paper with flour, salt and pepper. You can add herbs at this point.

- Thoroughly dry the piece of meat or fish you plan to sauté. Do this to avoid making a gooey mess when you dip it in flour.

- Heat the pan over medium-high heat. Add the oil to the pan.

- Start to brown the food.

Wait for the Sizzle

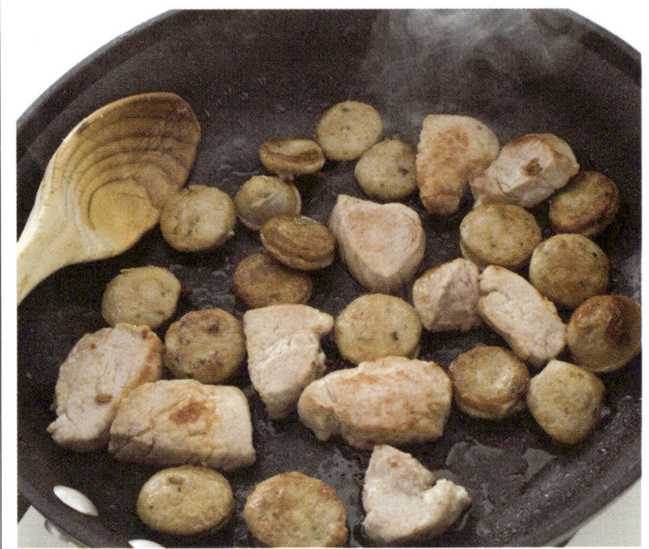

- Listen for the sizzle before lifting the food. When the meat or fish is sizzling, look under it by lifting a corner with your spatula.

- When you see that it's nicely golden on one side, turn the meat or fish.

- At this point, you will probably want to turn the heat down.

- Cooking time depends upon the thickness of the meat or fish.

means putting it in a very hot pan, which seals in the juices and gives it a nice colour. It's also called caramelization, as heat browns the food, bringing out the juices, starches and sugars. You need only enough olive or canola oil to coat the bottom of the pan.

Butter should not be used since it has a low burning-point and will not get as hot when cooked, whereas grapeseed oil can get hot without burning. The searing part of a sauté is enhanced by adding a dusting of flour to food. It forms an attractive crust when you do not want to use high heat.

Pan-frying

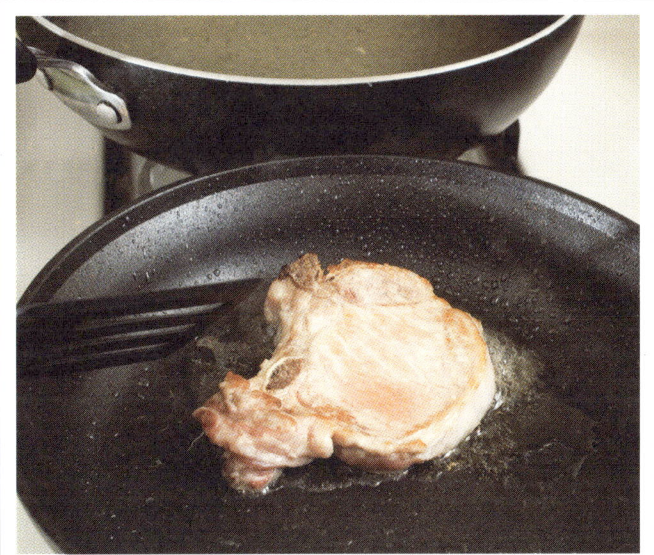

- It is quick to sauté thick pieces of meat on top of the stove. When you sauté or pan-fry meat, washing up is relatively easy.

- First, as with thin cuts, sear the meat on a medium-high to high flame. After you've turned it, reduce the heat to low.

- Cover the pan and let the steak or chop cook for 3 minutes. Turn and cook for another 3 minutes for medium rare.

- Give it 4 minutes more per side for well done. Always rest the meat in a warm place, covered, for at least 5 minutes.

Deglazing the Pan

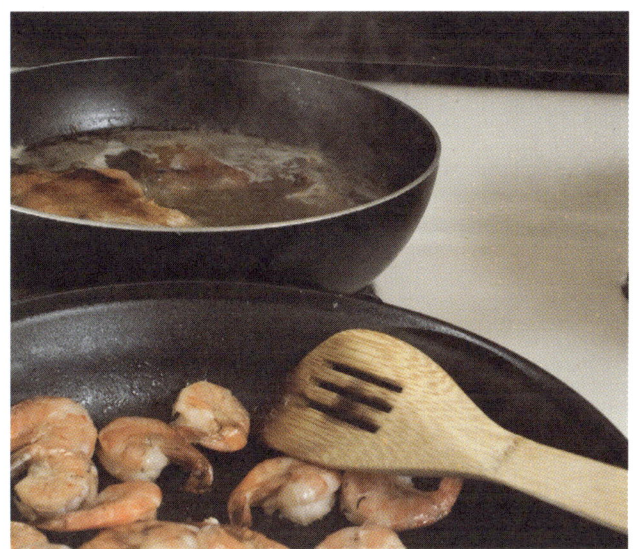

- Once you've finished sautéing, you'll see brown bits in the bottom of the pan. These are nuggets of flavour and the base for a sauce.

- If you've cooked chicken, add ½ cup of chicken stock; if veal, the same; for beef or a veal chop, add beef stock.

- With fish, add water or fish stock.

- Raise the heat to medium and simmer, stirring to scrape the residue off the pan. Add ¼ cup of red wine for beef or lamb, or ¼ cup of white wine for fish or chicken. Season with pepper and herbs.

BRAISING

This technique is a progression from sear and sauté to simmer

Braising is an age-old technique. It sears in the juices and then adds liquids and flavours for a long, slow simmer on top of the stove, in the oven or in the slow cooker. Braising produces warming comfort food, the stuff of cold winter nights and chilly days out-of-doors.

Chillies, stews, fricassees and pot roasts are all braised. When you make chilli, the liquids become gravy and carry the flavours of the dish. Everything is blended into a wonderful marriage. With stew, the pieces of meat retain some of their individuality. A pot roast is mostly meat with just enough gravy and vegetables to be delicious and moist. A chicken fricassee is made of pieces of chicken that have been browned, and then vegetables and lots of thickened gravy are incorporated.

Equipment for Braising

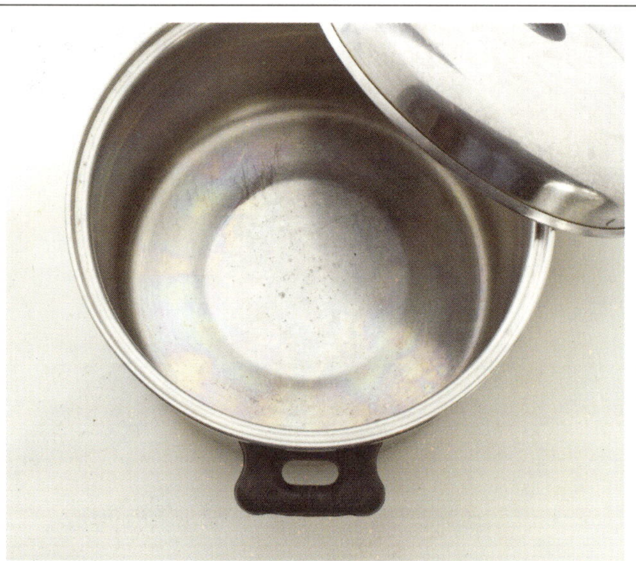

- Braising requires a heavy pot. It must take the heat of the first step – the sauté – and then the long simmer.

- A Dutch oven, either all metal or enamelled metal, works beautifully. The pot must have a tight lid to retain the steam.

- You can finish the braising process either on top of the stove or in the oven.

- A slow cooker is not suitable unless you sauté your food first and then add it to the pot.

Stews and Pot Roasts

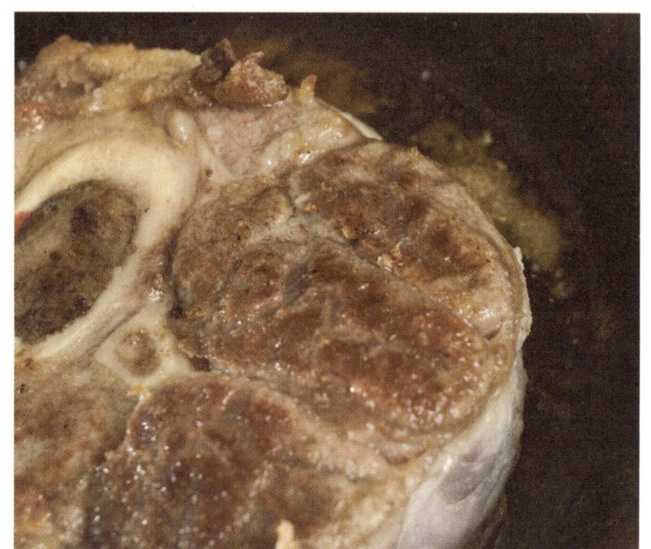

- Stews and pot roasts are braised. The beef, veal or lamb is seared until brown. It's pushed to the side, and then the vegetables are sautéed until softened.

- The liquids are added and the heat reduced to a very slow simmer.

- The stew is covered and allowed to cook very gently until the beef is tender.

- The stew can be thickened after removing the meat and vegetables by adding a mixture of flour or cornflour and water.

Remember, too much heat at the wrong time makes food tough and tired. The only blast of heat you give a braised dish is at the very outset. The sear is the one short exposure to high heat. If, once you have added the liquids, you let the chilli, stew, pot roast or fricassee boil, you will create a dry, tough dish.

After browning the meat, sauté aromatic vegetables, which include garlic, onions, and parsnips, to add essential flavour to the braised dish. Adding stock and wine will create deep, rich flavours. Add liquids as necessary, keeping an even level of wine, stock or tomato sauce to almost cover the meat. It takes time for the wine to mellow in the gravy or sauce. Other flavours can be added as you go along or towards the end of the cooking time. Give it an occasional stir.

Chilli

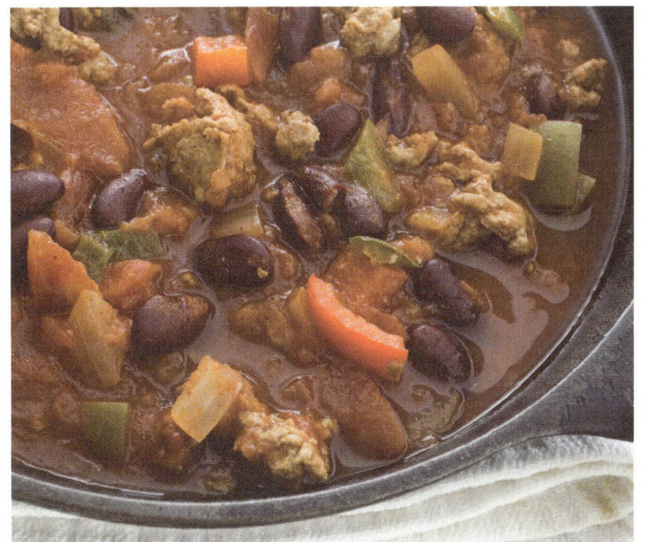

- Whether made with turkey, beef, pork or veal, chilli is braised.

- The meat is browned first. If you brown the vegetables first, they'll burn when you sauté the meat.

- The quantity and variety of vegetables can be quite a challenge, with onions, garlic and sweet and hot peppers.

- If there's too much liquid when the chilli is done, simply take the lid off and let it simmer down until it reaches the thickness you like. Timing depends on the quantity of extra liquid.

Chicken

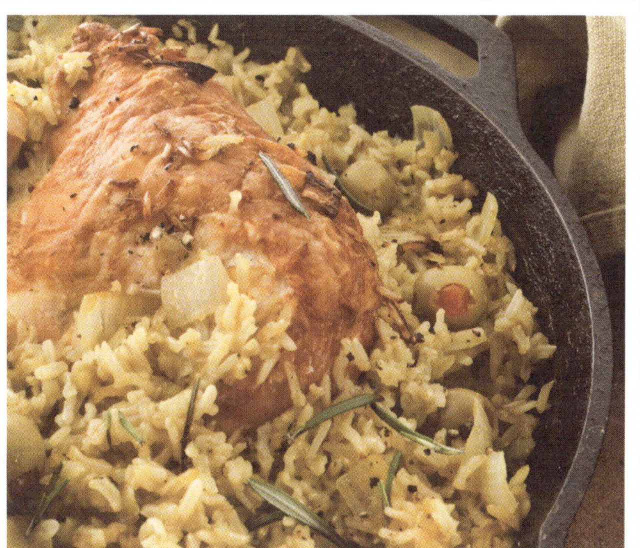

- When you braise chicken, it absorbs whatever flavours you add to the pot. The olives, herbs, garlic and onions all are incorporated.

- The wine and olives in this recipe clearly affect the flavours of the chicken, the rice and the liquid, which becomes the sauce.

- The method of sautéing (browning) the chicken gives it a very appetizing golden colour.

- The braising process ensures that the chicken is cooked through.

BOILING & STEAMING

These are two simple techniques that you will use often in cooking

Boiling and steaming are two basic techniques that all good cooks need to know. Boiling is used for dried foods, while steaming is used for foods such as vegetables and fish. Grains, beans, pulses and pasta are boiled because they are dry and hard, and must absorb moisture to soften enough to eat.

Boiling occurs in three stages. The first is the scald or simmer stage, when tiny bubbles appear around the side of the pan. The second stage is the slow boil, with gentle bubbles all over the surface of the liquid. The rolling boil is a full 100°C. All you need is a pan large enough to hold the cooking liquid.

Steaming exposes food to evaporating liquid. There are metal and bamboo steamers that you can use for this technique. The easiest steaming method is to put the food you want to steam in a glass or ceramic dish with some

Boiling in Extra Nutrition

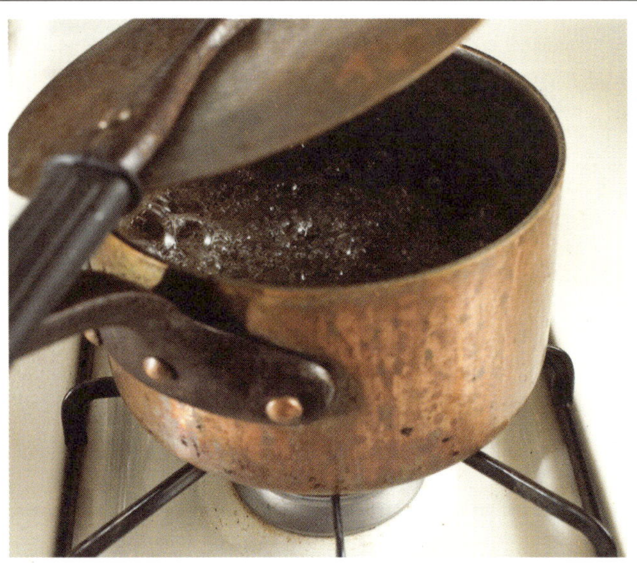

- You need a good 2- to 4-litre saucepan for boiling dried foods. Always use a pan that's big enough for the food to fit without overflowing. It can double as a soup pan.

- Your pot for boiling foods such as pasta must have two handles for gripping.

- Pasta pots with a removable colander make lifting and draining the food easier.

- When boiling polenta or rice, choose from vegetable, chicken or beef stock to enrich flavour and nutrition.

Microwave Steaming

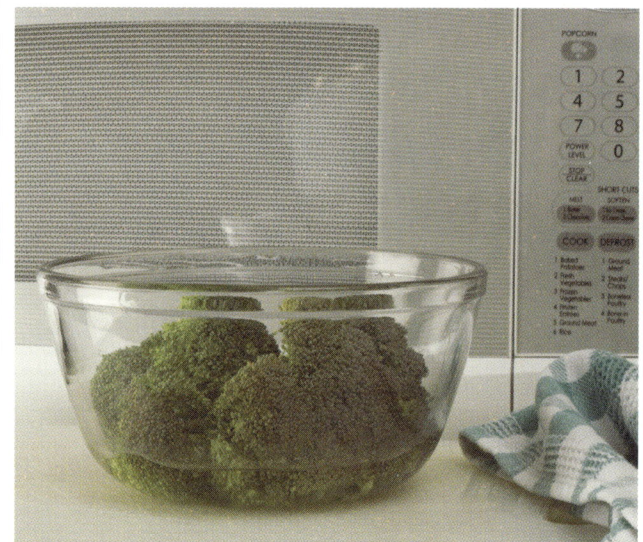

- Steamed broccoli is delicious and healthy to make. Rinse broccoli in a colander and toss in a large glass bowl with lemon juice.

- A Pyrex bowl is excellent for microwave steaming. You can put a lot of broccoli in the bowl.

- The vegetables are steamed in the microwave. Then they are finished in a sauce.

- Stock up on greaseproof paper, which works well for covering a bowl of vegetables to be microwaved.

water, cover it with paper, and place it in the microwave. Depending on the quantity of vegetables and whether you like them crisp-tender or soft, time will vary from 1 minute to 3–4 minutes.

So how do you know when to boil and when to steam? Boil vegetables only in soup. The reason for not boiling vegetables to be served at the table is that a great many of the nutrients end up in the water, not in the food. If vegetables are cooked in the soup, the goodness goes into the cooking liquid, not down the drain.

Carrots, broccoli, cauliflower and other stiff vegetables are best steamed in the microwave. Rinsed spinach that's moist actually steams as it is sautéed in olive oil. Bitter greens such as kale and turnip tops are best blanched: they are dropped in boiling water for a few seconds, then drained and sautéed. Frozen vegetables are best when microwaved. The bags they are sold in usually give timing instructions.

Whole artichokes are the exception; they are best boiled.

Pre-steaming Vegetables

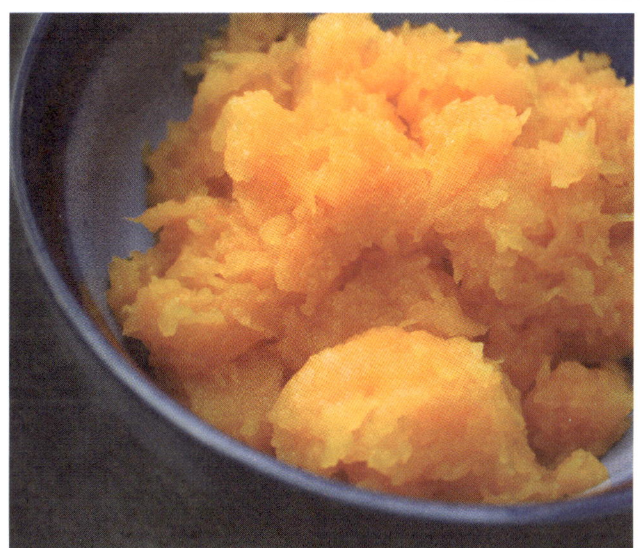

- The pre-steaming technique is good for butternut squash, turban squash and pumpkins.

- Winter squash is pre-steamed in the microwave prior to stuffing and roasting or mashing.

- You don't have to cut it in half; simply make slits with a knife so the steam can come out.

- Once the squash is steamed in the microwave, it can be cut up and mashed, cut in half and stuffed, or baked.

Boiling and Steaming on the Stove

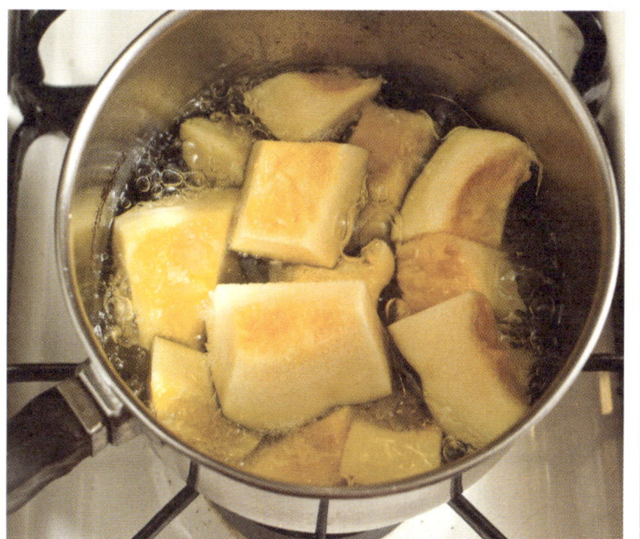

- When root vegetables and dried beans are boiled in a saucepan, the lid should be a good fit to stop the liquid boiling off.

- You need a good, heavy-bottomed saucepan or pot.

- Metal steamers that adapt to the size of a saucepan are useful for steaming on the stove, as they keep vegetables off the bottom of the pan.

- Adjust the cooking time to the size and thickness of the vegetables. You can always pull one out and test it.

BAKING DISHES & TINS

A few square and round glass and ceramic dishes are multifunctional in your kitchen

Certain metal tins and most glass dishes are excellent for baking, whether it's a delectable dessert or a hearty entrée. Casseroles can be cooked in 1- to 2-litre ceramic or glass dishes with lids, whereas gratins and baked pasta dishes such as lasagne are often baked in rectangular dishes: a 22 x 33 cm glass dish is a useful size. And, of course, baking sheets are an essential part of any kitchen, and can be used for far more than baking biscuits.

Pyrex toughened glass baking dishes go from the freezer to the microwave for defrosting or to the oven for baking. They are excellent for dishes that you can assemble in advance and then bake for dinner.

Ceramic Dishes

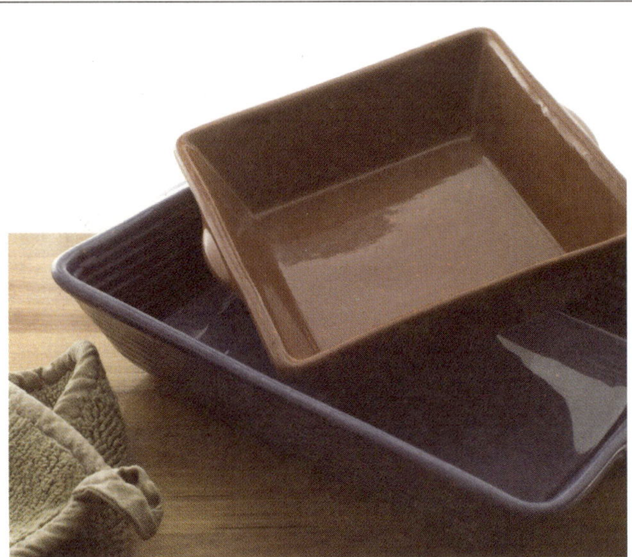

- Depending on their size, bake egg dishes in a ceramic gratin dish or a rectangular lasagne pan. Recipes with eggs in them will puff up nicely.

- Ceramic dishes can go in the microwave as well as the dishwasher.

- Many baked dishes can be assembled in advance, refrigerated, and baked just before serving.

Glass Baking Dishes

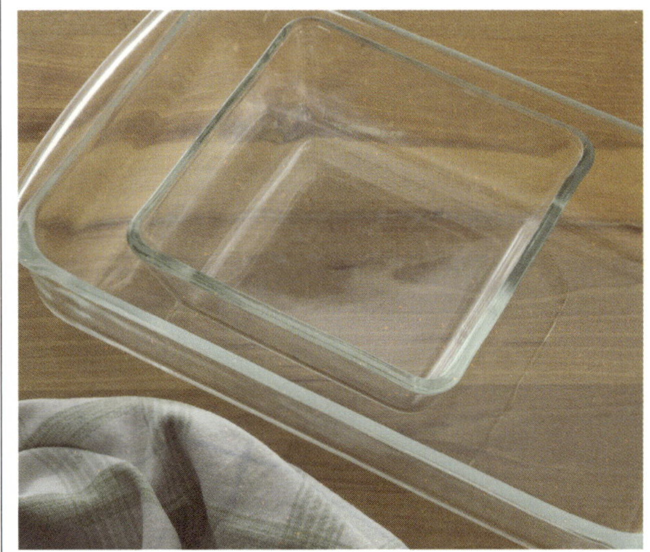

- Glass baking dishes will withstand a high oven temperature (but don't use Pyrex at temperatures over 225°C).

- Baked fruit, for example, is best made in these types of dishes. Try baking individual portions of fruit in glass custard cups.

- Most baking takes place at 170–180°C, though pastry should be baked at 200°C. Any hotter is likely to burn the food.

- Baking at below 170°C will dry out the food and it will take forever to cook.

You can use flameproof casseroles to soften vegetables and brown meat on the hob before cooking them in the oven. A flat-bottomed, straight-sided soufflé dish is essential for soufflés but can also be used for other wonderful dessert dishes.

Whenever you acquire kitchen equipment, look out for multipurpose pots, pans, muffin tins and dishes. You can buy online or at discount stores, but it's always worth browsing around kitchen shops and kitchen sections of department stores for inspiration and new ideas: some offer cooking classes and demonstrations.

When baking in glass or ceramic dishes, prevent food from sticking by buttering or oiling the dish, and then dusting it lightly with flour. This will make washing up much easier, even when food has browned in the dish. If the food is baked hard on to the empty dish, fill it with water with a little washing-up liquid and leave to soak, overnight if necessary, to loosen the deposits.

Baking Sheets

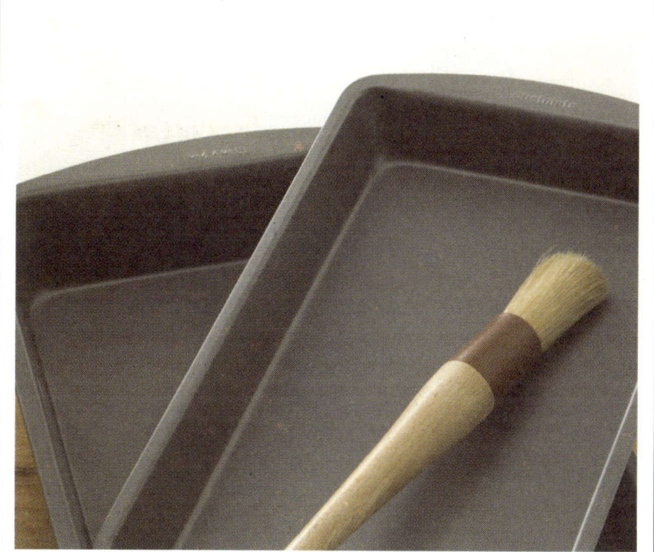

- Baking sheets are great multipurpose dishes to use in the kitchen, and there is a wide variety of foods that can be cooked on them.

- Meringues, for example, do well when cooked on baking sheets. They typically bake for a long time on low heat.

- Meringues can be baked on a flat baking sheet to make small, individual nests.

- Individual meringue nests are piped on to the baking sheet through a piping bag or heavy plastic bag.

Soufflé Dishes

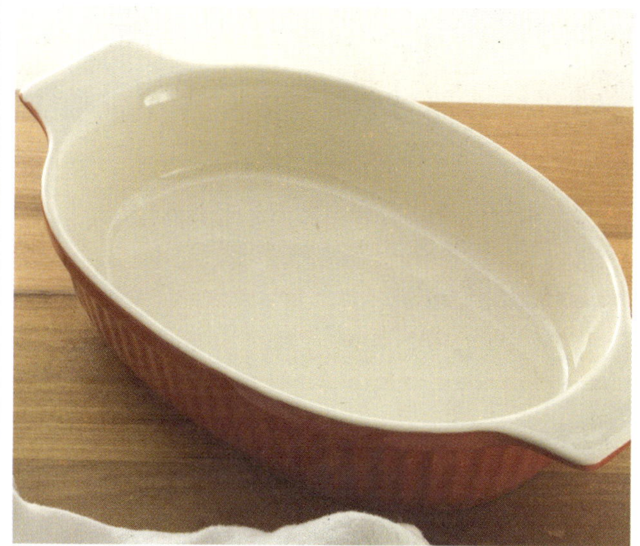

- To ensure a puffed soufflé, as opposed to a 'sou-flop', you need a real soufflé dish. These dishes come in various sizes and individual portion sizes, too.

- For a soufflé, preheat the oven to 200°C so that the egg whites get a blast of heat at the outset.

- After 15 minutes, turn the oven temperature down to 170°C.

- The soufflé dish uniformly distributes heat, and its high sides ensure that none of the gooey deliciousness of the dish spills out.

GRILLING

Grilling is a technique you will use often in the kitchen, and sometimes outdoors, on either a charcoal or gas barbecue, to produce tasty and flavourful results.

Cooking with an overhead grill supplies heat from above, using gas or electricity, while a barbecue or iron griddle supplies it from below, using gas, wood or charcoal. Grilling can be a great cooking technique to use when you are trying to

stick to a calorie-controlled diet, as much of the calorie-rich fat drips away from the meat during the cooking process.

Some kitchens are equipped with open-flame grills and may have charcoal-burning elements with excellent hoods to suck out the fumes. You should never use a charcoal grill indoors unless you have the proper venting equipment, and propane gas barbecues should never be brought indoors,

Grilling

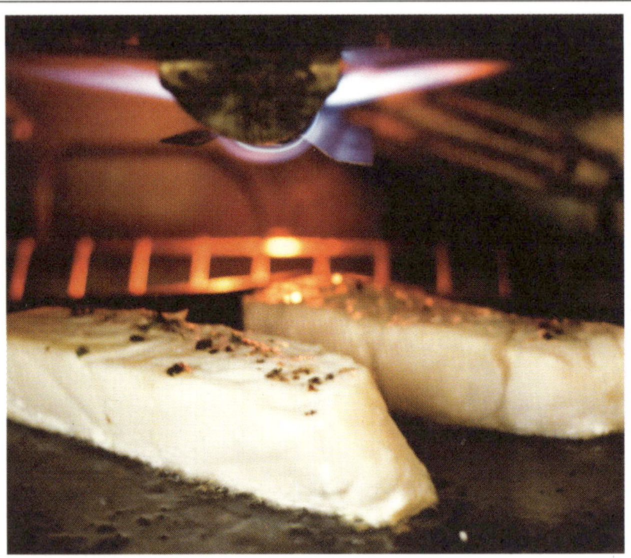

Chargrilling

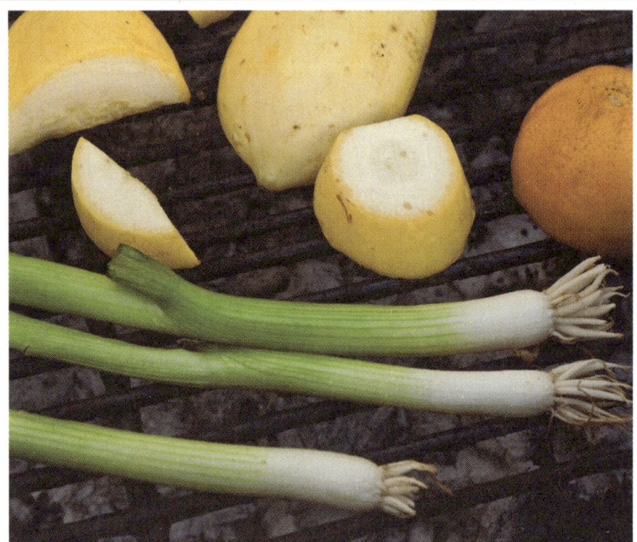

- An overhead grill sends the heat from the top down to the food. If you want to sear food, set the temperature of your oven grill to the maximum.

- To grill the food slowly, as with a thick piece of meat or fish, set the temperature between 150–200°C.

- Another method of slow grilling is to move the rack down to a lower level, between 10–30 cm from the flame.

- With a charcoal or gas barbecue, or a stovetop charcoal grill, heat comes from the bottom up.

- Stovetop grills are generally wrought iron or enamel-coated metal. You can control heat for searing and for slower cooking.

- When using a charcoal barbecue, you need to get used to letting it develop until the coals are a soft rose colour with a light coating of ash, not flaring.

- Simply set a gas barbecue to the desired temperature: high for searing, medium to cook food through.

even if it's raining outside. Carbon monoxide is a very dangerous, potentially deadly gas, and any kind of flame produces this gas, so keep your kitchen extractor fan working whenever you use the grill.

For grilling in the oven, use enamel or nonstick-coated metal pans, which should have racks to keep the meat off the bottom of the pan. Preheat the grill before cooking in order to get the food cooked through. With a thick piece of meat or fish, you can sear it on both sides using the grill then turn on the oven to finish cooking.

TECHNIQUES

Cleaning Grills

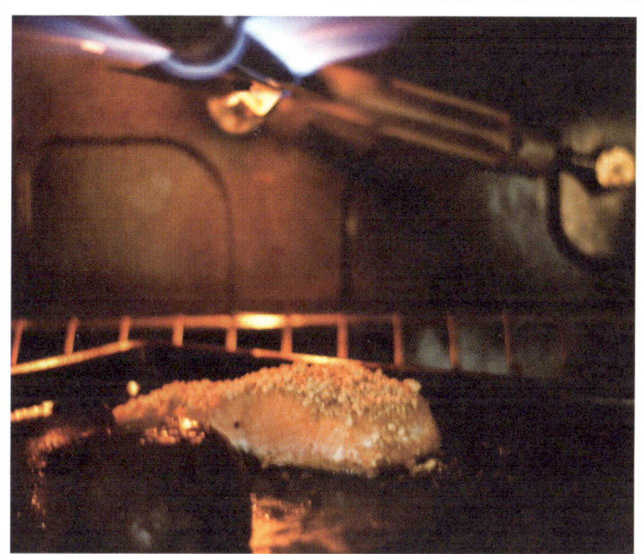

- Keep your barbecue, grill and oven very clean. Clean them often. You do not want a build-up of grease to taint the flavours of your food or start a fire.

- Cover grill pans with aluminium foil. Oil the rack before use.

- As soon as your barbecue is cool and you've finished dinner, spray it with a degreaser and rub it down with a wire brush.

- Be sure to keep food at least 15 cm from the flame.

Timing

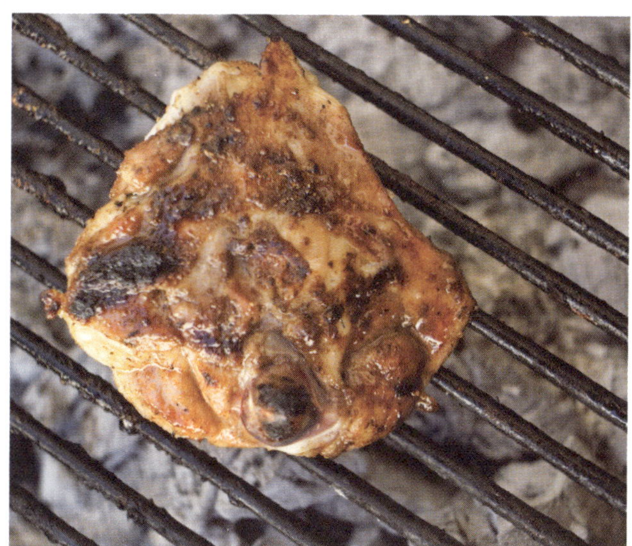

- Timing is of the essence when grilling, but a meat thermometer is far more reliable than a timer.

- Timing varies according to how you like your food done.

- Bone-in and skin-on meats will take longer to cook than boneless and skinless meat.

- If the food browns too fast under the grill, lower the temperature or move the meat further away from the heat.

- Chicken can dry out quickly on the barbecue or under the grill. Watch food carefully all the time and don't leave it.

ROASTING

Learn these techniques to help you cook a variety of healthy foods

Terms can get confusing when it comes to roasting. A roast is generally a large piece of meat or a whole chicken, turkey, duck or pheasant. But a pot roast is braised meat, browned and then slowly simmered in a small amount of liquid until it is very well done. A rib roast or top sirloin of beef may be basted but cooks in the oven uncovered; roast beef or lamb is often served rare to medium.

The best technique for roasting most joints of meat is to start cooking at a high temperature, and then reduce the heat for the remaining cooking time to let the joint cook through. This is true of beef, lamb and pork roasts. A pork roast with the bone in, for example, should also get a flash of heat to sear it and to crisp the skin, and then the heat should be lowered until the meat is done. The reverse is true of a large turkey, however. It

Lamb Roasts

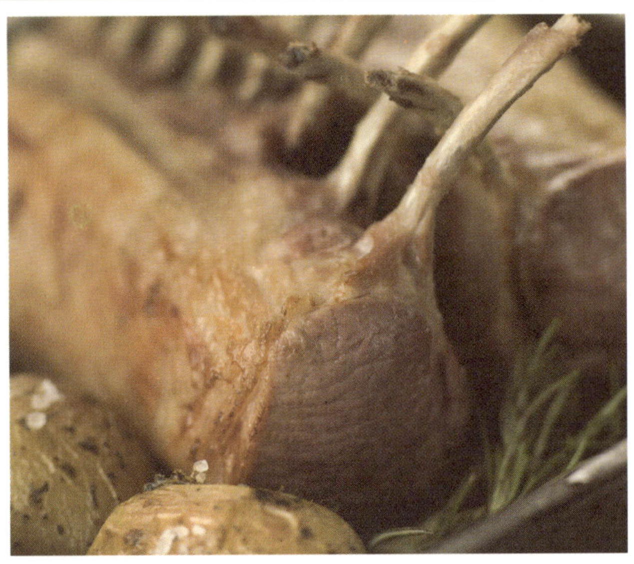

- With a lamb roast, you need to cut virtually all of the fat off the meat. The fat is strong and will affect the flavour of the meat.

- Young lamb is much more delicate in flavour than meat from a mature sheep, known as mutton.

- Marinating the lamb tenderizes it.

- Baby rack of lamb doesn't need marinating and needs very little trimming. It's grilled and then baked.

Roasting Equipment

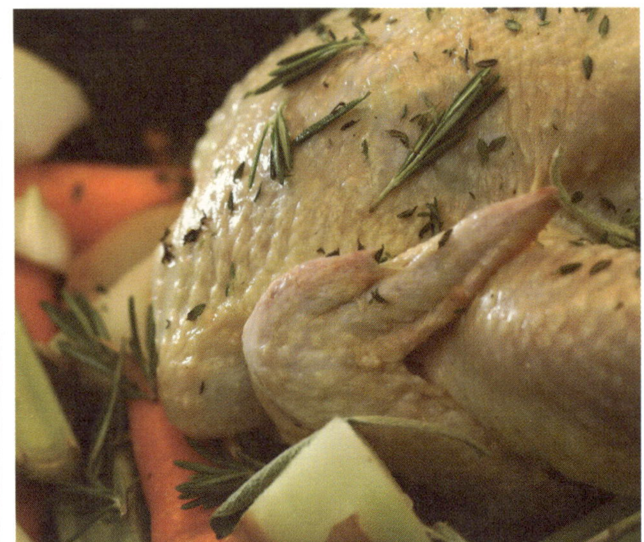

- The equipment you need is simple. If you can't afford a really great roasting tin, use an aluminium foil one.

- Meat thermometers also come in handy when cooking meat. Some thermometers are pushed into the meat, and others sit on the top of the oven, connected to the meat by a long cable.

- Cover the meat with foil or heavy kitchen towels to rest. This step is essential. If the meat does not rest, the juices will run out when it's carved. When it's rested, the juice returns to the meat.

should be covered and cooked slowly until the end, and then be uncovered to brown.

Essential equipment for roasting includes an enamel-covered metal roasting dish with a rack, or a disposable heavy-duty aluminium foil dish, and a meat thermometer.

Roasting Large Joints

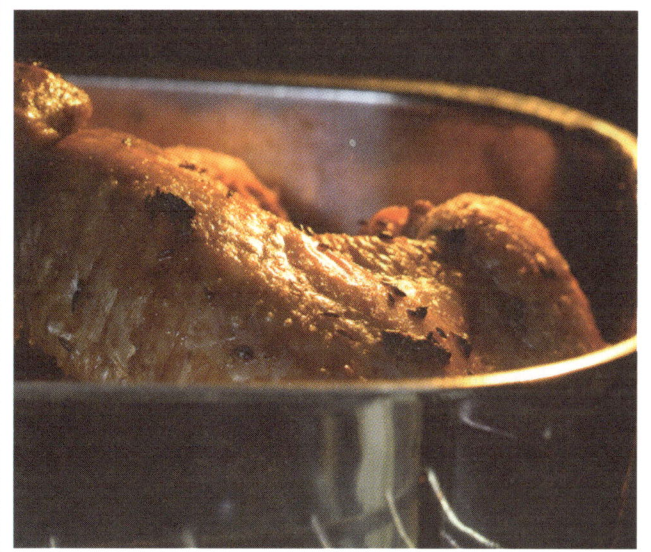

- In the case of a large rib roast or turkey, you may need to 'tent' it with aluminium foil to ensure that it will be cooked through.

- Tenting prevents meat from drying out and browning. Remove foil 30 minutes before the end of cooking time so the meat browns.

- Some cooks start turkeys, chickens, ducks and geese breast-down on a bed of celery and carrots. This sends juices into the breast.

- When roasting small birds such as ducks, pheasants or quail, wrap the drumsticks in foil to keep them from drying out.

Basting

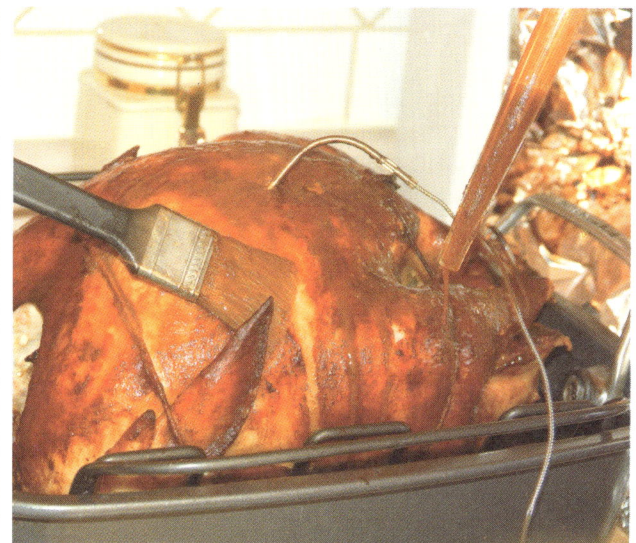

- Basting, or adding liquid to the meat, is an important technique in roasting. Use a variety of liquids or a mixture. For example, use chicken or vegetable stock on chicken.

- A mixture of red wine and beef stock works well on beef roasts.

- Herbs make a tasty addition to basting liquid. Add 1 tablespoon of rosemary to your chicken baste; add 1 teaspoon of sage leaves to your beef.

- Use a bulb baster, a small ladle or a pastry brush.

FAMILY FRITTATA

A frittata can be served hot, cold, or at room temperature

A frittata is an Italian open-faced omelette. It is versatile and delicious. Making a frittata is easier than making an omelette because you don't have to worry about it sticking to the pan or having to fold it in half.

This frittata is stuffed with caramelized onions, fresh tomatoes and basil. You can stuff a frittata with mushrooms or a combination of cheeses, and thinly sliced salami and favourite herbs can be added. Try a frittata with fresh baby spinach or frozen spinach and Gorgonzola cheese.

Kids love frittata, as do adults. They are a great way to use up the leftovers in your refrigerator: chop some cooked leftover broccoli, add cheese and eggs, and you've got lunch.

Ingredients

Serves 8

2 tablespoons olive oil

1 mild onion, white or yellow, peeled and thinly sliced

5 whole eggs

4 egg whites

Freshly ground black pepper to taste

25 g grated Parmesan cheese

1/4 teaspoon salt (optional)

1 medium tomato, cored and thinly sliced

10 large basil leaves, shredded, or 1 teaspoon dried basil

Calories 109, **Fat** 8 g, **Carbohydrates** 2 g, **Protein** 8 g, **Fibre** 0, **Saturated Fat** 2 g, **Cholesterol** 136 mg, **Sodium** 136 mg.

Family Frittata

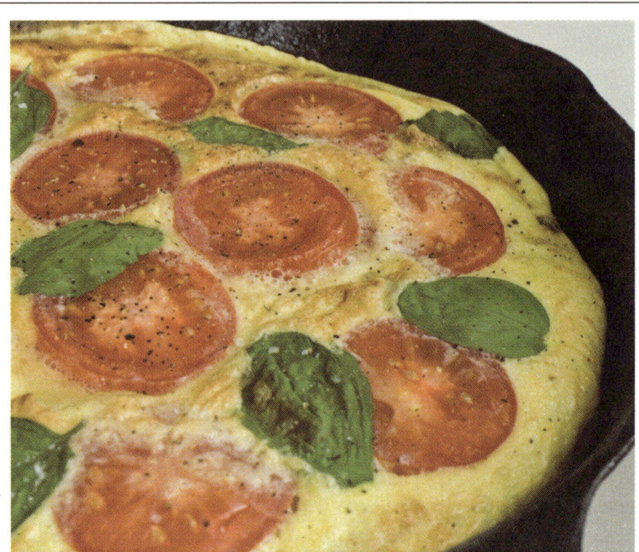

- Heat oil in large cast-iron pan. Add onions. Cook gently until softened. Remove from heat. Preheat grill.

- Place eggs and extra whites in a blender with pepper and Parmesan cheese. Add salt, if desired. Blend until smooth. Pour over onions and stir to distribute evenly.

- Arrange tomatoes and basil over the top. Place on low heat and cook until well set. Leave it a bit runny on top.

- Place under the grill until lightly browned, about 2 minutes. Cut into wedges to serve.

By cutting the number of egg yolks and using more egg whites, you reduce the calories and cholesterol drastically. You can also use other low-fat ingredients, such as mushrooms, spinach, herbs, tomatoes and other vegetables. Try adding barbecued vegetables for a wonderful boost of flavour.

• • • • • RECIPE VARIATION • • • • •

Experiment with new flavours: Try making the frittata with dill and salmon, or add some rosemary and 75 g crumbled turkey bacon. Fruit can be added to a frittata if you are making it for dessert. Use the basic egg recipe and top with a sliced peach and some berries. Sprinkle the top with Splenda when the frittata is done.

Cast-Iron Frying Pans

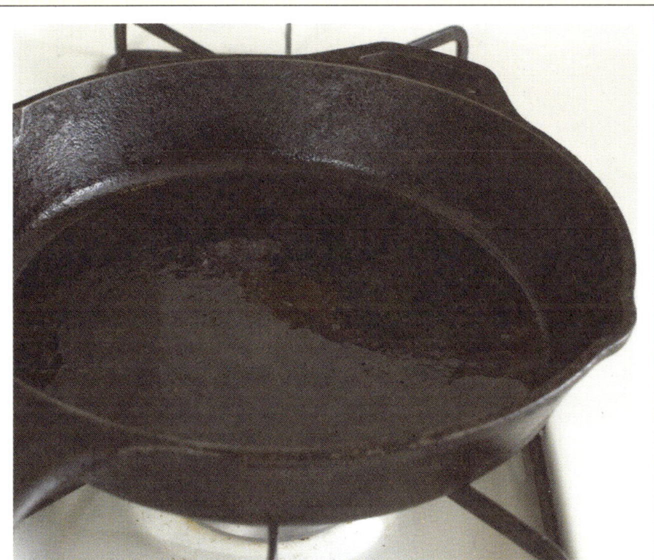

Seasoning Cast-Iron Pans

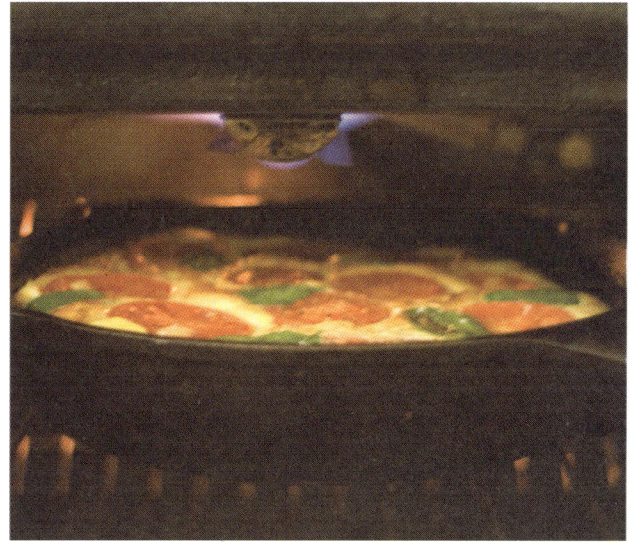

- Cast-iron pans are good for more than frying. Black and heavy, they are wonderful for all kinds of cooking. They hold the heat and distribute it evenly.

- These pans are perfect for using under the grill to brown food before serving. You can't do this with any pan that has a plastic handle.

- Be careful, however; use a potholder when picking up a hot cast-iron pan.

- Use cast-iron pans to make griddle cakes, simmer stew or fry chicken.

- These pans must be seasoned before using. First, heat the pan; then remove it from the heat and add cooking oil (not olive oil).

- Let the oil soak in while the pan cools, and then wipe it off with paper towels.

- Once the pan is seasoned, don't wash it with detergent or you will have to season it again.

- Just rinse the pan in hot water and wipe it dry with a paper towel after each use. You will have to reseason it occasionally.

PUFFY EGG WHITE OMELETTE

One bite of this delicious omelette, and you'll be a believer in the 'incredible edible egg'

Egg white omelettes are delicious, simple to make, and incredibly versatile. They cut absolutely all of the cholesterol out of the eggs.

This recipe is for a soufflé omelette. However, you can also make it in the traditional way. Avoid the 'puff' by whisking the eggs only gently.

This omelette, filled with lemon-flavoured ricotta and spinach, has a delightful tangy flavour. If you use frozen spinach thaw it completely before use and make sure you squeeze out all the extra moisture. Or make your filling with a couple of handfuls of fresh baby spinach, chopped and mixed in with the ricotta.

Ingredients

Serves 4

225 g low-fat ricotta cheese

275 g frozen chopped spinach or
100 g fresh baby spinach, chopped

$1/4$ teaspoon ground nutmeg

1 teaspoon lemon zest

25 g Parmesan cheese

10 egg whites

Calories 173, **Fat** 7 g, **Carbohydrates** 7 g, **Protein** 21 g,
Fibre 2 g, **Saturated Fat** 4 g, **Cholesterol** 25 mg, **Sodium** 263 mg.

Puffy Egg White Omelette

- Mix ricotta, spinach, nutmeg, lemon zest and Parmesan cheese in a bowl.

- Beat or whisk egg whites until they form high peaks (add a pinch of salt, if desired). Fold ricotta-spinach mixture into egg whites.

- Preheat grill and lightly oil a large cast-iron frying pan.

- Place pan over medium heat. Add egg mixture. Don't stir. Cook until mixture starts to brown on the sides. Place under the grill to brown the top, about 2 minutes. Serve immediately.

Puff and fill that omelette: you can get a nice puff in your omelette by beating the egg whites with an eggbeater or whisk. Fill the omelette by folding the goodies into the egg white mixture. For the full puff, start the omelette cooking in a nonstick pan on top of the stove and then finish it in the oven.

Add a bit of greenery: In addition to spinach, you can add chopped cooked broccoli, rocket or a combination of tomatoes and herbs. Another great filling for any omelette is asparagus, cooked and cut into 2.5 cm pieces. Or if you're splurging, just use the tips (save the rest of the spears for soup).

Separating Egg Whites

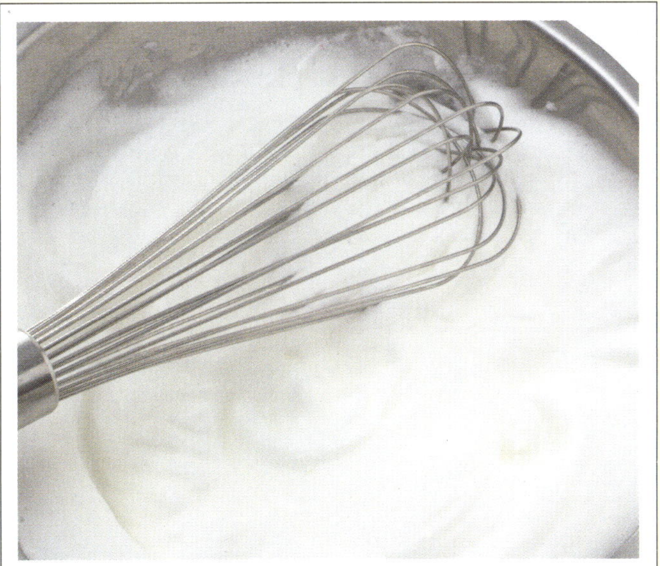

- If there is even a speck of egg yolk mixed with the whites, they will not whip properly.

- They will be foamy but not 'peaky', puffy or perky. Ensure that your whisk or eggbeater blades are completely degreased and clean.

- When you separate more than one or two eggs, it's prudent to use two glass bowls.

- Separate egg whites individually into a small bowl so that you can check each one for specks of yolk before adding it to the rest in the large bowl.

Cooking Under the Grill

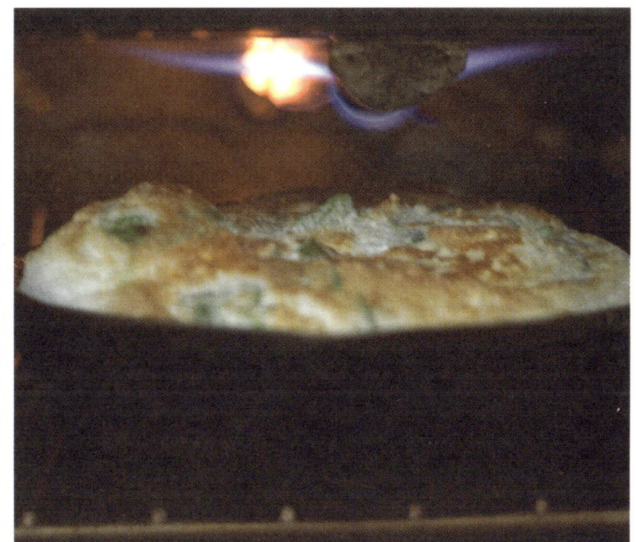

- Often a dish requires more than just cooking on top of the stove, which only cooks the bottom of the food.

- For this kind of thick omelette you need to cook the top using the overhead heat of the grill.

- Be vigilant with the grill. It's easy to burn the top of a dish and leave the inside raw.

- If the top browns too quickly, turn off the grill, close the oven door, and let the dish cook through in the low heat for a few more minutes.

HALF-YOLK OMELETTE WITH SALSA

This is a good way to retain a rich 'eggy' flavour while cutting the fat

You can make this recipe either in two batches, each serving two people, or as one big omelette to serve four people. If you have two matching nonstick pans it's easy to cook two omelettes at the same time.

Just be sure to prepare and place your fillings at the side of the stove before you start to cook the eggs. As soon as the eggs begin to set, you can add the fillings and fold the omelettes in half to finish cooking.

Some people like their omelettes soft and runny, while others like them well-set, almost stiff. It's simply a matter of timing. Just be sure to reduce the heat so that you don't burn the bottom of the more 'done' omelette.

Ingredients

Serves 4

4 whole eggs

6 egg whites

175 ml fresh tomato salsa (mild, medium or hot, to taste)

50 g low-fat Cheddar cheese, grated

4 tablespoons low-fat sour cream

Calories 157, **Fat** 8 g, **Carbohydrates** 5 g, **Protein** 16 g, **Fibre** 1 g, **Saturated Fat** 3 g, **Cholesterol** 220 mg, **Sodium** 536 mg.

Half-Yolk Omelette with Salsa

- Break whole eggs into a bowl. Add whites to the whole eggs. Whisk eggs until well blended.

- Lightly oil a 25-cm nonstick frying pan or two 17.5-cm pans.

- Pour the eggs in the pan(s); tip to spread eggs evenly.

- When the top is just set, spoon salsa on one side of the omelette and sprinkle with cheese.

- Fold the other half of the omelette(s) over the filling. Slip on to a plate and divide into servings. Spoon sour cream over the top of each serving.

Brunch, lunch or supper omelettes: An omelette can be as full of ingredients or as light as you wish – perfect for any meal. A medium-light omelette contains two whites for each yolk (e.g., four egg whites to two yolks), as opposed to all whole eggs. A light omelette consists of all egg whites. For light omelettes for big meals, try fruit fillings, low-fat cheese, and/or light meats, such as 50 g per person of smoked turkey or turkey sausage. Add 50 g per person small prawns for a flavourful lunchtime omelette. You can add asparagus, chopped artichoke hearts and roasted vegetables. If you serve an omelette for brunch or lunch, add a side salad to keep it light. If the omelette is for dinner, start with soup and serve hot multigrain bread on the side.

Don't Let It Dry Out

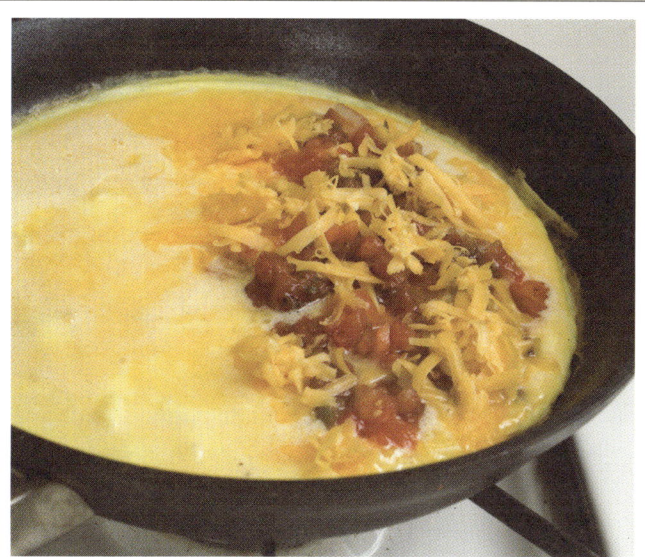

A Kitchen Sink Omelette

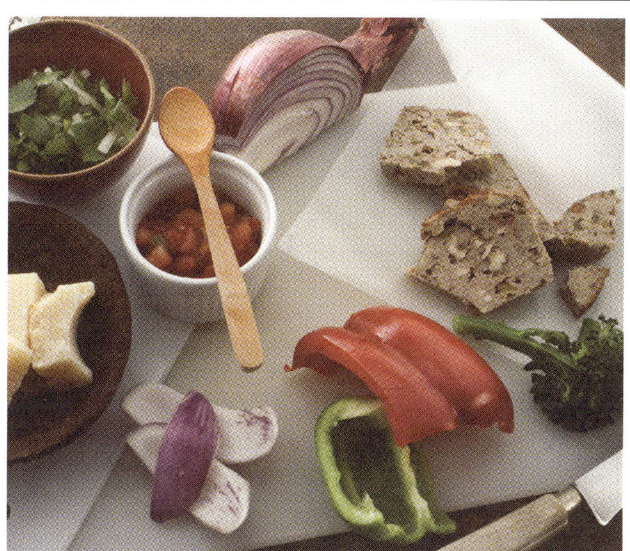

- Don't let the omelette get too dry; it will crack and be difficult to fold, and won't be good to eat.

- Place the filling on one side, then immediately turn the plain side on to it.

- Or spoon the filling down the middle of the omelette, then fold each side over the middle. Next, flip the omelette over, leaving the smooth side on top. This melds the sides together.

- Carefully remove the omelette to a warm platter. Cut into serving pieces and add extra salsa to each.

- When you're home alone, an omelette becomes the ultimate comfort food. It's quick and easy to make, and it's also easy on the digestive system.

- Try making a 'kitchen sink' omelette from leftovers. Start with an inventory of your fridge and freezer.

- Leftover salad vegetables work well, as do leftover cold cuts, steak, chicken or raw prawns.

- Use bits of cheese and whatever else you have. Whisk up a couple of eggs or one whole egg and two whites.

SALMON & EGG CASSEROLE

With this prepare-ahead dish, you can plan on a leisurely brunch

The delicious combination of salmon, cream cheese, eggs and spring onions makes a fabulous American-style brunch dish for friends and family.

Put the recipe together the day or night before for a quick meal. Pop it in the oven a little while before your guests arrive, and relax. This is best baked in a large, shallow oval or rectangular gratin dish, either metal or ceramic, which gives a lot of surface to brown to form a delicous crusty top. You can use multigrain white bread or a multigrain baguette instead of sourdough for extra texture.

Another important point about this recipe is that it tastes far richer and more caloric than it really is. Serve it with a crisp green salad on the side, or toss some frozen petit pois into the casserole with the onions and salmon.

Ingredients

Serves 8

500 ml semi-skimmed or skimmed milk

10 eggs

1 teaspoon homemade mustard (see recipe, page 204) or dry English mustard

$1/_2$ teaspoon cayenne pepper

225 g low-fat or light cream cheese, in chunks

1 loaf multigrain sourdough bread, cut in 2-cm cubes

1 bunch spring onions, trimmed and chopped into 6-mm pieces

115 g smoked salmon

Freshly ground black pepper to taste

Calories 325, **Fat** 8 g, **Carbohydrates** 43 g, **Protein** 20 g, **Fibre** 5 g, **Saturated Fat** 4 g, **Cholesterol** 21 mg, **Sodium** 709 mg.

Salmon & Egg Casserole

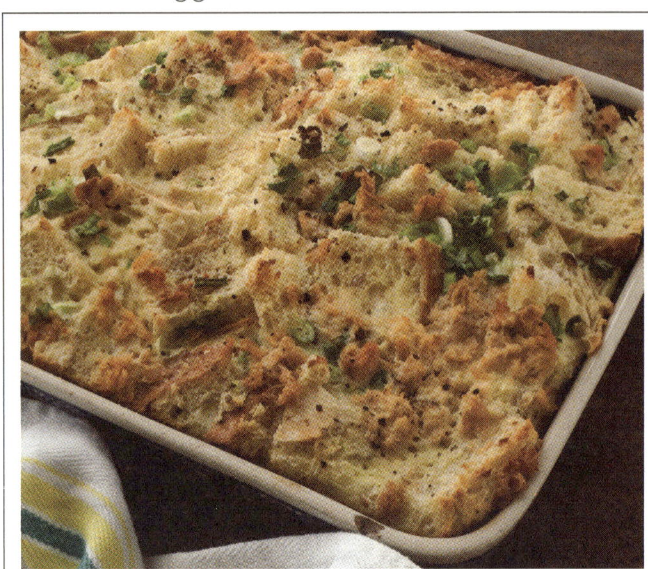

- Process milk, eggs, mustard and cayenne in blender for 1 minute. With blender on low, add cream cheese 1 teaspoonful at a time.

- Lightly oil baking dish. Spread bread cubes in dish. Pour in milk, egg and cheese mixture. Cover; refrigerate overnight.

- Remove from fridge 30 minutes before baking and preheat oven to 180°C. Mix spring onions and salmon into bread mixture.

- Sprinkle with black pepper; bake for 1 hour or until puffed and golden. Serve immediately.

Added nutrients: The multigrain sourdough bread provides fibre, B vitamins and other nutrients that are good for the diet. Serve the dish with a salad of roasted beetroot and mixed leaves. Or make a traditional Greek salad, but with only half the usual amount of feta cheese, as there is plenty of cheese in the casserole.

• • • • • RECIPE VARIATION • • • • •

For a different taste: Replace the salmon with the same quantity of ham, smoked turkey, cooked turkey bacon, or cooked turkey sausage. Use 225 g grated low-fat Cheddar or ricotta rather than the cream cheese. Thaw and drain 225 g frozen spinach to add, or use 115 g fresh baby spinach and roasted red pepper or green pepper for added nutrients.

Blender Secrets

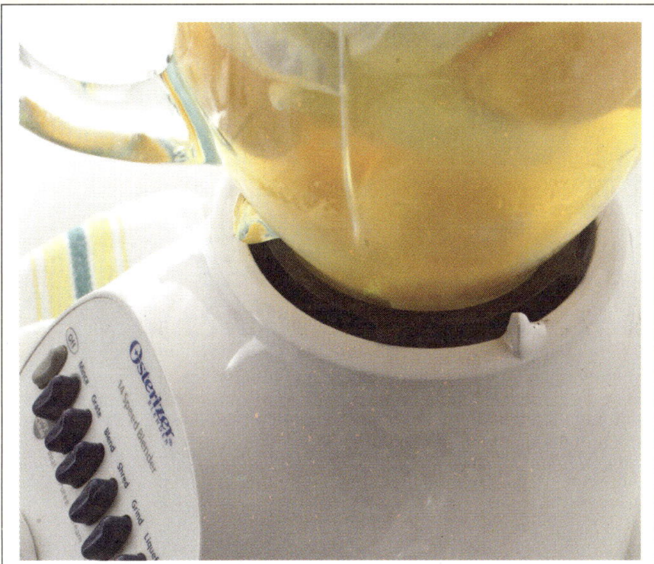

Fridge to Oven to Table

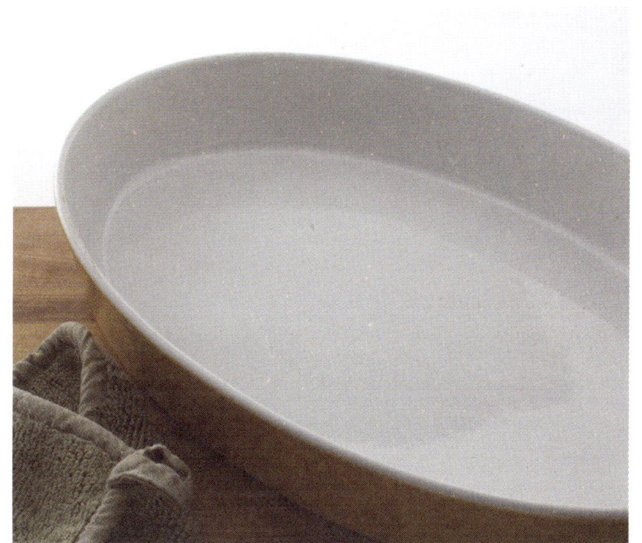

- Always start blending with the liquids in the recipe and make sure they are completely mixed; this can take about 2 minutes.

- When adding flour, cheese or sugar, do so slowly, with the motor on low.

- In between additions, give the liquids time to 'digest' the more solid ingredients.

- Turn the machine off from time to time and scrape down the sides with a rubber spatula. This ensures that everything is completely blended.

- Some manufacturers claim that their dishes can go from the refrigerator or freezer straight into a preheated oven.

- This isn't a good idea. The food will cook more evenly if it isn't frozen or icy cold. Bring it up to room temperature before baking.

- Ceramic or glass baking dishes can crack or even break in half, neither of which you want to have happen to your delicious food.

- Check that the dishes you buy can sustain both heat and cold.

CLAFOUTIS WITH PEACHES & HAM

The classic French dessert can be adapted for a special breakfast or brunch

Traditionally, clafoutis is made with fresh, stoned cherries, cream and a lot more sugar than in this recipe. You'll find that you can use Splenda, or eliminate most of the sugar entirely. Instead of cherries, try adding peaches, which should be blanched, peeled, stoned and sliced. You can use just about any fruit you like for this recipe, however, and the ham is optional. The dish looks very pretty baked in a white or decorated ceramic flan dish.

With this particular recipe, you get your dairy, carbohydrates and protein in one dish. You can also serve it with some fresh fruit compote, a dollop of low-fat sour cream, or a small scoop of sorbet for added flavour.

Ingredients

Serves 6

250 ml semi-skimmed milk

2 tablespoons Splenda for baking

5 eggs

1 teaspoon vanilla extract

$^1/_2$ teaspoon salt

75 g plain flour

4 large or 6 small peaches, blanched, peeled and sliced

115 g smoked or boiled ham, thinly sliced and shredded

Calories 204, **Fat** 7 g, **Carbohydrates** 23 g, **Protein** 13 g, **Fibre** 2 g, **Saturated Fat** 2 g, **Cholesterol** 189 mg, **Sodium** 454 mg.

Clafoutis with Peaches and Ham

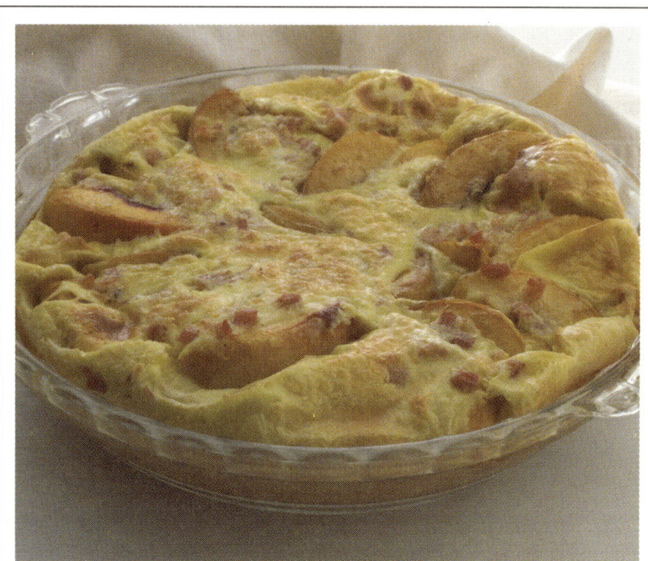

- Preheat oven to 180°C. Mix milk, Splenda, eggs, vanilla, salt and flour in blender until smooth, about 2 minutes.

- Lightly oil a flameproof flan dish. Pour in 6 mm depth of batter and place it over a very low heat.

- When it has set, add the peaches and ham, distributing them evenly on top.

- Pour the rest of the batter into the dish; bake in oven on middle shelf for about 30 minutes, until puffed and golden brown. Cut into wedges.

French country food: Classic clafoutis is a rustic pudding that originated in the Limousin region around Limoges in east-central France. It is a charming summer dessert that is still served in hotels in and around Paris.

Local farm shops and farmers' markets are a great source of fresh food that can be enjoyed all year-round. It doesn't take long to blanch, peel and freeze a box of peaches for winter pies; just add a little lemon juice and 1 teaspoon of sugar to the freezer container. You can then have fresh peach pies, clafoutis or omelettes all through the chilly months.

Blanching Fruit for Easy Peeling

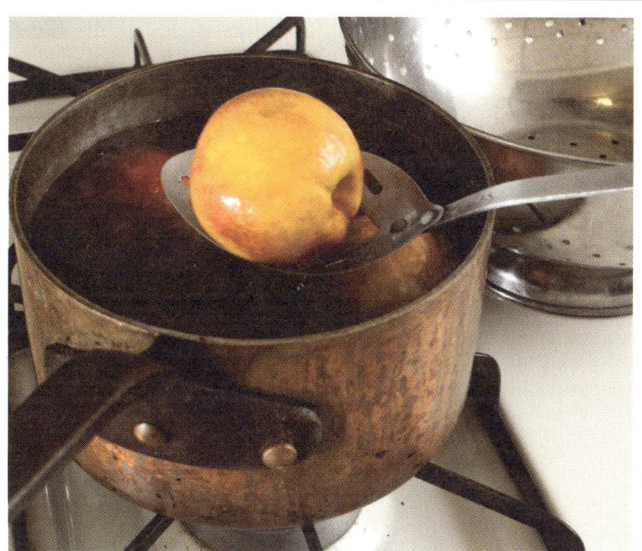

Slicing Blanched Fruit

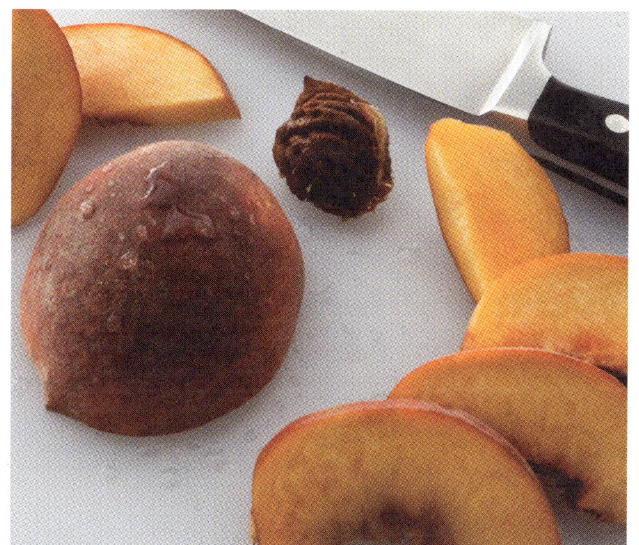

- Bring a large saucepan of water to the boil.

- Lower the fruit (peaches, apricots and nectarines) gently into the water. Turn the fruit to immerse fully.

- After about 2 minutes, remove the fruit. Place it in a colander and leave until cool enough to handle. Cold water can be run over the fruit to speed cooling and stop the cooking process.

- Slip off the skins. Cut the fruits in half; remove stones and slice.

- Rather than holding a slippery piece of blanched fruit in your hand, try this:

- Cut fruit in half. Remove the stone.

- Place cut-side down on a chopping board. Using a very sharp paring knife, slice lengthwise and place in a bowl.

- Add 1 teaspoon of lemon juice to the fruit to prevent it from turning brown. Use the same technique for preparing fresh fruit to be frozen.

45

WORLD-CLASS SCRAMBLED EGGS

Your friends and family will want to know the secret of this delicious way of cooking eggs

My mother brought this recipe home from a visit to the Scottish Highlands in the 1960s. She loved the scrambled eggs prepared this way, and couldn't believe how easy, simple and special the recipe was.

Ever since she gave me the recipe, I've been dong scrambled eggs in this way. People always ask for my secret.

It's simply a different formula: same fresh eggs, but much more milk than you'd normally use, and a very different and far gentler method of handling the eggs when they are in the pan. The results are truly amazing.

Ingredients

Serves 4

6 whole eggs

3 egg whites

150 ml semi-skimmed milk

Salt to taste

Freshly ground black pepper to taste

1 tablespoon butter or olive oil

Calories 166, **Fat** 11 g, **Carbohydrates** 3 g, **Protein** 14 g, **Fibre** 0, **Saturated Fat** 4 g, **Cholesterol** 327 mg, **Sodium** 164 mg.

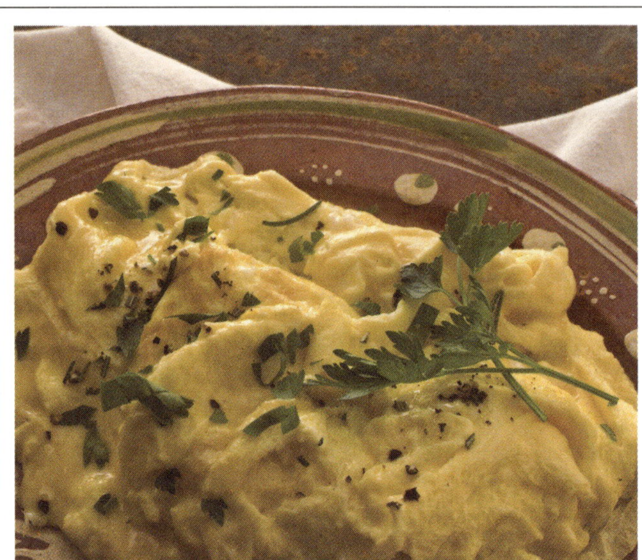

World-Class Scrambled Eggs

- Whisk or use an eggbeater to blend the whole eggs, egg whites, milk, salt and pepper.

- Place pan over medium-high heat and melt butter, or add oil. Add the eggs and reduce the heat to low.

- Let the eggs start to set, and then gently fold the eggs, once only, going around the sides of the pan with a rubber spatula.

- Cook to desired doneness and serve.

Embellishing your eggs: Au naturel is a popular way to serve this dish; however, you can enhance it with lots of different goodies. When the eggs are almost done, add a handful of chopped herbs. Or add 50 g crumbled Gorgonzola or Parmesan cheese. You can also add some chopped tomatoes, caramelized onions, or a little shredded smoked turkey or ham. Chopped roasted red peppers brighten up the eggs. A handful of chunkily chopped fresh mozzarella makes them chewy, while strips of processed cheese melt beautifully and give the eggs a creamy touch. One (400-g) can of unmarinated artichokes, drained, adds a lot of interest. Or add some blanched and drained asparagus tips combined with 1 teaspoon of lemon zest.

Adding Herbs

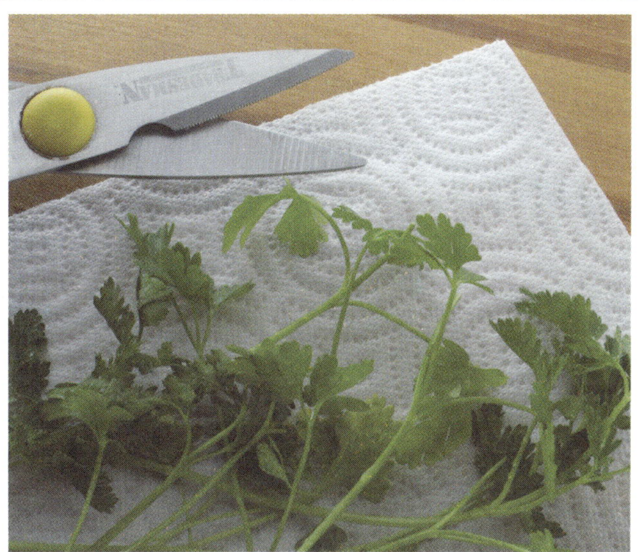

- Fresh herbs and eggs go very well together. Rather than mixing herbs into the eggs before cooking, try this method.

- Rinse and dry a small bunch of flat-leaf parsley, a bunch of chives and two or three sprigs of fresh oregano and basil leaves.

- Remove leaves from stems. Using kitchen shears, snip the parsley and chives on to a piece of greaseproof paper; add the oregano leaves and tear the basil. Sprinkle over the eggs.

Keeping Hot Food Hot

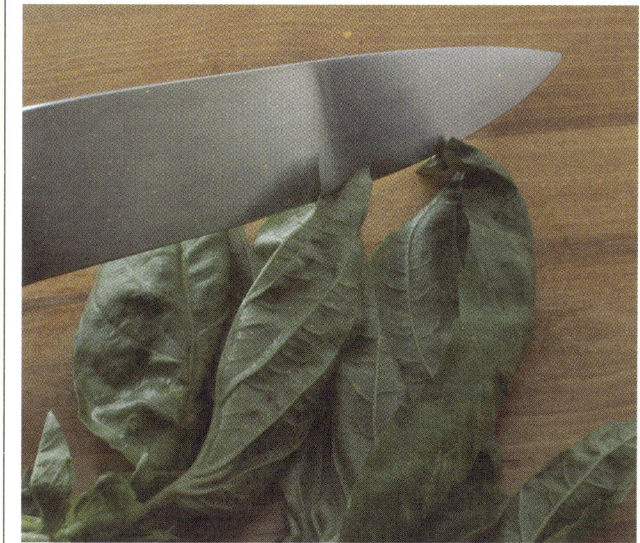

- Cold scrambled eggs are not appealing. Warm the plates either on a hot tray or in a slow oven for a few minutes so that the eggs won't pick up a chill from the plates.

- If you are making a large batch for a crowd, undercook the eggs slightly and keep them on a warm platter.

- The longer eggs wait to be eaten, the more done they will get if kept on a hot tray. They're best eaten the minute they're cooked.

BASIC PANCAKES

Fabulous and easy to make, pancakes can be savoury or sweet

Pancakes adapt wonderfully to almost any meal, whether it's a light lunch or a quick snack, a main course or a dessert. They're great either sweet or savoury, filled with whatever you desire.

Sweet pancakes can be filled with almost any fruit and/or creamy pudding mixture. They are festive when filled with slightly cooked berries.

Savory pancakes filled with asparagus and dressed with a warm mayonnaise and cheese sauce are delicious for lunch. They can be stuffed with spinach and ricotta cheese or chicken and mushrooms.

You can make pancakes a maximum of 3 days ahead and keep them in the refrigerator, or make them a week ahead and freeze them. Make three 15-cm pancakes per person.

Ingredients:

Serves 4

For the pancakes:

500 ml cold skimmed milk

2 whole eggs

3 egg whites

1/2 teaspoon salt

2 tablespoons Splenda (if making sweet pancakes)

175 g plain flour

50 g whole-wheat flour

2 tablespoons unsalted butter

1 tablespoon low-fat margarine

For the filling (sweet pancakes):

120 ml cold water

1 tablespoon cornflour

1 teaspoon Splenda

175 g fresh raspberries

175 g fresh blueberries

Calories 422, **Fat** 10 g, **Carbohydrates** 67 g, **Protein** 18 g, **Fibre** 6 g, **Saturated Fat** 5 g, **Cholesterol** 124 mg, **Sodium** 443 mg.

Berry Pancakes

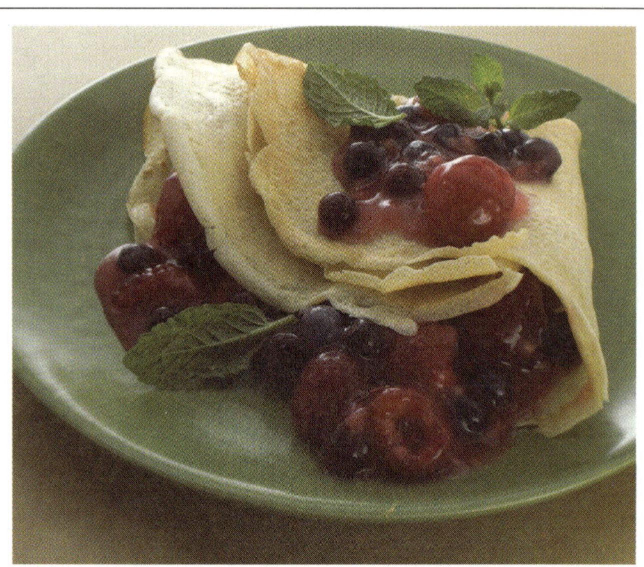

- Blend milk, eggs, salt and Splenda. On low, slowly add flour. Scrape bowl. Add butter and margarine; blend 1 minute. Refrigerate 2 hours.

- Heat a nonstick 18- or 20-cm pan over medium-high heat and oil lightly. Pour in 50 ml batter; swirl to make a 15-cm pancake.

- When brown on both sides, place pancake on waxed paper and repeat with rest of batter.

- Whisk water, cornflour, and Splenda in pan, and add berries. Boil, stirring until thickened. Spoon on to pancakes and fold or roll. Pour juice over all.

Stuffing for savoury pancakes: Omit the Splenda to make a perfect plain pancake to fill with chicken or other savoury stuffing. Mix together 1 (275-g) can low-fat cream of chicken soup and 225 g cooked chicken breast, diced. Add 25 g Parmesan cheese and enough skimmed milk to make a thick filling. Place 2 tablespoons of the filling in the middle of each pancake and roll carefully into a tube. Place the filled pancakes side by side in an oiled baking dish, seam side down. Thin the remaining sauce with more milk and pour over the top. Bake at 170°C until steaming hot and serve. Or mix 115 g each ricotta and spinach and 1 egg with 1 tablespoon of Parmesan, and stuff savoury pancakes. You can sauce these pancakes with low-fat cream of chicken soup.

How to Spread the Batter

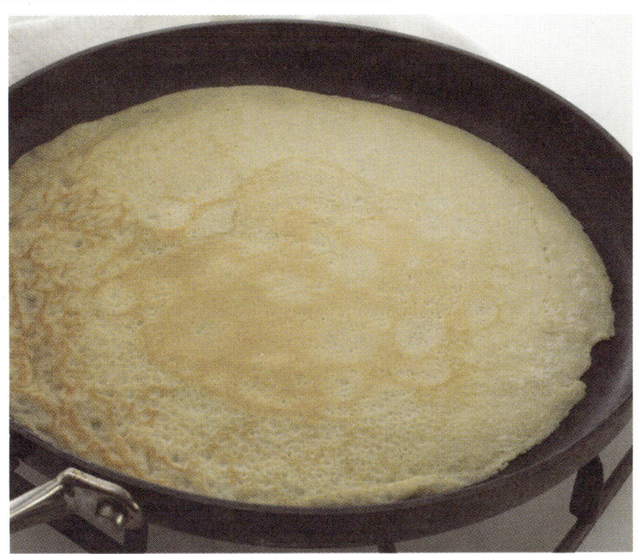

- Use a ladle, half full, to pour batter into the hot pan.

- As you add batter to the pan, lift the pan with your other hand and keep moving the batter around over the bottom of the pan to distribute it evenly.

- Lift the edges of the pancake with a heat-resistant spatula to prevent it from sticking. Turn the pancake as soon as it is lightly browned on the bottom. It may develop brown spots on the second side that is cooked.

Storing Pancakes

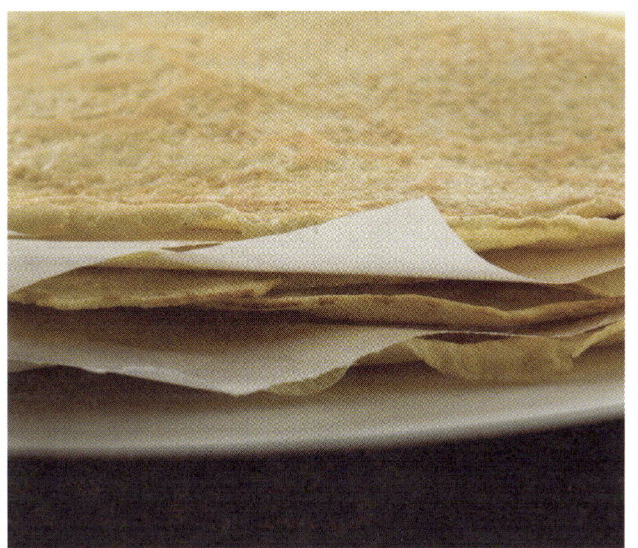

- As you cook the pancakes, remove them from the pan and place each one on an individual sheet of greaseproof paper. Leave to cool.

- Place the pancakes in a sealed bag and refrigerate. If you are freezing them, make a double quantity and freeze in groups of six.

- Remember they will be brittle when frozen, so pack paper plates around the batches of pancakes to be frozen to prevent them from breaking.

SPINACH-APPLE YOGURT SMOOTHIES

At breakfast or snack time, this quick smoothie can easily be part of a healthy eating plan

Smoothies can start your day with a real boost, giving you enough nourishment to last until lunch, even a late lunch. Since they can be high in carbohydrates, try to work them into your diet plan ahead of time.

With a smoothie, you can pack a bunch of healthy ingredients into one flavourful drink. Sneak cooked carrots or cauliflower into an orange-banana smoothie, and add a generous scoop of luscious Greek yogurt. Or, add a handful of fresh baby spinach to a blueberry-lemon smoothie for a delightful hidden vegetable mixture.

Ingredients

Serves 2

350 ml plain non-fat yogurt

2 tart eating apples

25 g fresh spinach leaves, rinsed

2.5-cm piece fresh ginger, peeled and chopped

2 tablespoons unprocessed bran

Juice of $\frac{1}{2}$ lemon

Salt to taste

2 ice cubes, crushed

Spinach-Apple Yogurt Smoothies

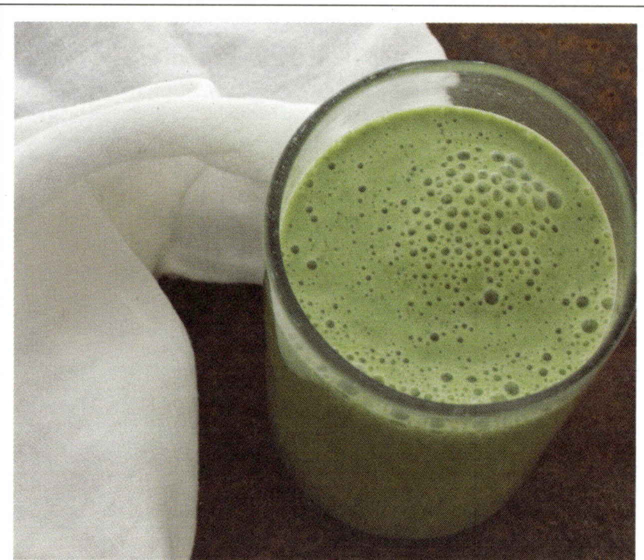

- Place all ingredients in a blender.

- Whirl until very smooth, stopping occasionally to scrape down the sides of the blender.

- Add 3–4 ice cubes for extra crushed ice. Add one cube at a time, to reach desired coldness.

Calories 203, **Fat** 3 g, **Carbohydrates** 36 g, **Protein** 12 g, **Fibre** 5 g, **Saturated Fat** 2 g, **Cholesterol** 11 mg, **Sodium** 143 mg.

It's amazing what nutrients you can conceal in a delicious smoothie. Try adding 1 scoop each of wheatgerm, unprocessed bran and multigrain cereal to smoothies. You could also add a serving of instant porridge, prepared in the microwave, to increase staying power.

Super smoothies: Besides spinach, you can add a scoop of protein powder or some leftover vegetables such as lima beans, sweetcorn or peppers, or leftover cooked rice. Equal amounts of chopped tomatoes and plain yogurt with a squirt of lemon juice makes a wonderful creamy smoothie; just add a celery stick and a few onion slices to the blender, and it's a fine lunch. You will find smoothies that your kids will love and want constantly – try variations.

Cut Fruit for Smoothies

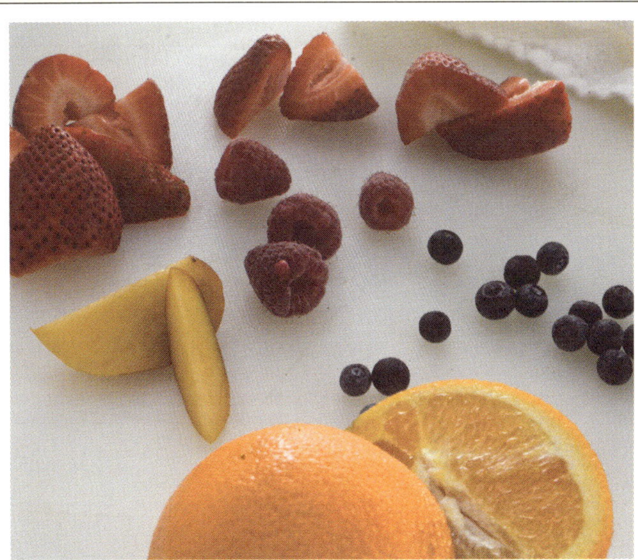

- Putting together a smoothie is a great way to use up ingredients in your fridge. Fruit in a smoothie is always a crowd favourite.

- Try using fresh or frozen blueberries or sliced apples. Or try bananas and strawberries with a squeeze of lemon juice.

- Cut fruit into smaller portions for a finer blend.

- For extra protein, add 120 ml more yogurt.

Adding Extra Flavour

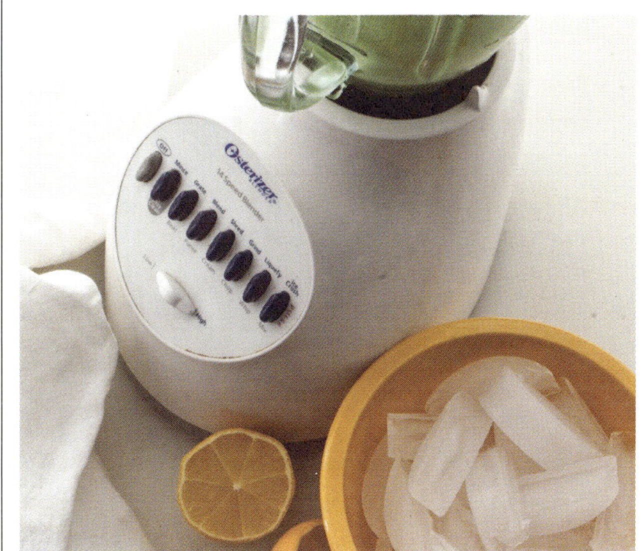

- Add even more flavour to your smoothie by mixing in extra ingredients.

- If it's that coffee or chocolate flavour you crave, blend 250 ml low-fat, sugar-free coffee yogurt with120 ml sugar-free chocolate ice cream, ½ banana, and 2 tablespoons unprocessed bran. Be warned, however, that this will increase the carbohydrate content.

- Add some coffee-flavoured liqueur or sugar-free chocolate syrup if you have a real chocolate craving.

STUFFED FRENCH TOAST

When cut into equal quarters, this 'breakfast' makes a perfect lunch

Stuffed French toast is good for breakfast, lunch or a light supper. It's totally versatile and can be made quickly with whatever ingredients you have in your fridge.

The particular stuffing given in this recipe is quick and easy to make, and it can be sweet or savoury. You can also add fresh or dried fruit, or slices of tomato, smoked meat or smoked salmon.

Forget about high-sugar maple syrup or other syrups; add fibre and freshness by making your own puréed fruit toppings and fruit coulis, which will contain more nutrients. You can use fresh blueberries, strawberries, raspberries, mangos, peaches or nectarines. Low-fat cheese tends to melt better than fat-free cheese. If your cholesterol count is healthy, go ahead and use the low-fat cheese rather than fat-free.

Ingredients

Serves 4

For the French toast:

2 whole large eggs

2 large egg whites

120 ml semi-skimmed milk

1 teaspoon lemon zest (optional)

$^1/_2$ teaspoon Worcestershire sauce

$^1/_2$ teaspoon hot pepper sauce, or to taste

8 slices slightly stale whole-grain bread

4 slices low-fat, low-sodium Cheddar cheese

8 slices low-sodium smoked ham

For the mustard sauce:

120 ml low-fat mayonnaise

1 tablespoon homemade mustard

1 tablespoon finely chopped onion

$^1/_2$ teaspoon curry powder

Calories 402, **Fat** 19 g, **Carbohydrates** 33 g, **Protein** 26 g, **Fibre** 4 g, **Saturated Fat** 7 g, **Cholesterol** 164 mg, **Sodium** 827 mg.

Stuffed French Toast

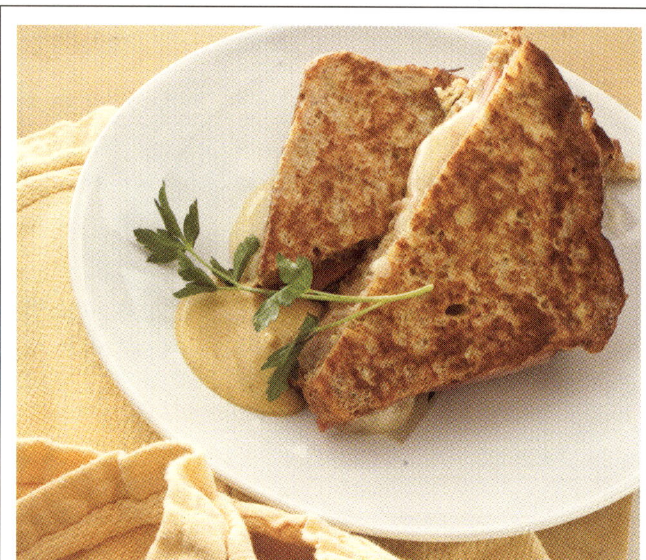

- Preheat pan over medium heat. In wide dish, whisk together eggs, milk, lemon zest, Worcestershire sauce and hot pepper sauce.

- Place cheese and ham on four slices of bread. Close sandwiches. Dip sandwiches in egg mixture, coating both sides.

- Oil pan lightly and sauté sandwiches 4 minutes each side, until bread is browned and cheese melted.

- Cut in quarters and place on a warm platter.

- Mix sauce ingredients in a bowl and serve by the teaspoonful.

French toast is versatile: The beauty of French toast is that you can use multigrain bread. If you are trying to keep your cholesterol intake down, reduce the egg yolks, replacing each omitted yolk with another egg white. This recipe calls for using 2 yolks, but you can cut that in half. It's important to use a nonstick pan, lightly oiled, to sauté your French toast.

French toast spreads: Make different spreads for French toast. Mix 4 heaped tablespoons low-fat ricotta cheese, 2 tablespoons Parmesan cheese and a dash of herbs. Or mix 1 tablespoon of chopped roasted red peppers with ricotta. Spread mixture on to bread and top with second slice to make a sandwich. Dip sandwich into beaten eggs and milk, and sauté.

Separating Egg Yolks from Whites

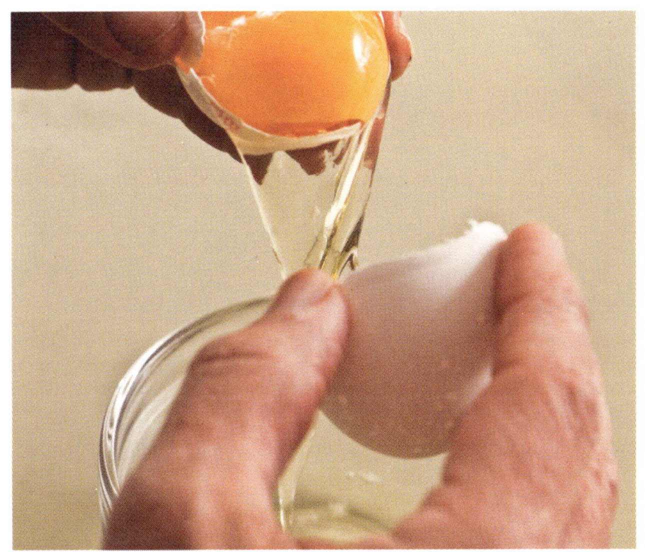

- Have two bowls ready, one for the egg whites and one for the yolks.

- Use a knife or the side of the bowl to crack the egg-shell; open it over one bowl, tipping it so that the yolk sits in one half of the shell.

- Let the egg white drop into the bowl. Now slide the yolk into the other shell and let the remaining white drop into the bowl.

- Drop the yolk into the empty second bowl.

Whisking Eggs

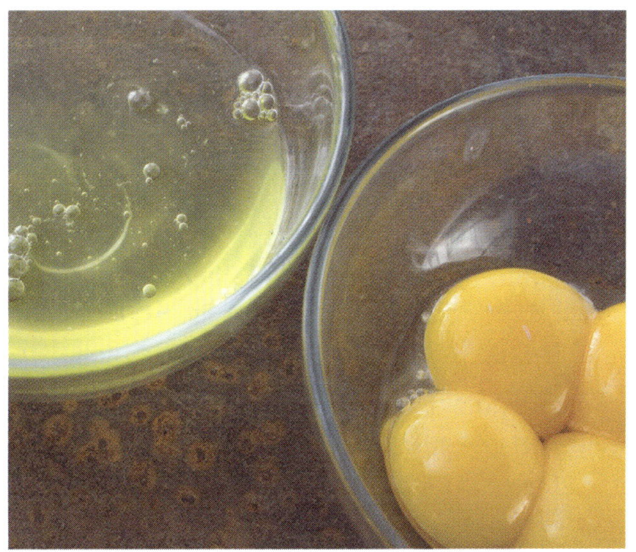

- It's important to whisk your eggs until emulsified. Then whisk in other ingredients.

- You can use a traditional whisk or a fork.

- Move the utensil in a small circular motion to get every bit beaten.

- Some cooks use an immersion blender or electric eggbeater for whisking. That's not necessary unless you are doing a very large number of eggs or are working with whites that have to be beaten stiffly.

QUINOA CAKES WITH BLUEBERRIES

Quinoa with fruit is just waiting to be discovered by health-conscious cooks

Quinoa is a carbohydrate that's higher in protein than most carbohydrate foods. It will keep the family feeling full all morning with slow-release carbs, plenty of protein and lots of fibre.

These blueberry-filled cakes are delectable and can include nuts, if desired, or you could also make a zestier version with chopped pepperoni, ham or roasted vegetables mixed in with the quinoa. The more you use quinoa, the more wonderful uses you'll find for it. Most health- and whole-foods stores stock quinoa. If you can't find it locally, go shopping on the Internet, and you'll have it at a great price in a day or two. Stay away from syrups for quinoa cakes; instead, dress them with a fresh fruit coulis.

Ingredients

Serves 4

2 large eggs, beaten

2 tablespoons plain flour

1 teaspoon baking powder

1 teaspoon salt

1 tablespoon lemon juice

1 teaspoon Splenda

$1/4$ teaspoon cinnamon

400 g cooked quinoa

50 g fresh or frozen blueberries, rinsed and dried if fresh

50 ml canola oil

Calories 507, **Fat** 22 g, **Carbohydrates** 64 g, **Protein** 16 g, **Fibre** 6 g, **Saturated Fat** 3 g, **Cholesterol** 138 mg, **Sodium** 787 mg.

Quinoa Cakes with Blueberries

- Whisk the eggs, flour, baking powder, salt and lemon juice together until well blended. Whisk in the Splenda and cinnamon. Fold in the quinoa and berries.

- Heat the oil in a nonstick pan over medium heat.

- Drop the batter into the oil, using about 2 tablespoons per cake.

- Let the cakes cook slowly; turn when nicely browned and hot through.

Plan ahead: Having a bowl of cooked quinoa in the refrigerator can solve myriad time problems such as, 'What's for breakfast? Lunch? Dinner?' Just make extra when you are home at the weekend, doing some additional cooking. Use it as a base, and mix in all kinds of yummy additions. Try it with chopped turkey and dried cranberries. Or add some leftover cold meat and Parmesan cheese to the recipe.

Enriched meatloaf: You can also add quinoa to your favourite meatball and meatloaf recipes, substituting it for breadcrumbs. Enriched meatloaf is delicious: add 200 g cooked quinoa instead of breadcrumbs to 450 g minced beef or veal. Stir in 120 ml tomato ketchup and 1 teaspoon Worcestershire sauce.

The Fine Art of Folding

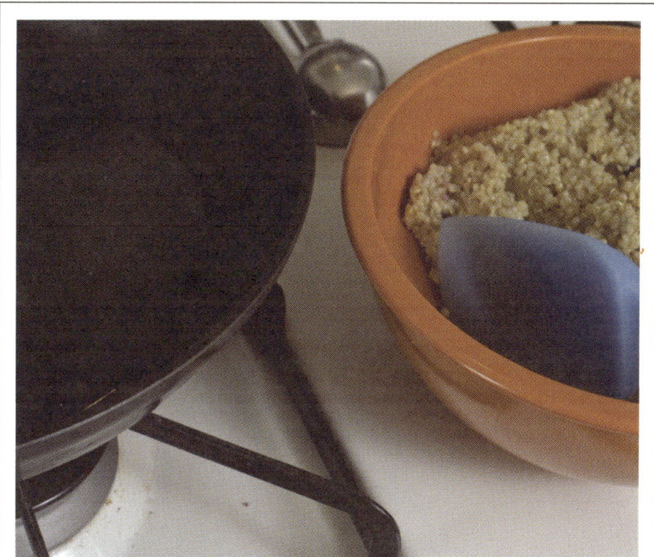

- Folding is a gentle form of mixing.

- To keep the quinoa, berries and batter mixture from turning into mush when mixed, put it all in a big bowl.

- Then, gently and carefully turn the food over with a rubber spatula until it is mixed.

- At no point should you swoosh or roughly mix it around. This will break the berries and make the whole thing much too wet.

'Dropping' Batter

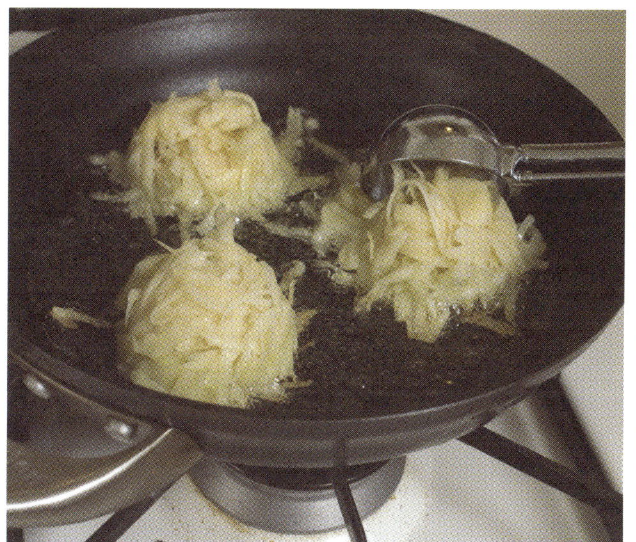

- Dropping batter into hot oil can cause a splash, which is not only messy but also potentially painful.

- For large cakes, use an ice cream scoop to place the batter into the pan. After you have carefully deposited the batter, gently push it down with the back of the scoop to flatten it out.

- Use a tablespoon for small cakes. Put one tablespoonful in the pan and place another tablespoonful on top. Then flatten it with the back of your spoon.

LIGHT LUNCHES

POTATO PANCAKES WITH ONIONS
Enjoy a light lunch with a wonderful crunch and taste

These delicious pancakes are quite easy to prepare. They make a nice light lunch, or you can serve them as a side dish with roast beef or poultry. The coarse grating gives the pancakes lots of texture and a dark golden-brown colour. Be careful not to burn the oil or the pancakes. Once they start to brown, they do so quite quickly. Using a kitchen thermometer, keep the oil at 170–180°C.

Do not make the batter in advance, because the potatoes will turn grey. You can, however, sauté the cakes in advance and reheat them just before serving.

Potato pancakes are traditionally served with sour cream and apple sauce. They are also excellent with gravy, chutney or fruit sauce. Leftover potato pancakes topped with salsa make good snacks.

Ingredients

Serves 4

2 extra-large Nicola potatoes, peeled and grated

1 medium onion, peeled and grated

2 large eggs, lightly beaten

50 g matzo meal

1 teaspoon salt

1/2 teaspoon freshly ground pepper

1/2 cup canola oil

Calories 242, **Fat** 16 g, **Carbohydrates** 22 g, **Protein** 4 g, **Fibre** 3 g, **Saturated Fat** 2 g, **Cholesterol** 67 mg, **Sodium** 31 mg.

Potato Pancakes with Onions

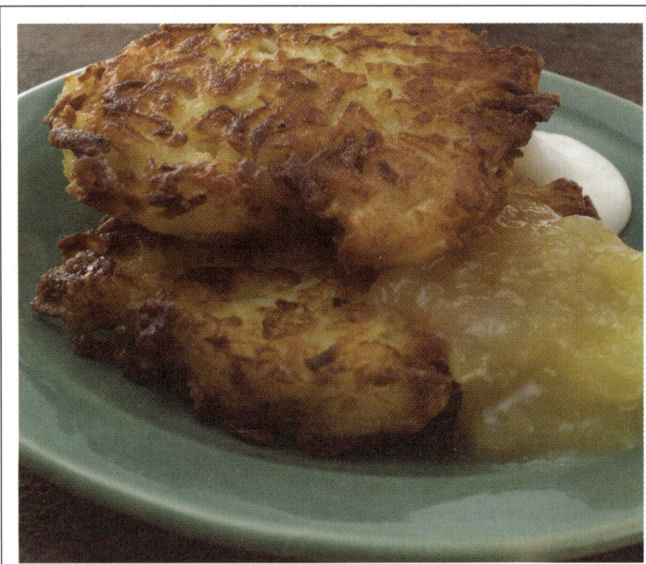

- Put the grated potato and onion in a large bowl. Whisk eggs and add to potatoes and onions; stir gently to coat.

- Stir in matzo meal, salt and pepper. In a large frying or sauté pan, heat the canola oil over medium heat.

- Gently spoon the cakes into the hot oil. Regular size should be about 2.5 cm in diameter. Minis should be about 12 mm in diameter.

- Drain pancakes on paper towels. Serve immediately.

The secret to wonderful potato pancakes – crunchy on the outside, savoury on the inside – is that the potatoes are coarsely grated, not boiled and mashed. You can use a box grater and grate by hand, or the grate/shred blade on your food processor. The same blade can be used for the onions. Just be sure that it all goes through and you don't have any big pieces in your batter.

Traditional spreads: Top pancakes with a spread of 4 thin slices smoked salmon, chopped, 1 tablespoon finely chopped spring onions and 250 ml low-fat cream cheese. Mash it all together; spread it on pancakes. Or, instead of apple sauce, use 6 peeled and chopped fresh pears, simmered until tender with a touch of lemon juice and a dash of ground cloves, then mixed.

Box Grater vs. Food Processor

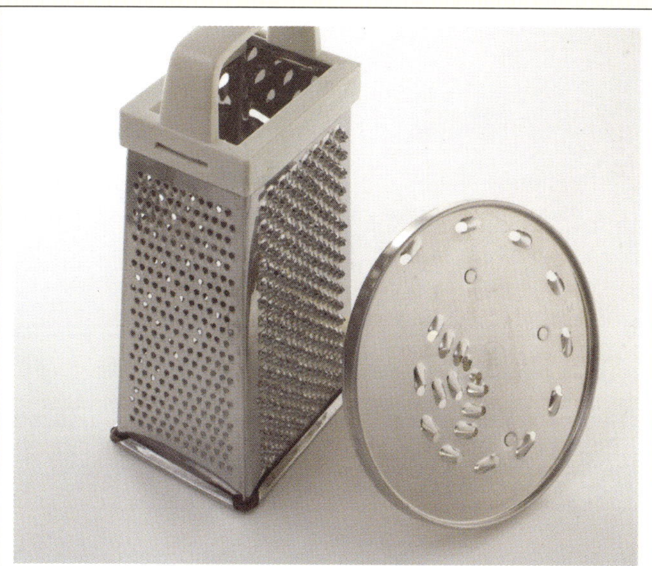

- When you use a box grater to grate potatoes, the job takes longer.

- When using a food processor, insert the grating tool. Then, cut the potatoes into long quarters so that they fit in the tube feeder.

- Using the plastic pushing tool that comes with the food processor, push the potato quarters through the tube. As the bowl fills, dump the potatoes into another bowl.

- You can use the grater or the processing blade to chop the onions, too.

Draining Fried and Sautéed Food

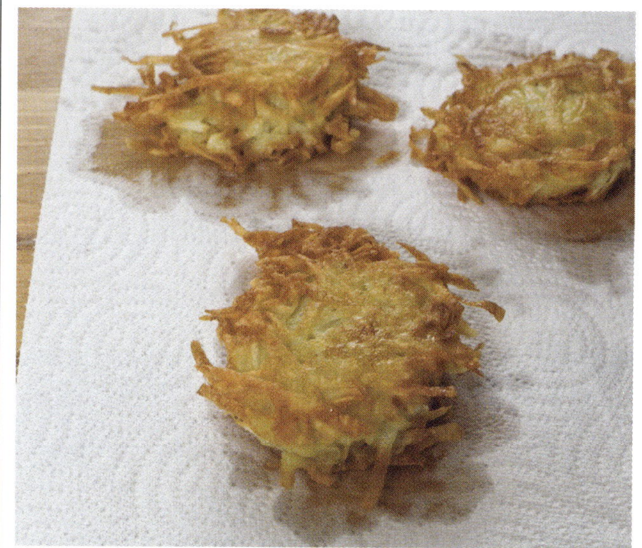

- It's important to get as much of the oil as possible off each potato pancake.

- If your frying pan is up to temperature, the food will not absorb as much oil as it would if using a pan that you did not preheat.

- Do not overload the frying pan; take pancakes out the minute they are brown.

- Place pancakes on a paper towel. Turn them in 1 minute to drain the other side.

STUFFED TOASTED CHALLAH BREAD

Jewish in origin, challah is a rich, yeasty bread for the whole world to enjoy

Challah is usually made on Thursdays and sold on Fridays for eating over the Jewish Sabbath. One taste, and you will find it a treat no matter what your religion.

The dough is egg-based and made with yeast. A long, thick rope of dough is braided, and the bread is glazed with an egg wash to give it a rich colour and high gloss.

This recipe is basically a panini, a small sandwich that is heated and pressed flat on a dual-contact grill or in a panini maker. If you do not have a panini maker, you can cook these on a ridged griddle or a heavy frying pan, using a second frying pan with a brick wrapped in aluminium foil to press down on the sandwiches.

Ingredients

Serves 2

4 thick slices challah bread

4 teaspoons low-fat mayonnaise

2 teaspoons homemade mustard (see recipe, page 204), optional

1 teaspoon dried thyme

6 rashers cooked turkey bacon

1 tart apple, such as Granny Smith, cored, peeled and sliced thinly

2 teaspoons extra-virgin olive oil

Calories 326, **Fat** 11 g, **Carbohydrates** 48 g, **Protein** 8 g, **Fibre** 1 g, **Saturated Fat** 1 g, **Cholesterol** 42 mg, **Sodium** 460 mg.

Stuffed Toasted Challah Bread

- Spread one side of each slice of bread with mayo, and mustard if desired. Sprinkle with thyme.

- Arrange three rashers of turkey bacon on two slices of bread; press into bread.

- Distribute apple slices over bacon. Close sandwiches.

- Heat a nonstick pan over medium flame and add olive oil.

- Put in sandwiches and press to brown first side. Turn; cook until second side is golden. Cut into quarters to serve.

Pressing Sandwiches

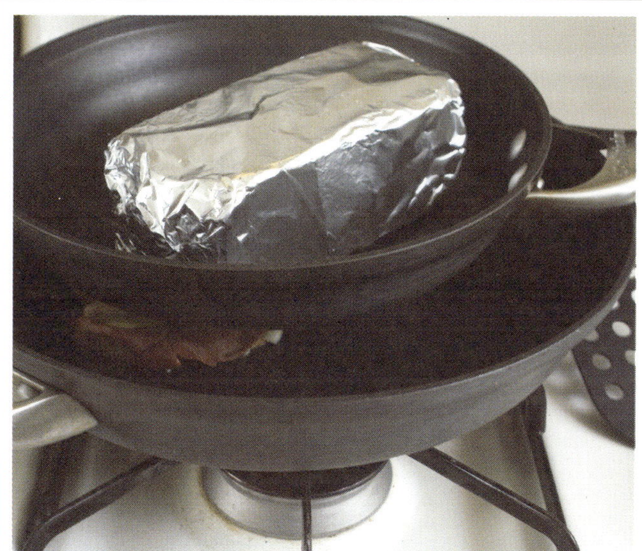

Browning Your Pressed Sandwich

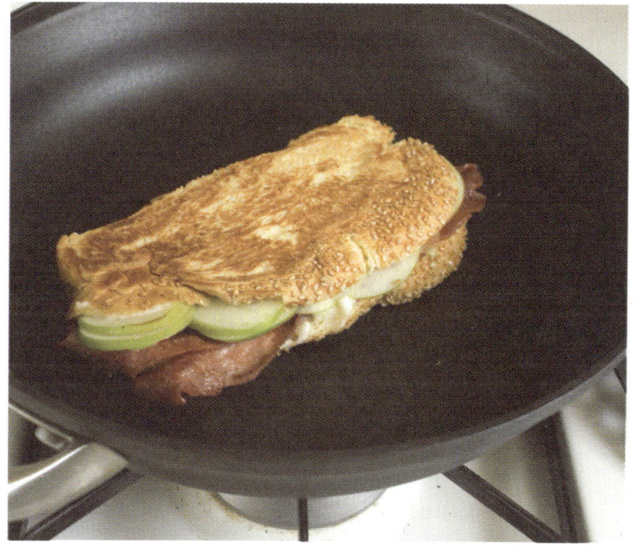

- Pressing a sandwich creates a magical transformation.

- It melds flavours, compressing them to the point of total flavour integration.

- If you don't have a panini press, improvise by using some kitchen staples. Use either the base of a heavy pan to press the sandwich, or the base of a smaller pan with a foil-wrapped brick weighing it down.

- Be sure your pans are clean inside and out before you use one as a press.

- If you use an electric panini maker, watch your sandwiches. Bread and fillings differ enough to make frequent checking important.

- When using a frying or sauté pan on top of the stove, you will need to turn the sandwiches from time to time to check on them.

- The outside of the sandwich should be very crisp and golden brown.

- If you need to add more olive oil, go ahead.

ASPARAGUS SOUP, HOT OR COLD

Once you try this velvety soup, you'll want to make it again and again

This is a beautiful and subtle 'green' soup that smells and tastes young and fresh. To add more colour to the soup, add 150 g frozen petits pois. To make it lighter in colour, substitute equal amounts of white asparagus and new potatoes for the green asparagus.

The base of the soup consists of sautéed aromatic vegetables and chicken stock. Aromatic vegetables include garlic, either roasted or fresh; onions, shallots and chives; celery, carrots and baby turnips; and parsnips and radishes. You can also use mustard greens, fennel, kohlrabi and celeriac.

As you adjust the ingredients to your liking, you will also adjust the taste, which makes this a tantalizing and always versatile summer soup.

Ingredients

Serves 6

450 g asparagus, rinsed, trimmed and cut into 5-cm pieces

300 ml chicken stock

2 tablespoons olive oil

4 shallots, peeled and chopped coarsely

1 tablespoon plus 1 teaspoon plain flour

250 ml skimmed milk, warmed

Juice of $1/2$ lemon

50 ml dry white wine (optional)

1 teaspoon lemon zest

$1/2$ teaspoon Worcestershire sauce

Salt and freshly ground black pepper to taste

Calories 78, **Fat** 4 g, **Carbohydrates** 7 g, **Protein** 3 g, **Fibre** 1 g, **Saturated Fat** 1 g, **Cholesterol** 4 mg, **Sodium** 145 mg.

Asparagus Soup, Hot or Cold

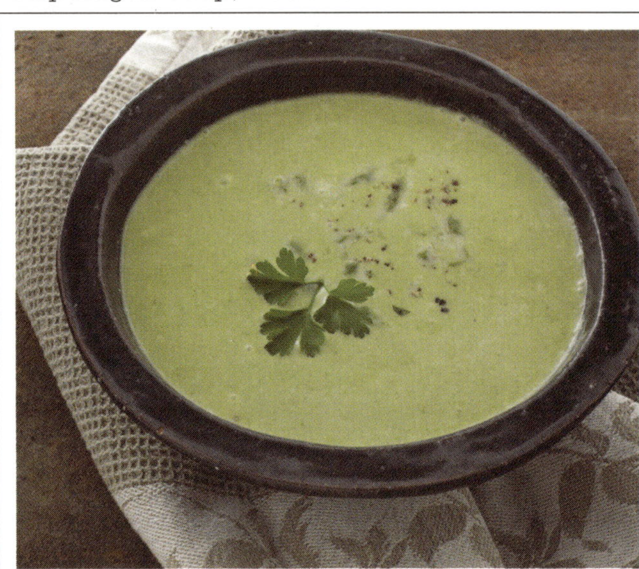

- Microwave the asparagus and 50 ml of the chicken stock in a non-metal bowl for 4 minutes. Set aside.

- Heat the olive oil at medium in a large nonstick pan; sauté the shallots.

- Stir in flour and cook 3 minutes, stirring constantly.

- Whisk in warm milk. Stir until very thick. Then whisk in remaining stock.

- Cook soup until thickened. Whisk in the remaining ingredients. Blend the soup and asparagus until smooth.

- Cover and refrigerate. Serve well-chilled or heated.

Cream soups and cholesterol: Be wary about using real, full-fat dairy products such as whole milk, butter, sour cream and ice cream, which are all high in saturated fat. Saturated fat raises cholesterol, while all types of fat (saturated or unsaturated) provide a lot of calories. If you choose to include some foods with saturated fat in your meals, these soups are great options. Consult your doctor to determine the best diet for you, depending on your cholesterol test readings. It's wise to make your own stock, cook your own fish and chicken, and use lots of fibre and olive oil in your diet.

Smooth Soup

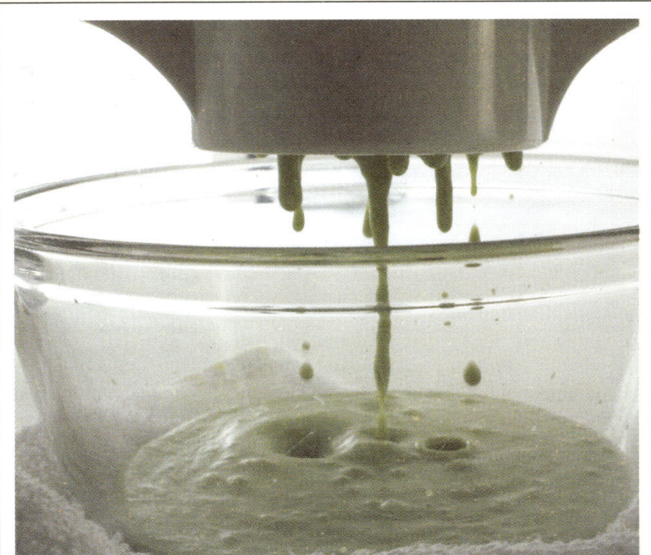

- A rough-textured soup can be rustic. However, if you want smooth soup, you need a fine blend.

- If blending doesn't get all the particles out of the soup, push it through a fine sieve.

- For people with digestive issues, a smooth soup is gentler on the body. The coarse texture affects the digestive system, slowing the absorption of carbohydrates.

- Keep in mind that the soup won't be completely smooth; some fibre will be there, no matter what.

Extra-Green Soup

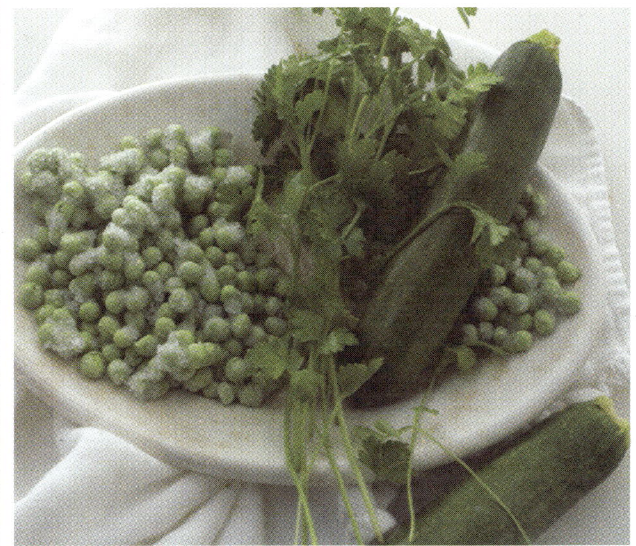

- The colour of the soup will change depending on the amount of green ingredients added to it.

- To make your soup very green, add 150 g frozen peas.

- Or add a few sprigs of parsley, chopped.

- If you want added colour but don't want to interfere with the flavour of the asparagus, add a medium-sized steamed courgette and purée with the soup.

SWEDISH FRUIT SOUP

Fresh raspberries are the crown jewels in this pretty and colourful fruit soup

In the past, during the long, cold winters when fresh summer fruit was impossible to get, Scandinavians made do with dried fruits, and fruit soup was eaten as a dessert. Today, a cold fruit soup is an excellent summer lunch dish.

Use dried apricots, fresh or dried peaches or a mixture of dried fruits, as was used in the 'old days'. Once you start making fruit soup, you can vary it with the seasons. Melon soup, made with honeydew or cantaloupe and spiked with lime juice and ginger, is delightful. Top with dried cherries or cranberries for a fine garnish. Garnish fruit soup with fresh mint leaves, basil leaves, toasted nuts or fresh berries. A dollop of low-fat yogurt or sour cream is also nice.

Ingredients

Serves 6

275–350 g dried apricots or peaches

6–8 medium fresh or dried cherries

1.5 litres water

1 tablespoon Splenda

1 teaspoon lemon zest

1 cinnamon stick

2 tablespoons tapioca

Juice of $^1/_2$ lemon

$^1/_2$ teaspoon salt

175 g fresh raspberries, rinsed

6 tablespoons low-fat sour cream or plain yogurt

Swedish Fruit Soup

- Place the first seven ingredients in a slow cooker or double boiler, covered, on low for 2 hours. Stir occasionally.

- When the fruit is tender, stir in the lemon juice and add a pinch of salt if necessary. Remove the cinnamon stick. Chill the soup.

- At this point, you can either purée the soup or serve it chunky – it's up to you.

- Serve topped with fresh raspberries and a spoonful of low-fat sour cream or yogurt.

Calories 78, **Fat** 2 g, **Carbohydrates** 15 g, **Protein** 1 g, **Fibre** 2 g, **Saturated Fat** 1 g, **Cholesterol** 6 mg, **Sodium** 7 mg.

ZOOM

Using dried fruit: When using dried fruit, such as apricots and peaches, start cooking the soup in a slow cooker. This is a great time-saver. Dried fruits do not have to be peeled or stoned, whereas fresh ones do need more attention. Recipes that practically cook themselves are wonderful for both family and entertaining.

• • • • • RECIPE VARIATION • • • • •

Fruit variety: Fruit soup can also be made with combinations of peaches and berries, such as using four blanched, puréed peaches to 350 g fresh blueberries. For creaminess, blend in 250 ml low-fat or fat-free yogurt, and add 1 teaspoon of Tabasco sauce for spiciness. Or, try cantaloupe melon and raspberries (275 g melon chunks to 400 g raspberries) with 250 ml fat-free or low-fat yogurt.

Using a Double Boiler

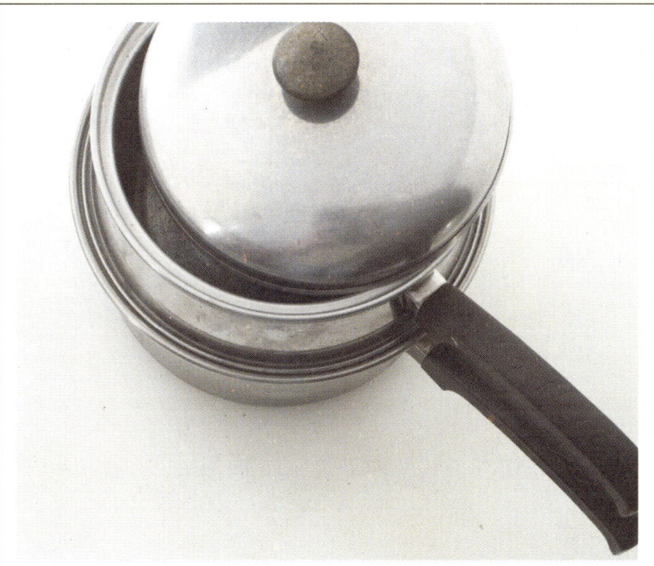

Freeze Your Soup

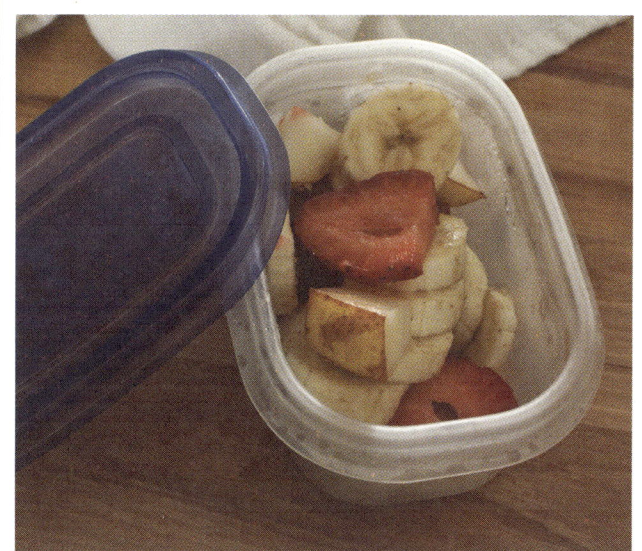

- The double boiler is wonderful for simmering sauce or soup over very low heat without burning it.

- The concept is a hot-water bath in the bottom pan and a tightly fitting top pot that sits over the boiling water.

- The boiling water should not touch the pot that sits on top.

- This is also a great way to make puddings that easily stick to the bottom of a pan on the stove.

- Local seasonal fruits are best for making the soup. They are less travelled and freshest when in season.

- Use lots of peaches, apricots, berries and melons – fruits in season in summer.

- Freeze the fruit for use in winter. Nothing is more refreshing on a winter evening than to serve a fruit soup when you have a chicken or turkey roasting in the oven.

- By freezing your soups, you can enjoy fresh 'summer soups' all year round.

COLD CUCUMBER SOUP

The busy cook's dream dish is this light and luscious soup that requires no cooking

Cold cucumber soup is not cooked on the stove. It actually cooks in the acid of the lemon juice. You make it the day before, so the taste can transform from being a bit harsh to very smooth and easy on the palate.

Hot pepper sauce goes into the recipe because it adds a bit of zing to this otherwise cool and refreshing soup. Fresh dill is far superior to dried dill, but if you can't get the fresh stuff, by all means use dried.

A small amount of crab or prawn salad on top is a nice touch. Even a little ready-made seafood salad is pretty when spooned on top. But use store-bought seafood salads sparingly because they are usually loaded with mayonnaise.

Ingredients

Serves 6

1 cucumber, rinsed and cut into 2.5-cm chunks

1 medium onion, peeled and coarsely chopped

1.2 litres non-fat plain yogurt

Juice of 1 fresh lemon

1 teaspoon lemon zest

2 tablespoons fresh dill plus sprigs for garnish, or 2 teaspoons dried dill

1 teaspoon hot pepper sauce

$^1/_2$ teaspoon salt, or to taste

Optional but recommended: 175 g crab, prawn or mixed seafood salad for garnishing the soup

Calories 117, **Fat** 3 g, **Carbohydrates** 15 g, **Protein** 9 g, **Fibre** 1 g, **Saturated Fat** 2 g, **Cholesterol** 10 mg, **Sodium** 121 mg.

Cold Cucumber Soup

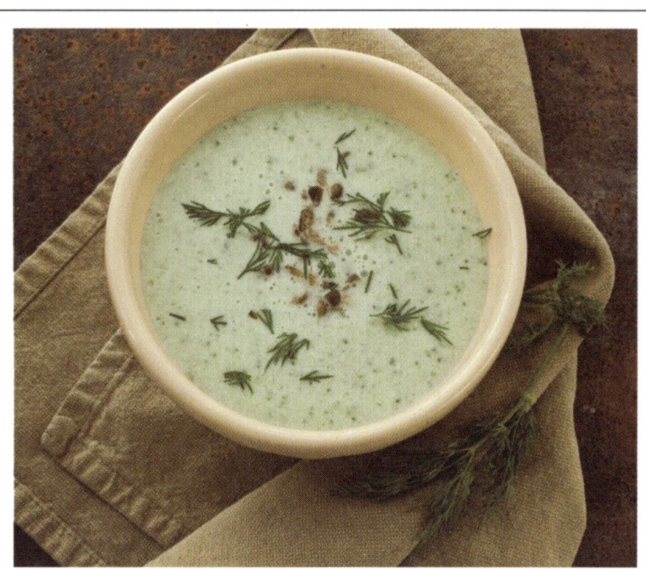

- Purée all ingredients, except for the optional seafood, in a blender or food processor.

- Scrape down the sides of the blender goblet from time to time, and process until very smooth.

- Chill overnight. Pour into chilled bowls, and top with a little seafood salad, if desired.

- Add sprigs of fresh dill for flavour and decoration.

MAKE IT EASY

Make soup in advance: There is something wonderful about opening the fridge on a hot day and pulling out some icy cold soup. And this soup has just about everything you need to be cooled and well fed at the same time. Because the soup cooks in the lemon-zest acid, making it a day ahead will ensure that the flavour has enough time to mellow.

ZOOM

Better ingredients mean better flavour. Try to get local, fresh organically grown cucumbers from a farm shop or farmers' market. Use the entire cucumber after rinsing. Remember, the fresher the ingredients, the more vibrant the flavour.

Squeeze, Ream and Zest

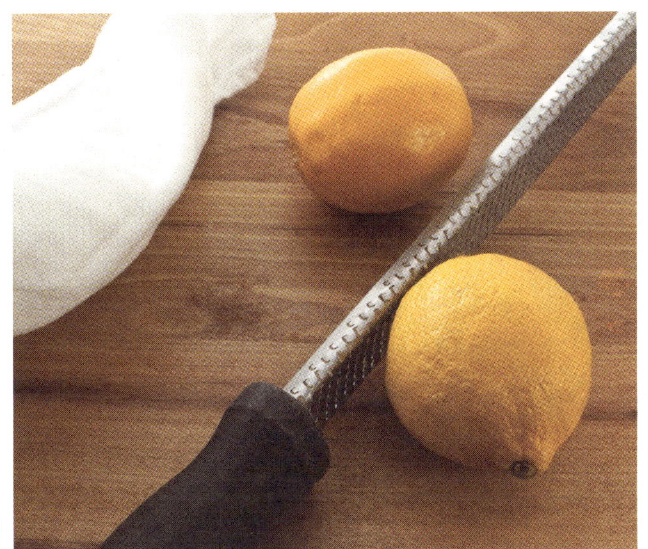

Playing with Garnishes

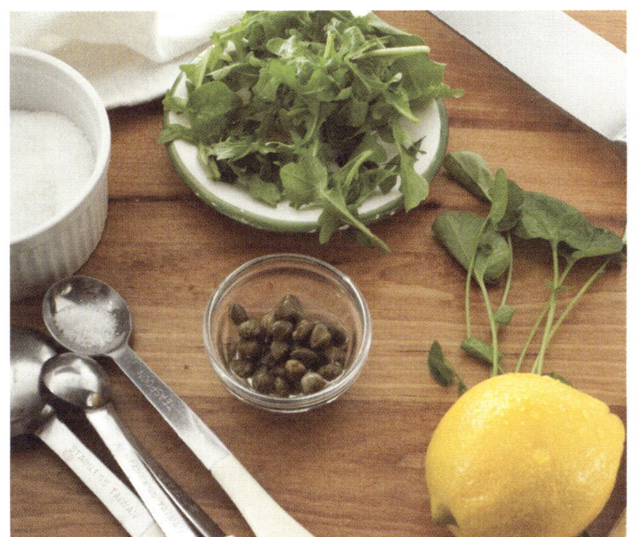

- Fresh lemons give you so much more than reconstituted juice in bottles. You get the zest, seeds for the kids to plant and, of course, lovely fresh juice.

- Zest the lemon before you cut it. You can use a rasp or box grater. Rinse the lemon before zesting.

- You can use a lemon juicer to get the juice out, but a reamer works just as well.

- To make the juices flow, press and roll the lemon around on the work surface.

- Garnishes are fun to experiment with on soups.

- Sprinkle capers or green peppercorns over the soup.

- Play with bitter greens such as rocket and watercress for an added boost of flavour. Rinse fresh herbs and salad leaves well in cold water, then dry on paper towels.

- For use later, roll the leaves in paper towels, put in a plastic bag and refrigerate. They will stay crisp and bright.

COLD GARDEN TOMATO SOUP

Capture the very essence of summer by making this soup with sun-ripened fresh tomatoes

If you buy tomatoes in quantity in August and freeze them, you can make fresh soups and sauces all year round. Nothing from a can compares with fresh.

This soup is made with some red wine and beef stock to make it a bit heartier than straight vegetable soup. But you can also make it strictly with vegetables, using vegetable stock instead of beef stock. The fun part is adding some crunchy favourites on top and then having a platter loaded with extra vegetables on the side.

You can make the soup spicy or mild. Like so many soups, it's best to make it the night before and let the flavours marry in the refrigerator for a more vibrant taste.

Ingredients

Serves 8

2 tablespoons olive oil

1 small onion, peeled and coarsely chopped

4 cloves garlic, smashed, peeled and coarsely chopped

6 cups chopped tomatoes, fresh or canned

400-g low-sodium beef stock

250 ml dry red wine

Juice of 1 lemon

1 teaspoon hot pepper sauce, or to taste

1 teaspoon Worcestershire sauce

50 g each carrots, celery, spring onions, radishes, celeriac, fennel and red and green peppers, all chopped, to accompany

Calories 116, **Fat** 4 g, **Carbohydrates** 14 g, **Protein** 3 g, **Fibre** 3 g, **Saturated Fat** 1 g, **Cholesterol** 0, **Sodium** 137 mg.

Cold Garden Tomato Soup

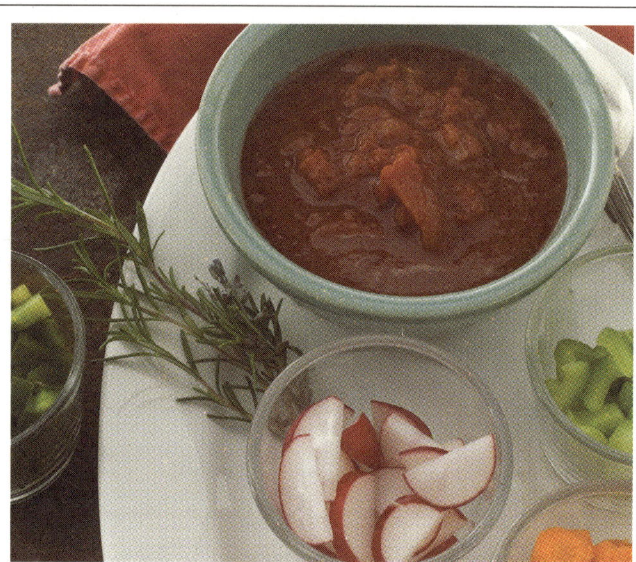

- Heat olive oil in a saucepan set over medium heat. Add onion and garlic and sauté, stirring, until softened.

- Add tomatoes and stock. Bring to the boil and reduce heat to a simmer.

- Add wine, lemon, hot pepper sauce and Worcestershire sauce. Cover and simmer for 15 minutes. Remove from heat and allow to cool. Transfer to a bowl and store in the fridge.

- Either mound the chopped vegetables on a platter or lazy Susan so that people can help themselves, or add them to the soup.

MAKE IT EASY

Food processor chopping: Using the food processor as a chopper is easy and works well for onions, garlic, carrots and other firm vegetables. It will coarsely chop tomatoes if you pulse it on and off, or it will purée them. Cut your onions, carrots, etc., into chunks, and always pulse to get an even chop.

• • • • RECIPE VARIATION • • • •

Adding celeriac or spinach: Try adding 150 g grated celeriac or 100 g shredded fresh baby spinach to the basic recipe for Cold Garden Tomato Soup. You will also change the character of the soup by adding one fennel bulb, trimmed and shaved paper-thin.

Smash That Garlic!

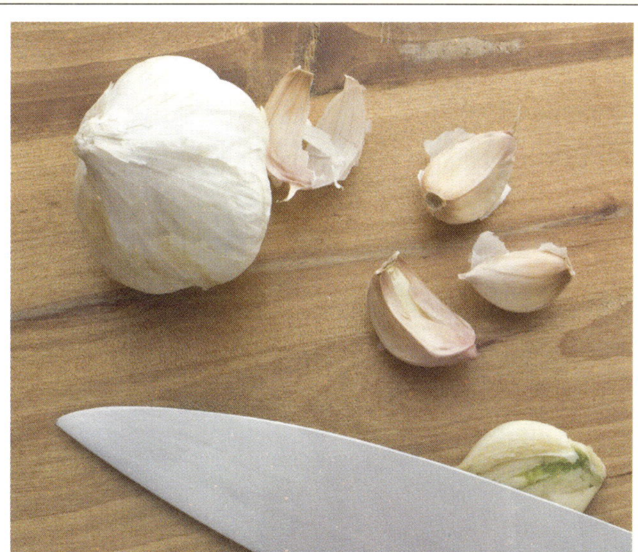

- The easiest way to prepare garlic is to smash it.

- Put the clove on a chopping board; press the flat side of a chef's knife down on the garlic and apply pressure.

- For a lot of cloves, spread them on a piece of greaseproof paper. Add another layer of greaseproof paper, then rock a heavy frying pan over the paper to smash.

- Once smashed, the garlic peels easily, and the split cloves are ready to go into the pan.

Marinating, Macerating and Marrying Flavours

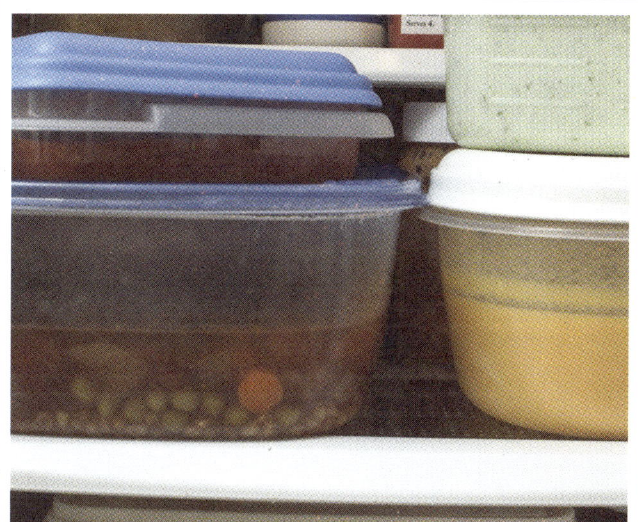

- This complex soup needs to spend time marinating so that the flavours can marry.

- When you combine flavours, they need to 'cook' in order for the process of marinating or macerating to work.

- Maceration is done mostly with fruit mixed with sugar, citrus and wine or liqueur, which becomes a sweet syrup after a period of time.

- Marinades have a special effect on meat – tenderizing it by breaking down the fibres and adding flavour.

FROSTY GREEK LEMON SOUP

Traditionally served hot, this soup can also be chilled and served cold the next day

When you are in a hurry, make this traditional everyday soup and serve it hot. Put together a green salad, toast a few slices of multigrain bread, and you've got a complete meal. When you have plenty of time, make the soup in advance and then chill it for a light lunch or to serve as the first course of an elegant dinner. It's light enough to be a starter and has enough protein to keep you going all afternoon if you eat it for lunch.

The wonderful thing about this soup is that you can add chopped fresh spinach, watercress or rocket to it. Any of these make a delicious foil for the lemony flavour. However, don't use frozen spinach for this recipe; it just doesn't cut it.

Ingredients

Serves 6

1.5 litres low-sodium chicken stock

Juice of 3 lemons

Salt and freshly ground black pepper to taste

3 eggs

Garnishes: a handful per serving of either baby spinach, watercress or rocket; try it with 75 g cooked prawns or shredded cooked chicken for extra protein.

Fresh mint leaves

Calories 91, **Fat** 3 g, **Carbohydrates** 3 g, **Protein** 13 g, **Fibre** 0, **Saturated Fat** 1 g, **Cholesterol** 143 mg, **Sodium** 695 mg.

Frosty Greek Lemon Soup

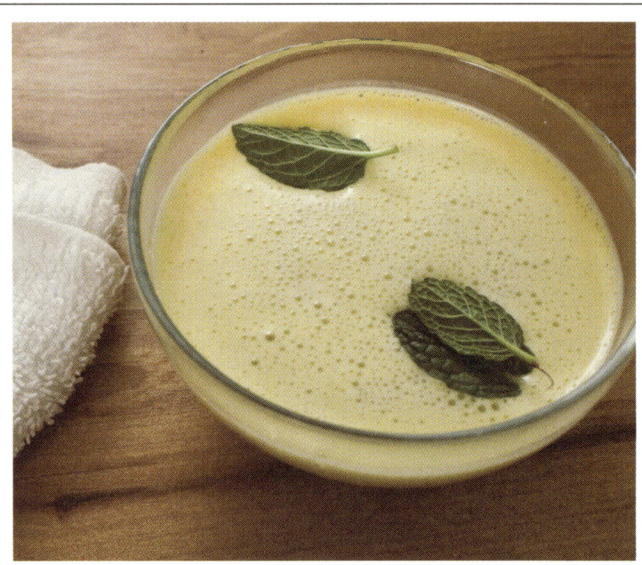

- Bring stock to the boil over high heat. Add lemon juice, salt and pepper. Reserve 250 ml of the hot soup; pour the rest into a large tureen or bowl for serving.

- Beat eggs in a separate bowl until pale yellow.

- When the soup has cooled slightly, whisk the reserved cup of hot soup into the egg mixture. Then, slowly whisk the mixture into the warm soup.

- Add garnishes; serve immediately, or chill for later. If chilled, give the soup a last whisk before serving, then add your garnishes.

Rescuing Curdled Soup

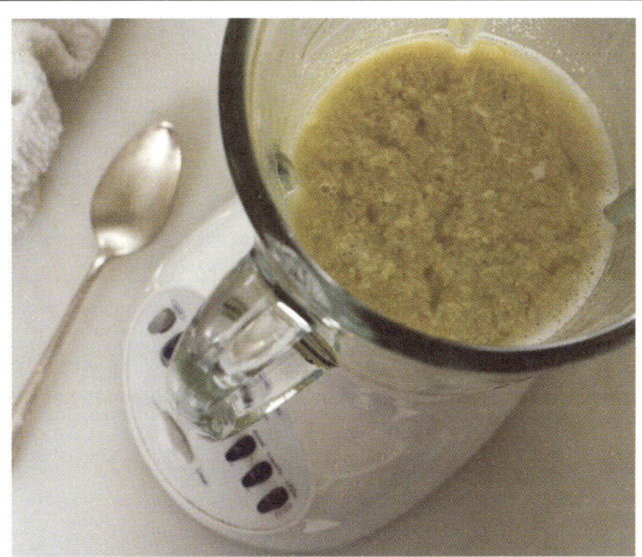

Tempering

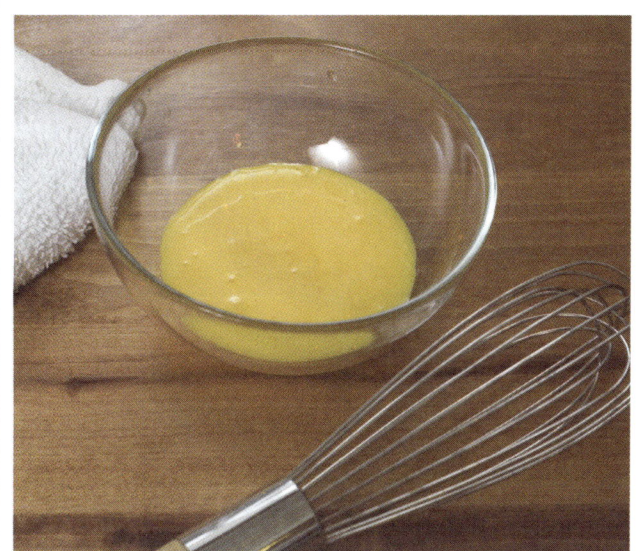

- If the egg and lemon sauce is added when the soup's too hot, it may curdle. This is unpleasant.

- However, it's simple to rescue. Immediately pour the soup and 2 tablespoons of boiling water into the blender and whirl until the curds are gone.

- Wash the bowl before returning the soup to it.

- This technique works well for curdled or lumpy custards, sauces and soups.

- It's important to temper ingredients that you want to meld and blend.

- Add a small bit of the egg or butter to the soup or sauce base. Then, slowly pour in the rest, bit by bit, stirring constantly.

- You can use an electric mixer or blender rather than hand stirring.

- Your goal is to achieve a coherent mixture, marrying the diverse ingredients into one smooth whole.

MEDITERRANEAN SEAFOOD SOUP

There are many recipes for seafood soup, and this is one of the healthiest

The combinations are almost endless when it comes to making seafood soup. You can make a soup base with fish stock, prawn-shell stock, or either of these mixed with tomatoes.

The seafood combinations are all based on what's fresh in the market and your personal preferences. Mix clams and scallops, prawns and clams, or lobster with anything you like.

Add fresh chunks of filleted fish, too. A great favourite is mussels with prawns, or use just mussels if you prefer. Mussels add a lot of liquor to the soup, which is a natural marriage with tomatoes. Vary the herbs you use, but always start with aromatic vegetables – garlic and onions sautéed in olive oil and then added to the stock.

Ingredients

Serves 4

2 tablespoons olive oil

4 shallots, peeled and chopped

2 cloves garlic, smashed and coarsely sliced

1 kg fresh tomatoes, chopped or 2 (400-g) cans chopped tomatoes

50 ml dry red or white wine

1 kg fresh mussels

1 teaspoon dried oregano

15 g parsley

Freshly ground black pepper

Calories 279, **Fat** 12 g, **Carbohydrates** 19 g, **Protein** 25 g, **Fibre** 3 g, **Saturated Fat** 2 g, **Cholesterol** 54 mg, **Sodium** 561 mg.

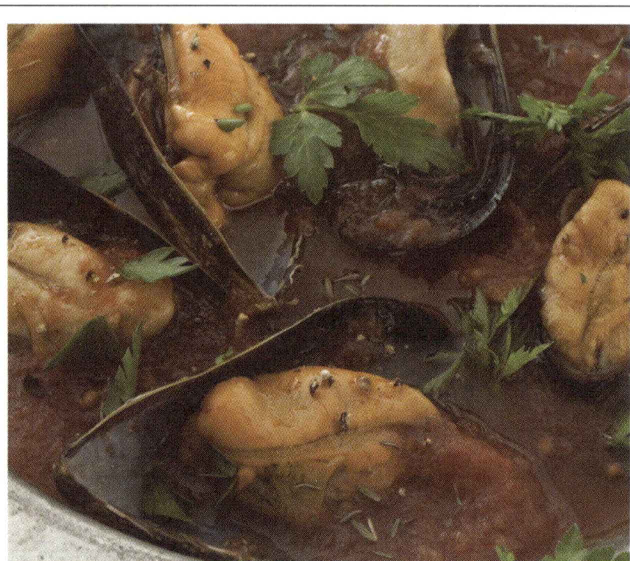

Mediterranean Seafood Soup

- Heat olive oil in a large pan set over medium heat. Add shallots and garlic; cook until softened. Be careful not to burn the garlic, which will then taste bitter.

- Add tomatoes, wine and mussels; bring to the boil. As the mussels open, remove them using a slotted spoon. Remove the top shell from each mussel, then place them on the half shell in a warmed tureen.

- Reduce heat to low; add oregano, parsley, and pepper.

- Pour the hot soup over the mussels in the tureen.

Cleaning Mussels

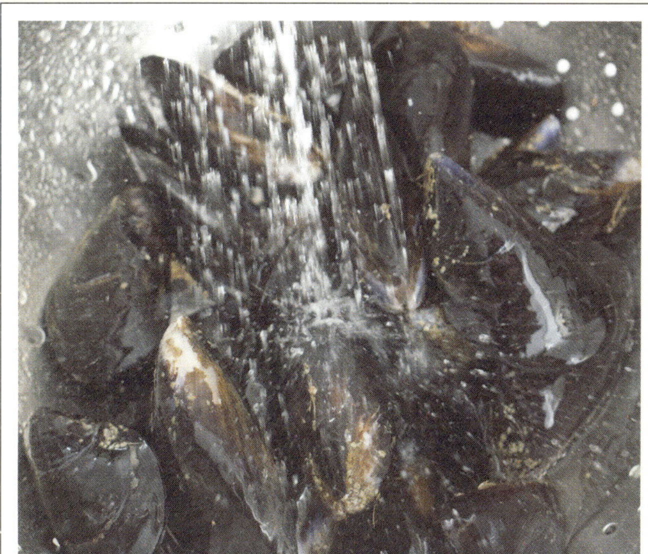

- Mussels from the market are farm raised. However, if you live on a rocky coastline with mussels thriving in clean water, you can gather them yourself.

- Farm-raised mussels are generally clean and free of sand.

- If you get wild mussels, soak them for 2 hours in fresh water with 50 g cornmeal. The mussels will pump it through their systems, expelling the sand.

- Pull off the beards (the curly threads that help the mussels cling to the rocks), and they're ready to use.

Tomatoes for Mediterranean Soup

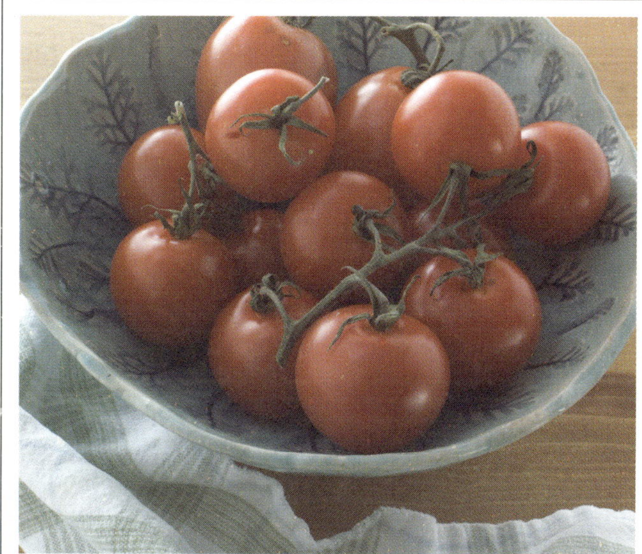

- For this recipe, you can use a variety of tomatoes, either fresh or frozen. Canned and bottled tomatoes are also of good quality.

- The best are imported from Italy and provide fresh flavour to add to your home-frozen tomatoes.

- If you're using fresh, choose ripe plum tomatoes or cherry tomatoes with good flavour.

- Remove the stem ends and blend the tomatoes, then strain to remove the seeds and pulp.

ITALIAN SAUSAGE & BEAN SOUP

This soup combines flavours that work together and marry well

You can prepare this soup any time because courgettes are available all year round. The courgettes should not go into the soup at the outset because they will get mushy; it's better to add them it towards the end of the cooking process.

Soak the dried beans overnight, then cook them for 3 hours or until tender. You can use canned beans, but drain and rinse them thoroughly before adding to the soup.

You can use spicy or mild turkey sausages for this recipe. If you are feeding young children, you probably won't want anything too hot. A good Italian sausage will have a nice amount of fennel in it, which imparts a luscious flavour to the soup. This recipe is best used in moderation with the rest of your diet.

Ingredients

Serves 8

900 g Italian-style turkey sausages

120 ml water

2 tablespoons olive oil, if needed

2 medium sweet onions, red or white, peeled and chopped

4 cloves garlic, smashed and peeled

2.4 litres chicken stock

450 g dried cannellini beans, soaked overnight, or 2 (375-g) cans cannellini beans, drained and rinsed

4 medium-size courgettes, trimmed, halved lengthwise and cut into 2.5-cm chunks

1 tablespoon dried rosemary or 3 tablespoons fresh rosemary

1 tablespoon dried oregano or 2 tablespoons fresh oregano

15 g chopped fresh parsley

Salt and freshly ground black pepper to taste

Calories 438, **Fat** 22 g, **Carbohydrates** 37 g, **Protein** 26 g, **Fibre** 8 g, **Saturated Fat** 7 g, **Cholesterol** 37 mg, **Sodium** 1345 mg.

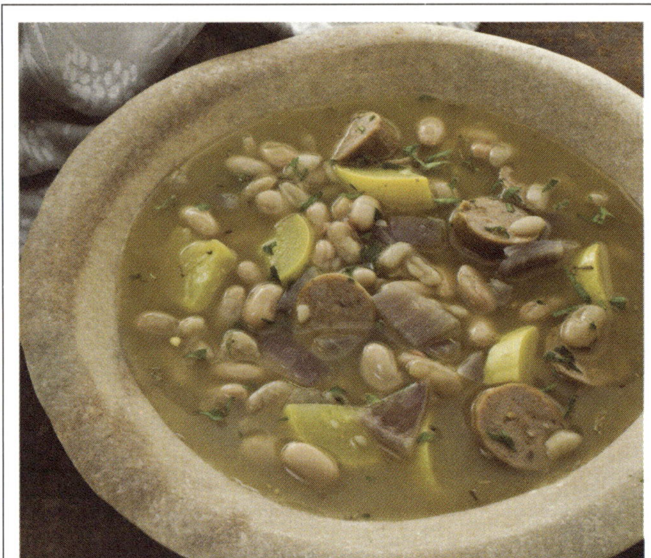

Italian Sausage and Bean Soup

- Place sausages in a large saucepan with water. Bring to the boil; cook, turning occasionally, until water is gone and sausages are firm to the touch. Drain on paper towels.

- Reduce heat to low. If pot is dry, add olive oil. Sauté onions and garlic until tender. Add stock and beans. Slice sausages into bite-size chunks and add them to the pan.

- Cook for 30 minutes. Add rest of ingredients and simmer, covered, 30 minutes more or until beans are tender. Dried beans will take longer than canned beans.

Herbs in soup: Add various dried herbs to this or any soup, but fresh herbs should be added near the end of the cooking process. Keep in mind that, when cooked too long, herbs lose flavour. Start with a few, and add more when soup is closer to being done. Rosemary, oregano and basil are used in Italian cooking. Fennel seeds and bulbs sliced thinly are tasty additions, as are fennel leaves.

Vegetable substitutions: As an alternative to green courgettes, use the same quantity of yellow courgettes, which have a slightly buttery flavour. Add them towards the end of cooking. Add green beans or grated carrots, which add a nice colour boost. For a subtle change in flavour, replace chicken stock with vegetable, beef or turkey stock. Chopped parsley and chives are delicious garnishes.

Cooking Italian Sausages

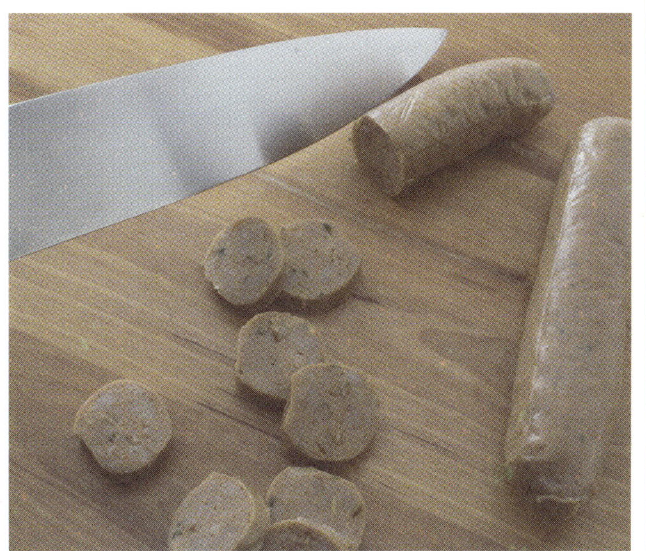

Cutting Courgettes

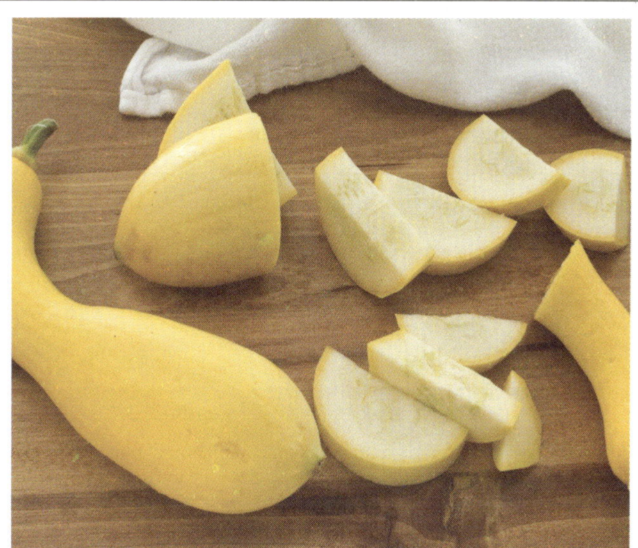

- Buy sausages that are at least 90 per cent meat.

- Once the sausages have started cooking in the water and begin to plump, prick them with a fork so that any fat runs out.

- Some turkey sausages are so lean that you may need to add a little olive oil. If there is some fat in the sausages, drain the fat before returning the sausages to the pan.

- The cooked sausages cut nicely into bite-size rounds.

- Yellow courgettes are quite bland but very pretty.

- You can cut them in various ways to make your soup more attractive.

- Try cutting them in julienne strips, which cook almost instantly. Cutting them crosswise in coins is very easy and attractive.

- Half-coins are also very pretty and easy. Simply cut the courgettes lengthwise and then, holding them together, cut crosswise.

PUMPKIN SOUP WITH ALMONDS
The almonds are toasted and used as a topping for this festive soup

Fresh pumpkins are a delicious food source. Small pumpkins are very sweet and are great for making pies and soups, and as a side vegetable. The huge pumpkins used for carving jack-o-lanterns are not so sweet but are a good source of food.

Although the recipe below calls for a garnish of toasted almonds, you can use toasted walnuts, pecans, peanuts or hazelnuts for variety. Just be sure to toast them first.

A little finely sliced or chopped tart apple can also be sprinkled over the hot soup to add a nice, crunchy contrast. The most interesting dishes feature contrasts in both flavour and texture – sweet and tart, soft and crunchy.

Ingredients

Serves 6

2 tablespoons low-fat margarine, or canola or olive oil

2 medium onions, peeled and finely chopped

800 g freshly roasted pumpkin, puréed

1/4 teaspoon ground nutmeg

Juice of 1 fresh lemon

1 teaspoon grated lemon zest

1 litre chicken stock

Hot pepper sauce to taste

Salt to taste

120 ml single cream (optional)

Garnish: 115 g slivered almonds

Calories 244, **Fat** 5 g, **Carbohydrates** 50 g, **Protein** 4 g, **Fibre** 15 g, **Saturated Fat** 1 g, **Cholesterol** 0, **Sodium** 743 mg.

Pumpkin Soup with Almonds

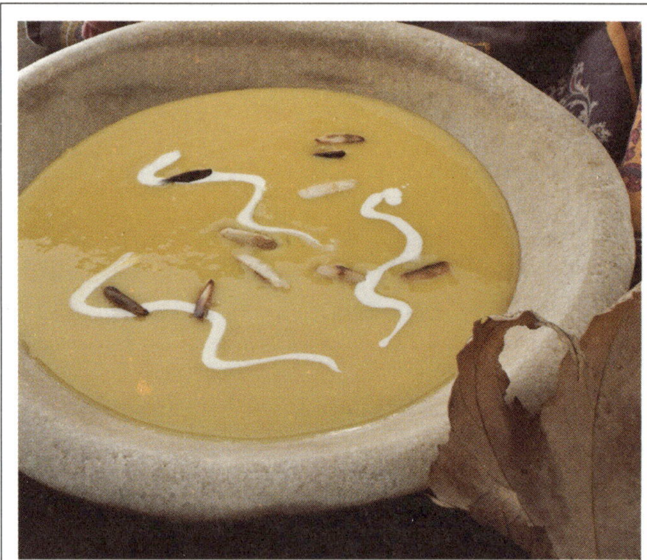

- Melt margarine or heat oil in a large saucepan over medium heat.

- Sauté onions until softened, about 4–5 minutes. Slowly whisk in all the remaining ingredients, except the cream and almonds.

- Reduce heat, cover, and simmer for 15 minutes. Meanwhile, toast almonds under the grill.

- When soup is done, whisk in the cream, if using.

- Serve the soup in warmed bowls; sprinkle the almonds on top just before serving.

• • • • • RECIPE VARIATION • • • • •

Butternut squash soup with almonds: The flavours of pumpkin and butternut squash are similar, so you can substitute butternut squash for the pumpkin in this recipe. Using butternut squash will provide less carbohydrate. Roast it in the same way as pumpkin.

Working with Fresh Pumpkin

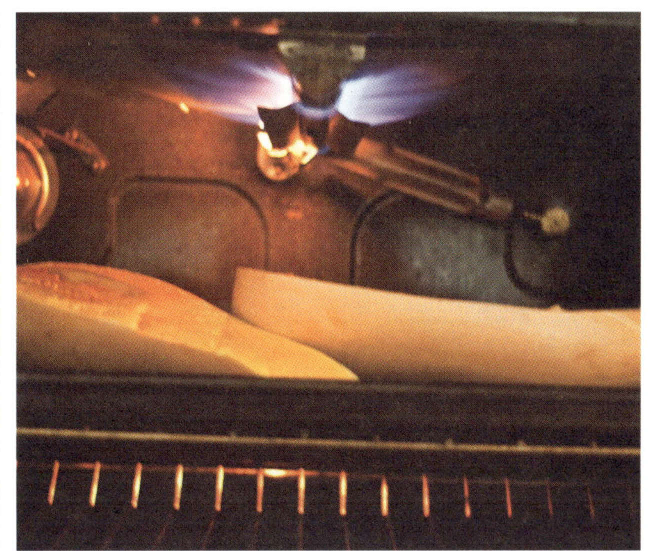

- Some cooks insist that you first peel and cube a fresh pumpkin, and then boil it to soften it.

- Drain boiled pumpkin in a colander to get the moisture out before roasting.

- Alternatively, put peeled, cubed pumpkin in a roasting tin with 250 ml water and roast it, covered with aluminium foil, at 150°C until fork tender.

- Or just cut the pumpkin in half, remove seeds and roast it in a tin with 250 ml water until tender, then scoop out the flesh.

Roasting Almonds

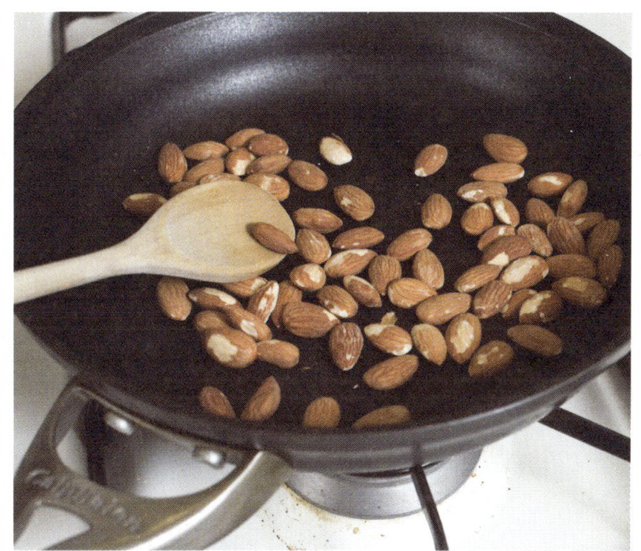

- You can roast almonds either in a pan on the hob or under the grill.

- You must watch them carefully so they don't burn, and shake the pan often to turn them.

- Slivered almonds make a very good garnish and save you the trouble or blanching and chopping whole almonds.

- Toast walnut and pecan pieces in the same way.

MUSHROOM VEGETABLE SOUP

Whole wheat grains make this a very hearty soup that requires a little patience from the cook

For this recipe, it's important to precook the wheat grains for 2–3 hours. If you don't have time to do this, substitute cooked wild rice, brown rice or quinoa.

Using a mixture of mushrooms enriches this soup. It seems that the darker the mushrooms, the more flavourful they are. White mushrooms are the least tasty in soup. If you have an Asian market handy, buy dried black mushrooms. Soak them according to the packet directions and add to the soup for a particularly rich flavour. Fresh chopped sage leaves are an excellent herb for this soup. Of course, you can use thyme or rosemary; however, fresh parsley is almost always the herb of choice to add as a garnish.

Ingredients

Serves 6

80 ml olive oil

2 medium onions, peeled and chopped

4 garlic cloves, smashed, peeled and chopped

2 carrots, peeled and grated

115 g frozen petits pois

175 g chopped fresh tomatoes (skin on is fine)

175 g cooked whole wheat grains, wild rice, quinoa or brown rice

1.5 litres beef stock

120 ml dry red wine

275 g fresh mushrooms, mixed varieties

5 fresh sage leaves, shredded

Calories 266, **Fat** 15 g, **Carbohydrates** 23 g, **Protein** 8 g, **Fibre** 4 g, **Saturated Fat** 2 g, **Cholesterol** 0, **Sodium** 28 mg.

Mushroom Vegetable Soup

- Heat 50 ml of the olive oil in a large saucepan over medium heat. Add onions and garlic and cook, stirring frequently.

- When onions and garlic are softened, add carrots, peas, tomatoes, wheat or other grain, stock and wine.

- Cover and cook over low heat for 30 minutes. While soup is cooking, heat remaining olive oil and sauté mushrooms in a separate pan.

- Add mushrooms and sage to soup, bring to the boil and serve hot.

More on mushrooms: Mushrooms may taste meaty, but they offer very little protein. They have an earthy quality that marries well with other flavours. Wild mushrooms, such as chanterelles and morels, have distinctive flavours and are very expensive. If you can find them, chickens-of-the-woods are absolutely delicious. Shiitake mushrooms are delicate and rich-flavoured. Mushrooms also absorb the flavours of the aromatic vegetables, herbs and sauces that surround them in any dish. If you want pure, unadulterated mushroom flavour, sauté them in olive oil.

Gathering and Cleaning Mushrooms

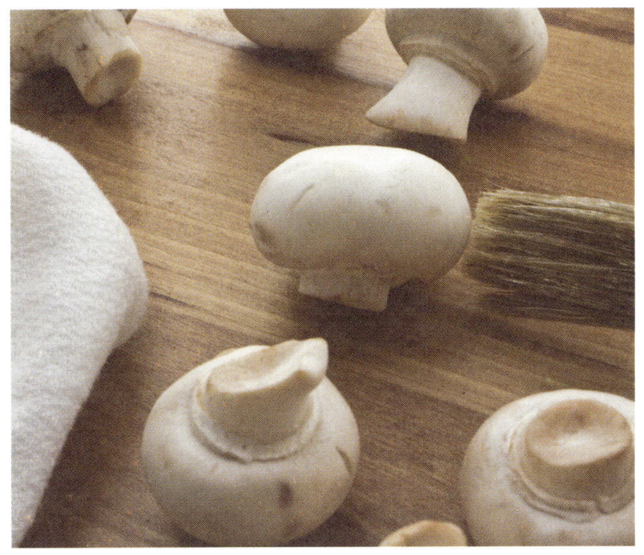

- Mushrooms should first be brushed clean or wiped with a paper towel.

- Mushrooms are commercially grown in horse manure. Before use, the manure is treated with thermophyllic bacteria, which is then burned away, purifying the manure.

- If you collect wild mushrooms, go with an expert mycologist, who can direct you to the safe ones.

- Remember that for every safe mushroom, there is a poisonous one that looks similar. To be safe, buy your mushrooms at the supermarket.

Cooking Wheat Grains and Wild Rice

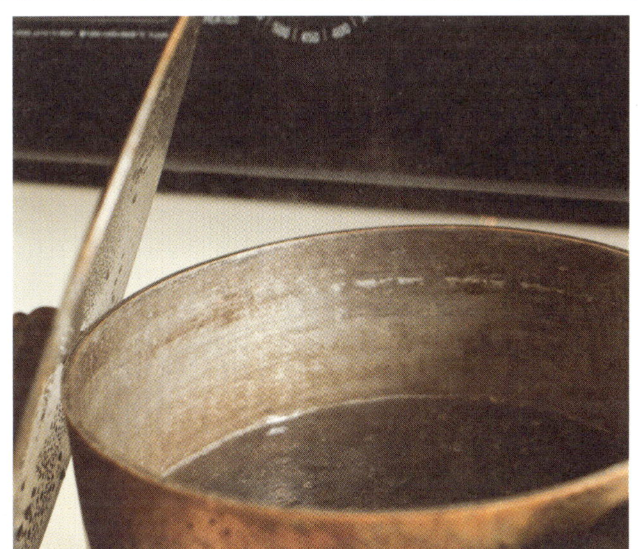

- Whole wheat grains and wild rice require a good deal of cooking time.

- Wheat must simmer for 3 hours over low heat, covered. The grains are done when they are chewable.

- Wild rice needs to simmer for 60–100 minutes.

- Wild rice morphs from little brown spikes into 'blooms' when done. The kernel grows, softens and pops the hulls apart.

IRISH LEEK & POTATO SOUP

Low-fat milk replaces the cream in this classic dish with pleasing results

The Irish are famous for their dairy products as well as potatoes and green vegetables, such as leeks. Those ingredients come together here to make a classic soup, but this one is lower in fat.

The traditional version of this recipe calls for both leeks and onions. You'll find that the flavour is more delicate when only leeks are used. If you'd like to include onions, use a mild variety such as Vidalia, which has a fine, sweet flavour. You can use any baking potato in this soup, but don't use new potatoes because they are too waxy and can become sticky.

Ingredients

Serves 6

4 large baking potatoes, peeled and cut into chunks

1 litre chicken stock

50 g low-fat margarine

6 leeks, white parts, cleaned and chopped

3 tablespoons plain flour

500 ml semi-skimmed milk, warmed

Salt and freshly ground pepper to taste

Calories 304, **Fat** 2 g, **Carbohydrates** 62 g, **Protein** 11 g, **Fibre** 6 g, **Saturated Fat** 1 g, **Cholesterol** 4 mg, **Sodium** 494 mg.

Irish Leek and Potato Soup

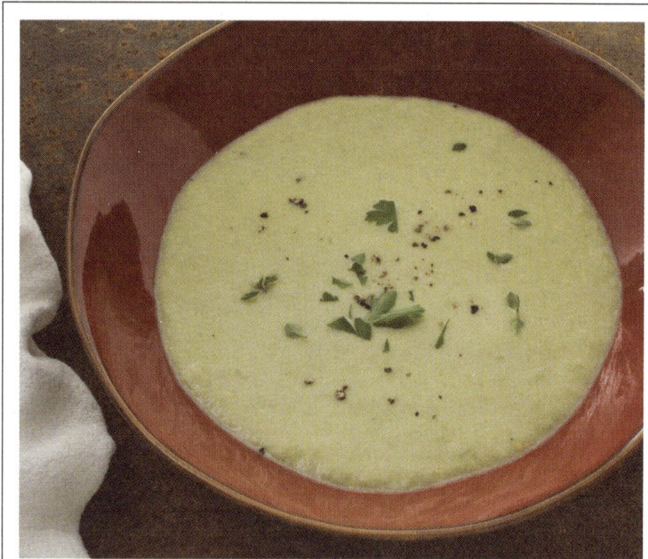

- Put potatoes in large saucepan with chicken stock. Bring to the boil; reduce heat, cover and simmer until potatoes are tender, about 20 minutes.

- Melt margarine over medium heat in a separate pan. Add leeks, cook until soft; add flour and mix well.

- Drain potatoes, saving the stock in which they were cooked. Whisk the hot stock into the leek and flour mixture, then whisk in the warm milk.

- Mash potatoes with a potato masher or ricer and add to soup. Season to taste.

MAKE IT EASY

For the recipe below, choose any good baking potato. Then mash it using a potato masher. Many cooks and chefs use a gadget called a 'ricer' to process the potato. You basically press a cooked potato through small holes in the ricer. This makes perfect rice-shaped pieces of potato ready to go into the soup.

ZOOM

More on potatoes: Potatoes are one of the most interesting tubers. Most new potato varieties are round and small. The thin skin can be either yellow, brown, purple or red. If you can find unusual old varieties such as Peruvian blue potatoes, which are a rich shade of purple, add them to mashed potatoes for extra colour. These potatoes taste exactly like the brown-, yellow- and red-skinned varieties.

A Good, Sharp Peeler

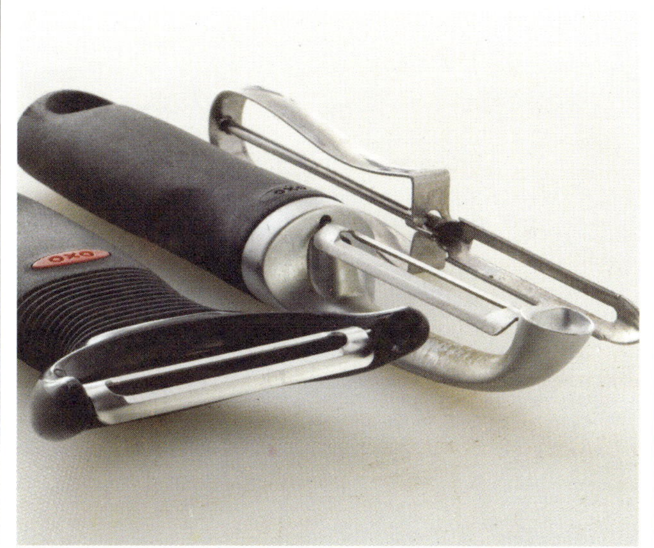

Exciting Potato Starch

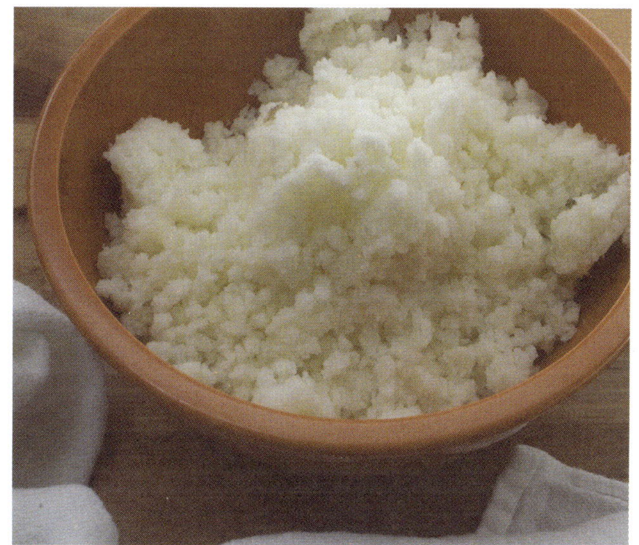

- A sharp vegetable peeler is an essential, invaluable tool. It will save you time and frustration, and it will save you food.

- If you use a knife to peel, even a very sharp one, you will waste quite a bit of potato.

- When your peeler gets blunt, throw it out. It should be comfortable to hold with a firm grip.

- When you find one you like, buy extras. Then your family and friends can help with the peeling.

- Have you ever made gluey or pasty mashed potatoes? This is the result of the starch in the potatoes getting 'excited' and changing its nature.

- Those shy potatoes must be mashed carefully. If you blend or process potatoes for use in soup, the starch will get sticky, with the consistency of wallpaper paste.

- Handling your potato starch carefully will prevent it from turning to a gluey mess.

TURKEY MEATBALL SOUP

A healthy version of the classic Italian wedding soup, complete with tiny meatballs

Spicy little meatballs, made with minced turkey instead of the more usual beef, are a perfect addition to nutritious soups. This recipe, a variation on a traditional Italian wedding soup containing pasta and meatballs, offers reduced amounts of fat and cholesterol. Tiny pearl onions are lovely in this soup. You can buy them peeled and frozen to save time and effort.

The more vegetables you add, the better the soup. Add a can of cannellini beans and extra stock to stretch the soup.

Plenty of herbs are another essential addition. Use rosemary, oregano and/or sage, and sprinkle snipped chives and chopped parsley on top. Another masterful touch is a sprinkle of Italian chilli flakes.

Ingredients

Serves 8

For the meatballs:

450 g minced turkey

2 eggs, beaten

50 ml chilli sauce

1 teaspoon Worcestershire sauce

25 g breadcrumbs

40 g finely grated Parmesan cheese

1 teaspoon each dried oregano and fennel seeds

Salt and pepper to taste

For the soup:

50 ml olive or canola oil

24 tiny pearl onions

4 cloves garlic, peeled and sliced

3 medium onions, peeled and chopped

225 g baby carrots

225 g green beans, trimmed and cut into 2.5-cm pieces

1.75 litres low-sodium chicken stock

2 (400-g) cans chopped Italian tomatoes

2 teaspoons dried or 2 tablespoons fresh oregano

1 bay leaf

$^1/_2$ teaspoon fennel seeds

Calories 250, **Fat** 13 g, **Carbohydrates** 18 g, **Protein** 17 g, **Fibre** 3 g, **Saturated Fat** 3 g, **Cholesterol** 34 mg, **Sodium** 775 mg.

Turkey Meatball Soup

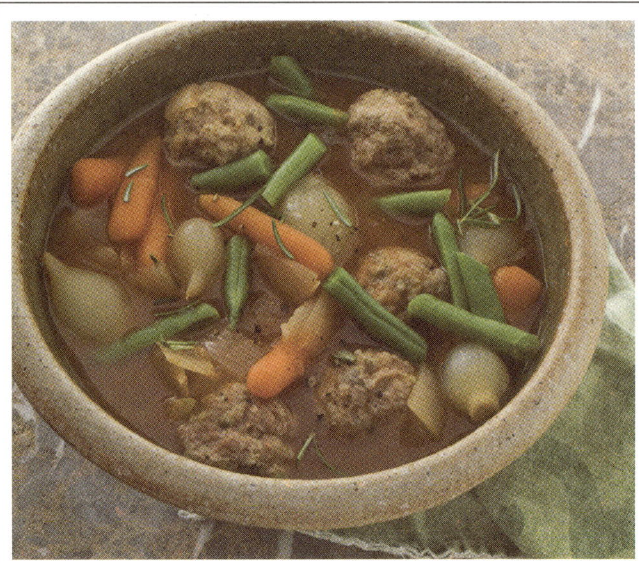

- Preheat oven to 180°C. Cover a baking sheet with aluminium foil and oil lightly.

- Thoroughly mix all the meatball ingredients. Form small meatballs; place on baking sheet. Bake 20–30 minutes. Drain meatballs on paper towels; cool.

- Heat oil in a large saucepan over medium heat. Add pearl onions, garlic, and chopped onions; sauté until soft.

- Stir in remaining ingredients, one at a time. Bring soup to the boil, and cook until carrots are tender. Add meatballs.

The meat in your meatballs: Turkey is recommended for this recipe; however, you can use an equivalent amount of lean minced beef if you prefer to make traditional meatballs for this soup. A mixture of minced beef, veal and pork also makes very tasty meatballs. However, weight for weight, turkey is lower in calories than beef.

If you are concerned about reducing fat, cholesterol and your caloric intake, it's advisable to use the turkey with the spices and herbs recommended in this recipe. Also, if you bake the meatballs as opposed to frying them, and then drain them on paper towels, you'll eliminate much of the fat.

How to Make Meatballs

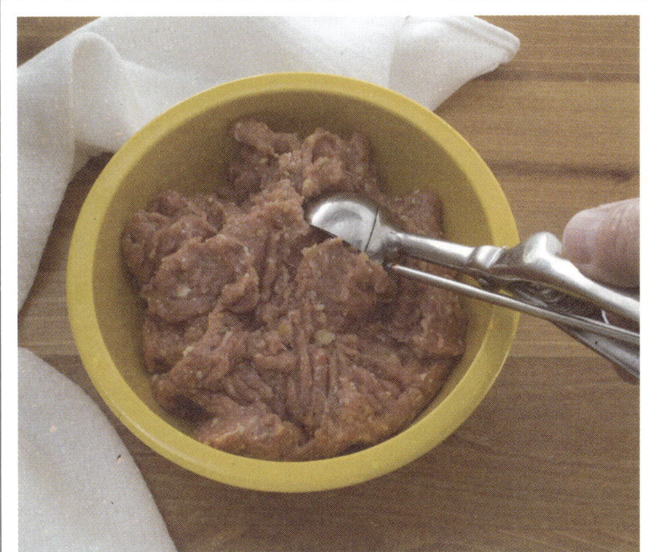

- For tiny meatballs, use a small measuring spoon to scoop up the meat mixture. For extra-tiny ones, use a melon baller.

- When making large meatballs for spaghetti sauce, use a small ice-cream scoop.

- Roll the meatballs around between your palms to compress them so they don't fall apart.

- If your meatballs are all the same size, they will cook at the same rate if your oven temperature is even from front to back.

Frying vs. Baking Meatballs

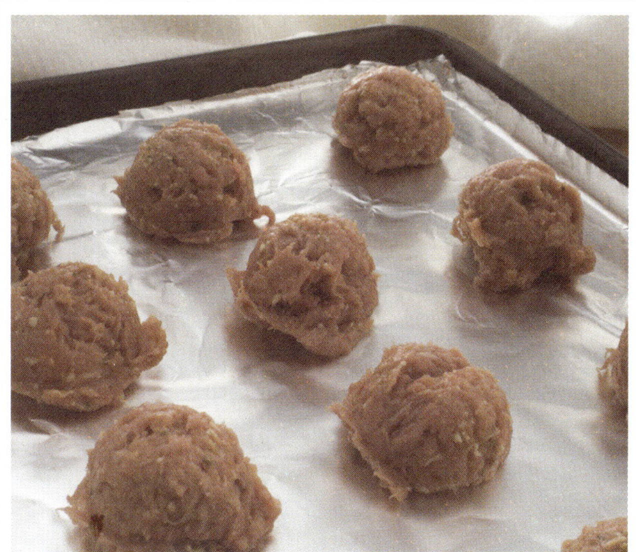

- For years cooks fried meatballs in deep fat, using lots of oil, and there is a slight advantage to that method.

- The outside of the meatball will sear, and the inside will stay moister than when baked.

- However, baking does not require the constant attention that frying does.

- By the time you add them to a pot of soup or pasta sauce, the meatballs will come out pretty much the same. Just be sure to season them well.

HOMEMADE STOCK

Making your own fresh stock is a great way to save money, and it's naturally low in sodium

When making stock, the basic techniques differ slightly depending on whether you use meat or poultry.

The classic stock, and probably the easiest, is that made from leftover Christmas turkey for turkey soup. It's also easy to make chicken stock from the remains of a large roasted chicken. Or you can ask your butcher for chicken necks and carcasses, which make wonderful stock and lots of it. Just add aromatic vegetables and herbs.

If your friendly butcher will also save you some meaty beef bones, you're in luck. Otherwise you can buy short ribs or oxtails for beef stock. Or, if you've done a large standing rib roast, you have the basis for excellent beef stock.

Ingredients

Makes 2 litres

About 2 kg chicken necks and carcasses, or beef bones such as oxtail, neck bones or short ribs

1 carrot, cut into chunks

2 sticks celery, cut into chunks

6 peppercorns

1 teaspoon Worcestershire sauce

Homemade Stock

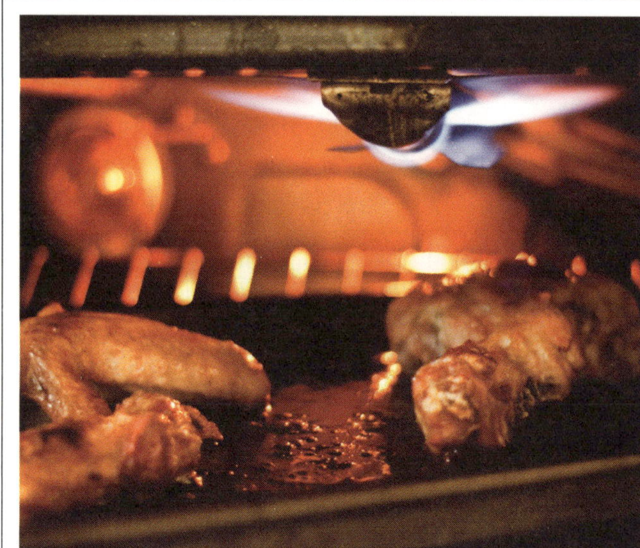

- Place chicken or beef bones in a roasting tin. Brown under the grill, then turn to brown the other side.

- Place browned bones in a stockpot. Deglaze the roasting pan with enough water to dissolve and scrape bits off the bottom; add to stockpot.

- Add remaining ingredients to stockpot and top up with water to cover bones.

- Bring to the boil then reduce heat, cover and simmer for 2–3 hours.

- Cool stock and skim off any fat. Remove bones. Strain; freeze for future use.

Stocking your freezer with stock: You can freeze stock in ice cube trays or 250-ml containers for use in sauces, or by the litre for soups and risottos. After you've frozen a couple of ice cube trays' worth, place the cubes in plastic ziplock bags. Then, when making sauces, you can add the cubes as you need them. Try to keep a couple of litres of chicken stock and beef stock in your freezer for making quick soup. You will then just need a few vegetables, any leftover meat and some pasta or rice. You can actually make a lunch of leftovers added to stock. And, if you need more sustenance, just thaw and cut up a frozen boneless chicken breast and toss it into the soup.

Why Brown the Bones?

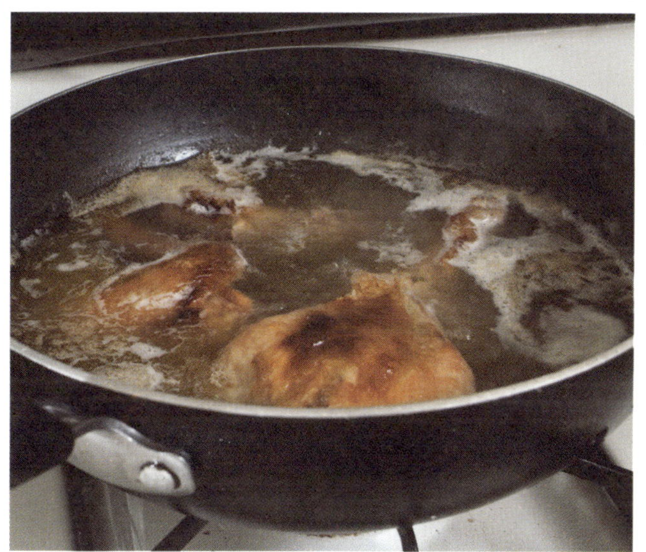

- When you brown the bones for stock, it creates a nice, rich colour.

- You will also get 'fonds' or meat essences – the brown bits on the bottom of the pan, which are concentrated nuggets of flavour.

- These blend into the stock when water is added.

- They should be scraped up with a wooden spoon as the warm water is added. Then add them to your stock for a rich flavour.

Stock Tips

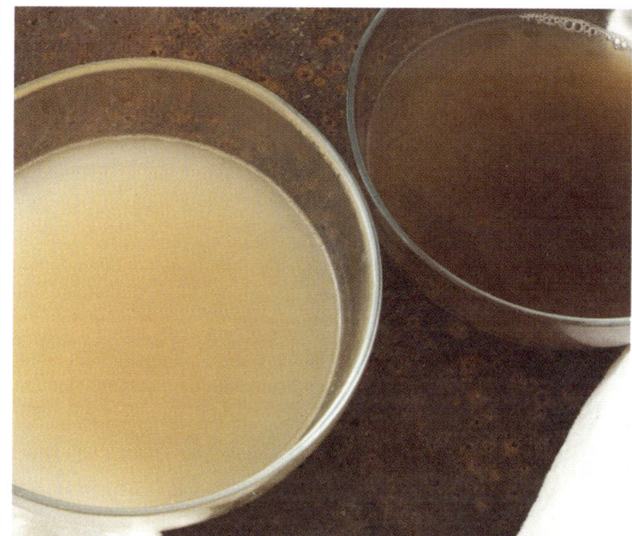

- Strong, rich homemade stock has great depth of flavour and is essential for making good sauces.

- Concentrate stock by cooking it down at high heat, uncovered.

- Don't add salt when making stock, as the reduction can make it too salty: season the soup or sauce to taste later.

- You can add red wine to beef stock and white wine to poultry stock.

- Bones from roasting a duck or chicken make a truly delicious stock for soup.

CURRIED CHICKEN SALAD

Served with rice and grapes, this salad makes a great summer lunch

Curry is a marvellous combination of spices. It enhances meat, poultry, seafood, eggs and vegetables. It can be whisked into salad dressings, mixed with mayonnaise, whirled into gravies and sauces – curry goes with just about everything.

Ready-made curry powders and pastes are excellent when mixed with mustard and then added to mayonnaise to be served with cold meats.

One way of getting a flavour that suits you is to buy a mild curry powder and then make it as hot as you like with cayenne pepper. Many people find curry quite entrancing, but for first-timers it's wise not to overdo it.

Ingredients

Serves 4

For the dressing:

1 egg

Juice of 1 lemon

2 teaspoons curry powder, or to taste

Few drops hot pepper sauce

Pinch of salt

50 ml extra-virgin olive oil

For the salad:

2 tablespoons olive oil

450 g boneless, skinless chicken breasts

50 ml dry white wine

350 g cooked basmati rice

100 g green or red grapes, halved

50 g unsalted roasted peanuts, almonds or walnuts

Salad leaves, enough for 4 generous servings

1 avocado, sliced, for garnish (optional)

Calories 525, **Fat** 28 g, **Carbohydrates** 34 g, **Protein** 31 g, **Fibre** 2 g, **Saturated Fat** 4 g, **Cholesterol** 110 mg, **Sodium** 85 mg.

Curried Chicken Salad

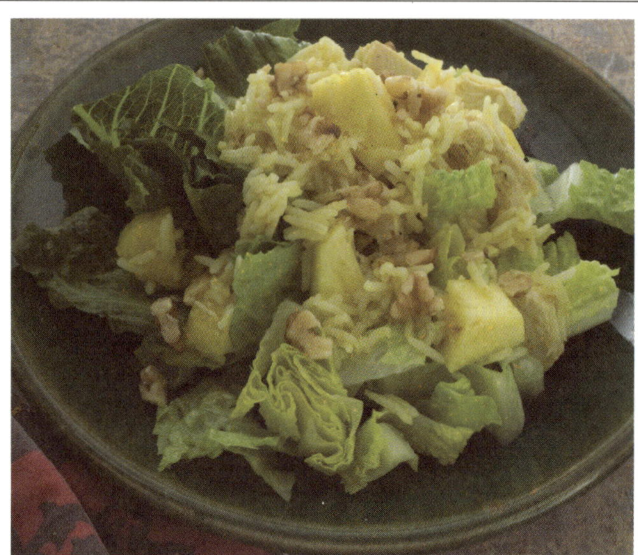

- To make dressing, blend all but olive oil in a blender. Slowly add oil, a few drops at a time. Set aside.

- Pour oil into a nonstick sauté pan over medium heat. Add chicken; brown on both sides.

- Pour in wine, reduce heat.

- Simmer until chicken is done, 8–10 minutes depending on thickness.

- Slice chicken. Add cooking liquid to rice in bowl. Combine all ingredients except salad leaves in bowl. Stir in dressing; serve on leaves and garnish with avocado.

Garnishes and substitutions: Although this recipe calls for whisking curry powder and hot pepper sauce into an oil-based dressing, you can also mix it with a base of low-fat mayonnaise instead of the oil. Vary the fruit used in the recipe. Grapes and melon balls are quite lovely, but pineapple is also excellent. Be careful to eat fruit in moderation and follow your specific diet.

Make your own chutney: Fresh mango chutney is particularly good with curried chicken, prawns or any cold meat. Combine the chopped flesh of 1 ripe mango, 1 teaspoon fresh grated ginger, the juice of half a lime, and 1 teaspoon hot sauce. Mash all together with a fork.

Chicken for Salad

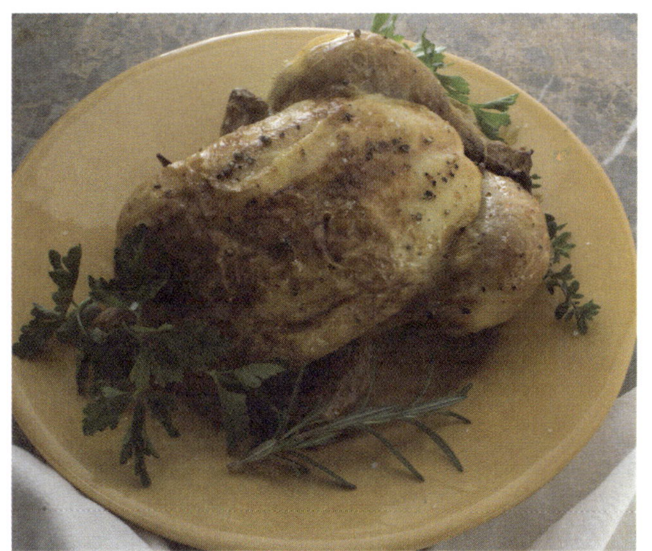

Removing an Avocado Stone

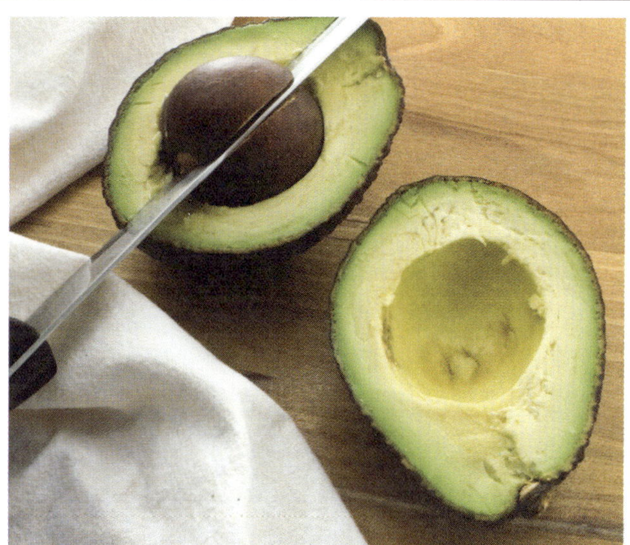

- As an alternative to cooking the chicken, use last night's leftover roast chicken or rotisserie chicken from the supermarket.

- These supermarket chickens are easy on the home cook but are often dried out, tough and tasteless.

- To avoid this, try to get one just as it comes off the spit.

- Save money by using one roast chicken for several different meals.

- Your final meal from this bird could be a rich chicken soup.

- To remove the stone, cut the avocado in half and twist the two sides apart.

- To get the stone out without mashing the avocado, place the side with the stone on a board, stone side up. Using a sharp chef's knife, carefully hit the stone.

- The knife should go partway into the stone and stick. Then, just pull the stone out with the knife.

- If you are holding the avocado while removing the stone, be careful not to stab through the avocado and into your hand.

ORANGE-GLAZED CHICKEN SALAD

This lovely salad has a tropical aroma and goes well with fresh, spicy rocket

For this meal, you can use boneless, skinless chicken breasts or, for a bit more flavour, chicken thighs. Either way, a glaze is a delicious way to enhance the chicken.

Some of the more luscious garnishes for this salad include sliced water chestnuts, mandarin oranges, toasted nuts or all of the above. You will also find that a bed of cold wild rice sets off the chicken and rocket perfectly. This salad is great for people with diabetes; although it does have a sweet flavour, the jam is sugar free and the orange juice is freshly squeezed. Brown or wild rice is a high-quality complex carbohydrate that slows the digestive process. The protein from the chicken adds staying power to the meal.

Ingredients

Serves 4

120 ml sugar-free orange marmalade

2 tablespoons light soy sauce

Juice of $^1/_2$ orange, freshly squeezed

1 teaspoon freshly grated ginger

$^1/_2$ teaspoon chilli flakes, or to taste

450 g boneless, skinless chicken breasts or thighs

40 g rocket or other salad leaves

120 ml citrus dressing or vinaigrette

175 g cooked wild or brown rice (optional)

Optional garnishes: dried cranberries; toasted pine nuts; water chestnuts, drained and rinsed; canned mandarin oranges, drained and rinsed

Calories 305, **Fat** 8 g, **Carbohydrates** 15 g, **Protein** 30 g, **Fibre** 1 g, **Saturated Fat** 2 g, **Cholesterol** 82 mg, **Sodium** 395 mg.

Orange-Glazed Chicken Salad

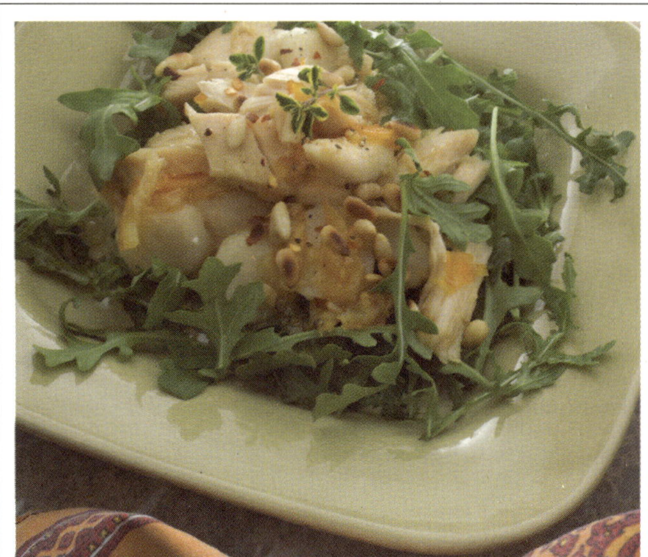

- Preheat grill to 180°C and set shelf 20–25 cm below it. Mix first five ingredients; warm in small bowl in microwave for 90 seconds, or in pan over low heat, until marmalade is melted.

- Place chicken on grill rack and coat with orange glaze. Grill for 5 minutes, being careful not to burn it. Turn; brush glaze on second side and grill for another 5 minutes.

- Cut chicken into strips; arrange rocket on platter. Pour dressing over rocket. Mix rice with chicken. Spoon chicken over rocket; garnish as desired.

Various glazes: You can also glaze chicken with fresh raspberries mixed with sugar-free raspberry jam. Or make a very nice cranberry glaze by reducing cranberry juice and adding dried cranberries. The glaze will also drizzle into and add flavour to the salad dressing. You can mix extra reduced juice with the dressing, or add it to cooked brown or wild rice to give your salad body. Finally, you can easily mix glazes such as cranberry and orange, or prune and orange. All are very good.

Switching the leaves: The fresher and crisper the salad leaves, the better. Rocket is suggested here, but you could also use mixed leaves, baby spinach or lettuce.

The Slow Grill

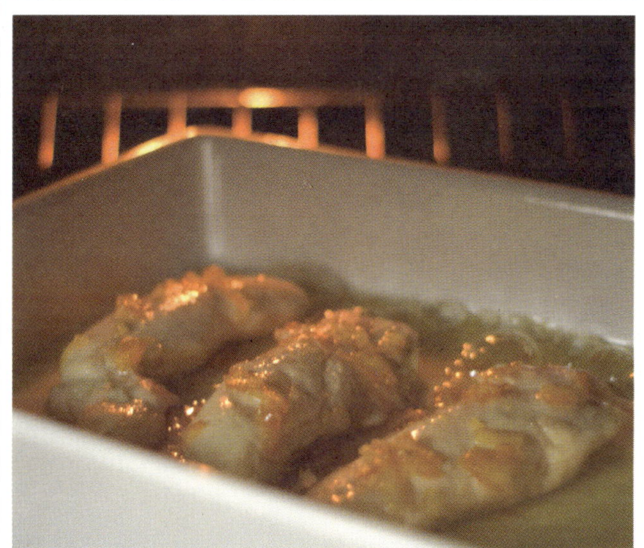

- Slow-grilling glazed meat or poultry has some advantages, the first being that it prevents the outside from burning while the meat is cooked through.

- You do not want to see any pink meat in poultry.

- You can get slow-grill results on a charcoal grill by banking the coals to one side and placing the chicken on the other, away from the direct heat.

- Cover the barbecue so that the inside of the chicken cooks thoroughly.

Alternative to Grilling

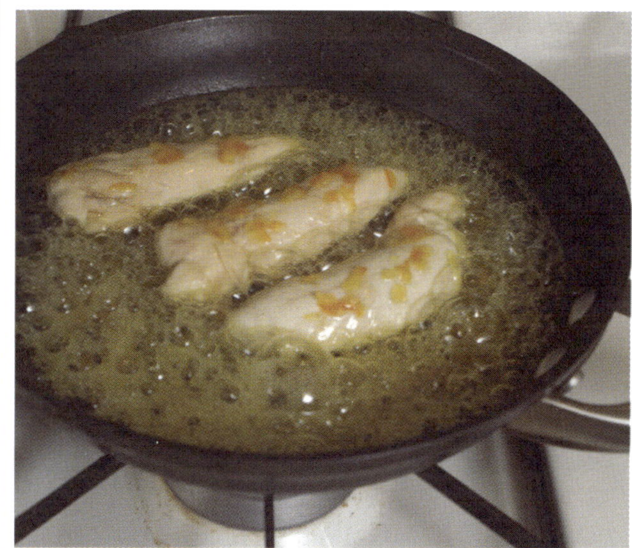

- As an alternative to grilling, poach the chicken in the glaze used in this recipe.

- Bring the glaze to a simmer in a pan on top of the stove. Cut the chicken into chunks and add them to the glaze; cover, keeping the heat very low.

- Let the chicken poach for 8–10 minutes, covered. This ensures that your chicken will be cooked through.

- If you are serving the salad with rice, drizzle the salad with the poaching liquid.

MEDITERRANEAN SEAFOOD SALAD

At lunch or dinner, this salad epitomizes the healthy Mediterranean diet

With this recipe, the more varieties of seafood you use, the better it tastes. Be sure to save the cooking liquids to add to rice or cooked small pasta shells for added flavour.

You can choose any combination of molluscs and crustaceans. Serve clams and mussels in their shells. You are not likely to find oysters in a seafood salad; somehow, they just don't quite fit. There is no law, though, that says you can't add a few shucked oysters, raw or poached, to the salad. Be careful, however, when you consume raw shellfish, as bad ones can lead to illness. You don't need to buy jumbo prawns or king scallops. Medium prawns and queen scallops are just fine and far less expensive.

Ingredients

Serves 4

75 ml fresh lemon juice

75 ml olive oil

1 teaspoon Worcestershire sauce

15 g fresh parsley, finely chopped

Salt and pepper to taste

12 clams

16 mussels

225 g queen scallops

16 medium raw prawns, shelled and deveined

225 g small shell pasta, cooked, or 200 g brown rice

115 g lettuce leaves

Garnish: avocados, capers or fennel leaves

Calories 552, **Fat** 22 g, **Carbohydrates** 49 g, **Protein** 38 g, **Fibre** 2 g, **Saturated Fat** 3 g, **Cholesterol** 168 mg, **Sodium** 689 mg.

Mediterranean Seafood Salad

- Mix first five ingredients together to make dressing.

- Scrub clams and mussels under cold running water. Discard open shellfish. Place 120 ml water in a pan over high heat. Add shellfish; cover and allow them to steam open. Transfer them to a separate bowl.

- Reduce heat to medium; add scallops and prawns. Cook for 2 minutes, removing when prawns turn pink.

- Combine cooked seafood. Pour half of dressing over seafood. Add rest to cooked pasta or rice. Top salad leaves with pasta or rice, then seafood. Garnish.

Artichoke heart salad: A delicious variation of this recipe is to add 275 g frozen baby artichoke hearts. Cook them according to the directions on the pack, but acidulate the water by adding 1 tablespoon of lemon juice to the cooking liquid to remove any bitterness in the artichokes. Marinate the artichokes in citrus dressing and let them 'cook' overnight in the fridge. Add to salad the next day.

Avocado salad: Another excellent addition to this main-course salad would be avocados. Just slice 2 ripe avocados over the top or arrange slices around the salad. Remember to brush them with fresh lemon or lime juice to prevent them from browning.

Use Safe Seafood

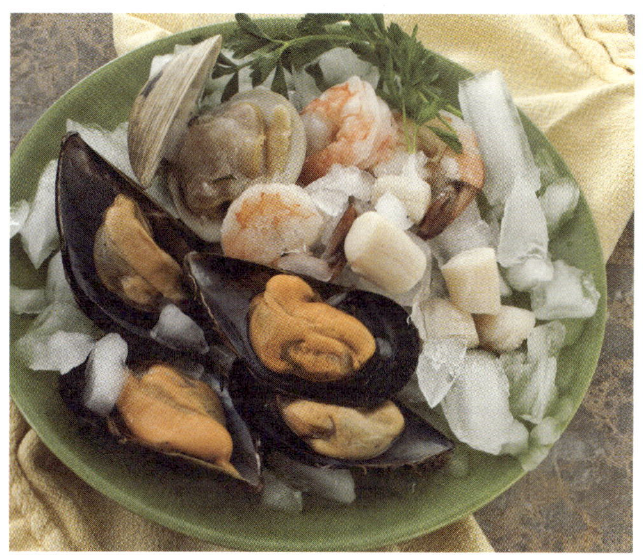

Overcooked Seafood

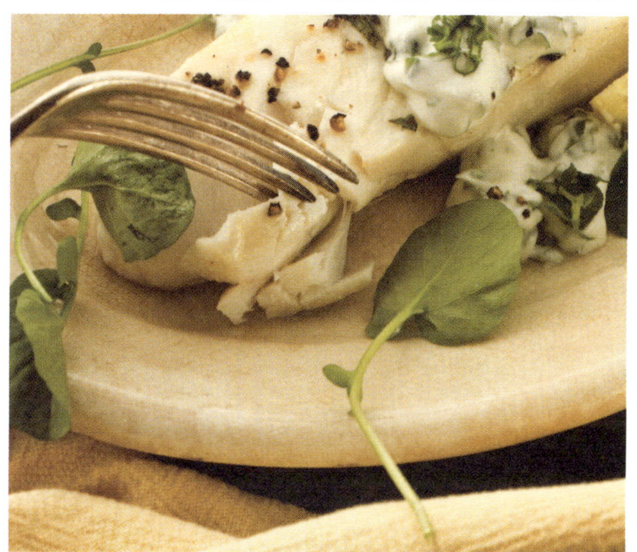

MAIN-COURSE SALADS

- When cooking with seafood, the first rule is never to use anything that smells even slightly sour or 'off'.

- Find a really good fish market or a supermarket with a knowledgeable fish department.

- Tap the clams and mussels together to make sure they close up tightly.

- If a clam or mussel makes a dull thud or hollow sound more than once, discard it.

- If you overcook fish, it will disintegrate into tiny flakes. This is not attractive and has a mushy texture if poached. When grilled, overcooked fish will dry out.

- Tuna hardens and salmon loses flavour and moisture when overcooked. Cook until it just begins to flake.

- If you overcook scallops, prawns, mussels, oysters or lobster, they become rubbery.

- Squid must be cooked only until just barely hot, or for a long time – up to 4 hours in a sauce – to prevent it being tough.

CHARGRILLED VEGETABLE SALAD

Whenever you fire up the barbecue, chargrill lots of vegetables to have on hand for later

Vegetables can be treated with lots of herbs and spices when grilled. They must first be brushed with a little olive oil before going on the barbecue – that's mandatory.

When working with vegetables, look for the small varieties of aubergine. Some are actually the size of eggs, while others are about 15 cm long and skinny. Although all aubergine skins are edible, the large ones can be tough, while the small varieties have tender skins. Red and green peppers need to be peeled if they char. Green and yellow courgettes are just fine – skin and all. Tomatoes are terrific on the barbecue, but should have some foil underneath to keep the juices from running into the fire.

Ingredients

Serves 6

2 tablespoons olive oil

2 cloves garlic, smashed and chopped

1 tablespoon dried basil or 3 tablespoons fresh basil

1 tablespoon dried oregano or 3 tablespoons fresh oregano

1 teaspoon hot pepper sauce, or to taste

50 ml red wine vinegar

2 red peppers, cut into quarters and cleaned

3 small courgettes, trimmed and cut lengthwise

3 small aubergines, trimmed and cut in half lengthwise

3 tomatoes, cored and cut into thick slices

18 thin asparagus stalks, trimmed

1 large head romaine lettuce, washed, dried and shredded

18 Italian or Greek olives

12 marble-sized balls fresh mozzarella cheese

Calories 176, **Fat** 10 g, **Carbohydrates** 18 g, **Protein** 9 g, **Fibre** 8 g, **Saturated Fat** 3 g, **Cholesterol** 8 mg, **Sodium** 219 mg.

Chargrilled Vegetable Salad

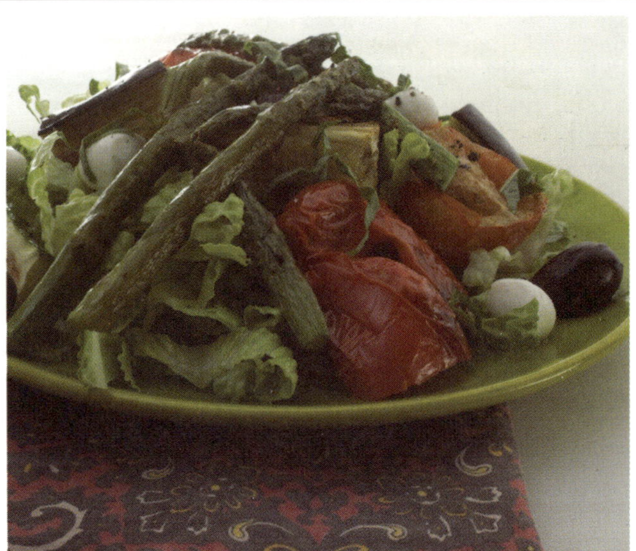

- Fire up the barbecue or preheat the grill. Whisk first six ingredients together to make dressing.

- Prepare vegetables, brushing lightly with dressing. Carve tracks into aubergines so dressing can soak in. Place tomato slices on heavy-duty aluminium foil.

- Grill vegetables until crisp-tender. Timing depends on barbecue or grill. If peppers are charred, peel them.

- Make a generous bed of salad leaves on a platter; arrange vegetables on top. Garnish with olives and fresh mozzarella. Pour any leftover dressing over top.

The health benefits of asparagus: Asparagus offers plenty of health benefits for people with diabetes. It is high in vitamin K and folate. Its high amounts of folic acid may help prevent some forms of heart disease and strokes. Eating asparagus regularly may also help you lower your cholesterol and fight off high blood pressure.

You may want to place all your vegetables in a colander in the sink to rinse them, rather than rinsing each individually. It is best to use a brush to gently scrub the skin of each vegetable to ensure that all dirt and residue come off, but don't use soap to wash your vegetables. Also avoid using either extremely warm or extremely cold water.

Washing and Drying Vegetables

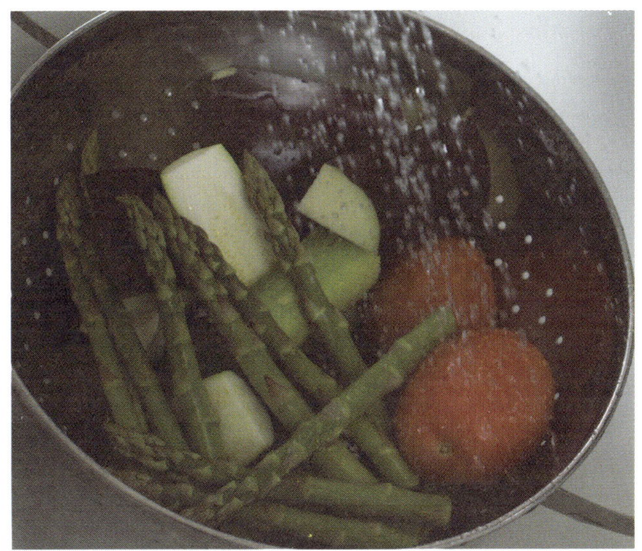

Storing Grilled Vegetables

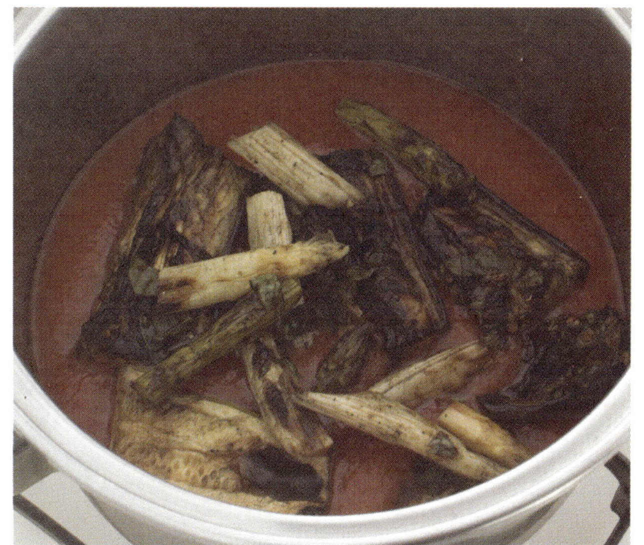

- Wash uncooked vegetables to remove germs and dirt, pesticides or fertilizer clinging to them.

- Dry the vegetables (air-dry or with paper towels) before cooking them so that the oil and herbs cling.

- Otherwise, the dressing will simply slide off and puddle into your barbecue or under your grill.

- All the vegetables in this recipe can be placed directly on the barbecue or grill rack.

- Grilled vegetables should be used within a day or two. You can keep them in the refrigerator for a couple days, but freezing them will turn them mushy.

- You can actually chop the grilled vegetables and add them to pasta sauce or soup. That will freeze quite well.

- However, the taste of vegetables fresh from the barbecue is unbeatable.

MAIN-COURSE SALADS

TOFU & BROCCOLI SALAD

An Asian-style dressing takes this vegetarian salad from ordinary to extraordinary

The more you cook with tofu, the easier it becomes. And when you add the crunch of nuts and broccoli to the satiny quality of tofu, the meal just gets better.

This Asian-style dressing is easy to make and adds the finishing touch to the dish. However, you can vary the ingredients and come up with something more Italian if you prefer.

Broccoli is one of the so-called power foods, and it is simple to prepare. Tofu is packed with protein, as it comes from soybeans. It is available in firm, extra firm and silken varieties. For this recipe, try using the silken style. For frying and cooking, use firm or extra firm.

Serve this salad warm or chilled.

Ingredients

Serves 6

2 tablespoons groundnut oil

1 tablespoon sesame seed oil

Juice of $^1/_2$ fresh lemon

2 tablespoons sherry vinegar

1 teaspoon homemade mustard (see recipe, page 204)

1 teaspoon grated fresh ginger

3 tablespoons light soy sauce

1 medium sweet onion, finely chopped

1 broccoli crown, divided into florets, microwaved in 120 ml water for 4 minutes on high, then drained

450 g silken tofu, cubed

40 g toasted pine nuts

115 g pasta spirals, cooked (optional)

Calories 306, **Fat** 22 g, **Carbohydrates** 17 g, **Protein** 16 g, **Fibre** 5 g, **Saturated Fat** 3 g, **Cholesterol** 0, **Sodium** 359 mg.

Tofu and Broccoli Salad

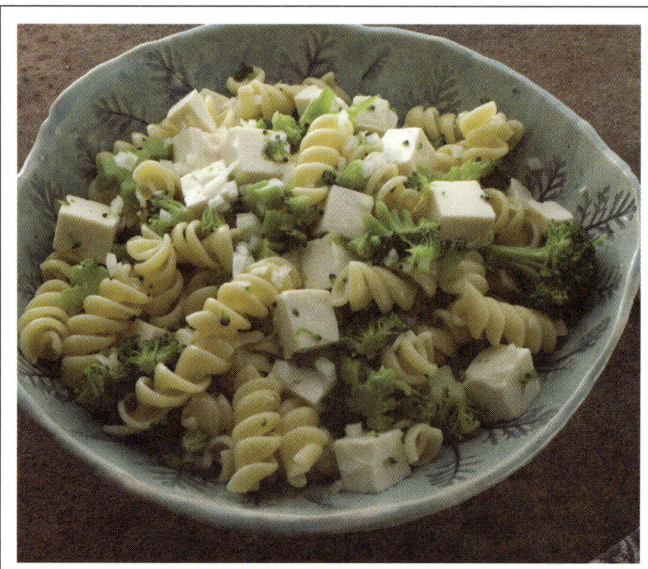

- Whisk first seven ingredients together to make dressing.

- Place all salad ingredients in a large serving bowl and pour on the dressing. Mix well.

- Serve immediately if you want to eat it warm, or chill to serve later.

Tofu with Chinese leaves and prawns: Shred Chinese leaves for a crunchy alternative. Mix 120 ml light mayonnaise with the Asian dressing. For added variety, add 225 g cooked prawns to the tofu and Chinese leaves. If you prefer, add 225 g chicken or crabmeat. Garnish the salad with 115 g sugar snap peas, blanched, rinsed, dried and cut diagonally into thick slices.

Italian-style: For the Italian version of this recipe, you can totally change the flavour of the salad simply by changing the dressing. Use basic red wine vinaigrette or a vinaigrette made with champagne or other white wine. With the broccoli, add some chopped roasted red pepper and 50 g crumbled Gorgonzola cheese.

Broccoli for Salad or as a Side Dish

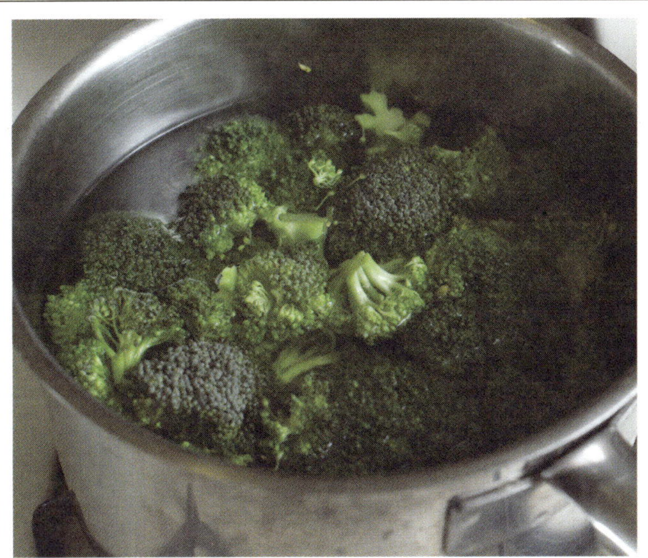

Pasta and Noodles in Salad

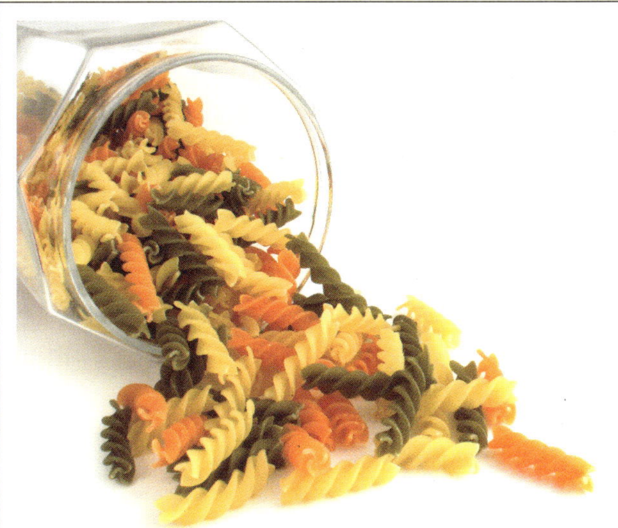

- When preparing broccoli for salad, you should generally cook it for a shorter time than for a side dish, to maintain the crunch.

- Uncooked broccoli can be harsh on the digestive system, producing stomach-aches and gas.

- If you are serving older adults or very young children, it's best to cook the broccoli until crisp-tender.

- Or if your dinner table includes elderly people, cook the broccoli for an extra 5 minutes.

- Check out the various kinds of Asian noodles available, and learn to enjoy many different types.

- Asian bean-thread noodles are much more delicate than regular noodles or pasta. They are often labelled 'glass' or 'cellophane' noodles.

- Of course, you can use any noodle or pasta that you like in a salad. However, cook the pasta al dente because it will absorb dressing and get softer as it does so.

MAIN-COURSE SALADS

PRAWN SALAD WITH CASHEWS

You can use other nuts in this recipe, but cashews go especially well with prawns

This delicious combination will take any home cook a long way. Serve it to a friend for lunch or dinner, or as part of a buffet at a family party, whenever you need a lovely dish that's easy to make the day before.

Lime juice is essential in this recipe to counterbalance the sweetness of the cashews. The counterpoint of sweet and tart is what makes food interesting. Make this recipe with cold cooked rice or small pasta shells. However, whenever you use a starchy food such as rice or pasta, make extra sauce and dress it well before serving, as the noodles or rice will soak up the dressing – remember to count the carbohydrates in your meal plan.

Ingredients

Serves 4

150 ml low-fat mayonnaise

Juice of 1 fresh lime

1 teaspoon mustard

Salt and freshly ground pepper to taste

15 g fresh parsley, finely chopped

450 g medium cooked prawns, shelled

2 sticks celery, finely chopped

50 g unsalted roasted cashew nuts

175 g salad leaves, such as romaine or iceberg lettuce or baby spinach

Calories 313, **Fat** 17 g, **Carbohydrates** 15 g, **Protein** 26 g, **Fibre** 2 g, **Saturated Fat** 3 g, **Cholesterol** 173 mg, **Sodium** 345 mg.

Prawn Salad with Cashews

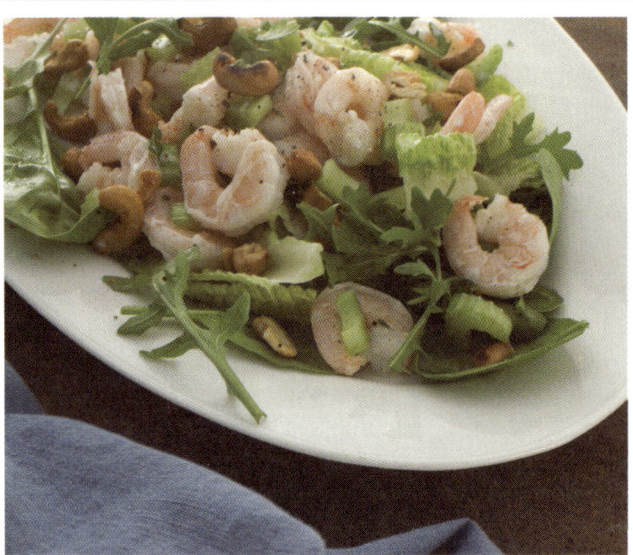

- Mix the mayonnaise, lime juice, mustard, parsley, salt, and pepper together in a bowl.

- If prawns are frozen, defrost under cool running water and check for remaining shells. Dry thoroughly.

- Mix together all the ingredients except the salad leaves.

- Cover and chill for serving later, or arrange over salad leaves and serve immediately.

Cooking with cashews: Cashews have a mellow, sweet flavour. They are great chopped and pressed into salmon that's to be grilled or barbecued, or you can grind them up and sprinkle them over peaches before you barbecue them. Cashews also are an excellent counterpoint to prawns, as in this salad. Don't buy salted cashews. The last thing anyone, much less a person with diabetes, needs to consume is extra salt. Just get raw or roasted cashews and add them to other salads, meat and vegetable dishes. Try adding cashews to any chicken dish, such as chicken salad. Baked chicken, even chicken pie, will benefit greatly from the addition of a handful of cashews. They add crunch and interest to what could otherwise be a bland dish.

Choosing Prawns for Salad

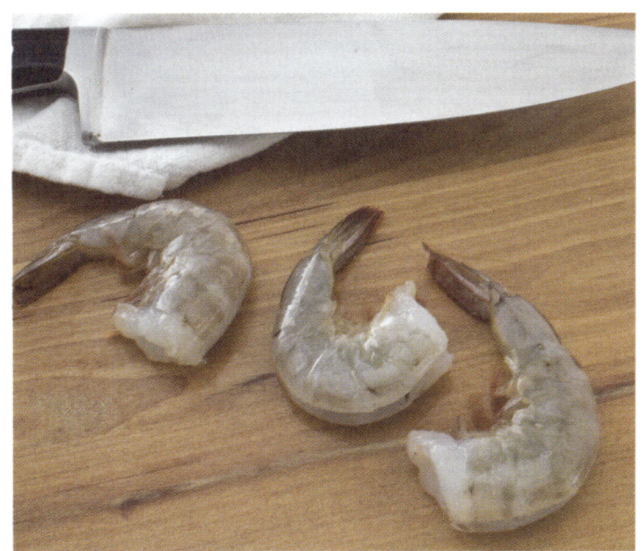

- Freshly netted and cooked prawns are a rare luxury unless you live by the sea, but they are the sweetest of all.

- Extra-large prawns should be cut into bite-size pieces for a salad.

- Although prawns have a bad reputation because they are high in dietary cholesterol, they are very low in saturated fat, so are a great source of lean protein. Just don't eat them every day.

Peeling and Cleaning Prawns

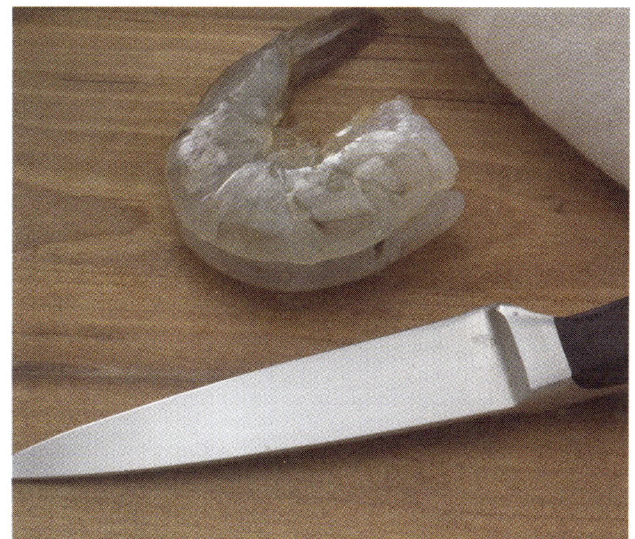

- Fresh or defrosted frozen prawns are easy to peel.

- First, pull off the legs and remove the shell.

- Then, with a very sharp knife, make a shallow cut along the back and remove any black intestines.

- Rinse the prawn thoroughly to remove any grit.

- Poach prawns (in wine or beer) until they turn pink. Drain, chill and use in your salad.

MAIN-COURSE SALADS

BARBECUED ASPARAGUS

You can make the same grilled asparagus that is served in many upscale restaurants

Antioxidants are incredibly important to your health because they kill cancer-causing free radicals. All green vegetables, including asparagus, provide antioxidants.

Asparagus can be grilled indoors or barbecued outside. If you are cooking it on a charcoal or gas barbecue, skewer the spears together with metal or wooden skewers. If you use wooden skewers, soak them in water for an hour, or the heat of the grill will burn them.

Asparagus is especially nice with either melted butter and lemon vinaigrette or Hollandaise sauce. Or eat it plain with low-fat mayo. Thick asparagus is tender and juicy but needs its ends peeled. Thin asparagus does not need peeling.

Ingredients

Serves 4

16–24 fresh asparagus spears

250 ml of your favourite vinaigrette

Calories 64, **Fat** 4 g, **Carbohydrates** 7 g, **Protein** 2 g, **Fibre** 2 g, **Saturated Fat** 0, **Cholesterol** 4 mg, **Sodium** 822 mg.

Grilled Asparagus

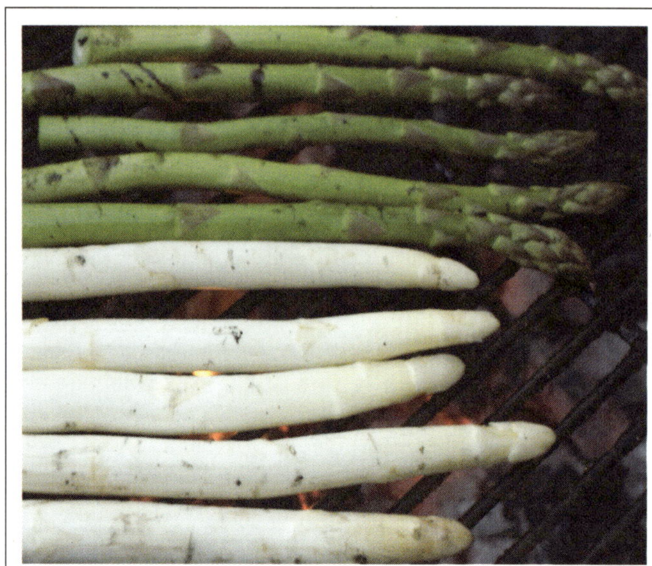

- Break off and discard the tough ends of the asparagus. Wash and dry on paper towels.

- Place the asparagus in a flat dish and add the vinaigrette.

- Marinate the asparagus for 30 minutes to 2 hours.

- Prepare barbecue or preheat grill to 180°C. Grill asparagus quickly, until just beginning to brown. Serve hot, at room temperature or cold.

Use asparagus in soups, salads or as a side dish. Or wrap it in light whole-wheat bread with a cheese spread, cut in small pieces, and bake for appetizers. Cook it quickly in the microwave. Cut it in lengths that fit your bowl. Add 2 tablespoons water, 1 tablespoon low-fat margarine and some lemon juice. Cover with paper. Depending on how well cooked you like it, microwave 2–5 minutes on high.

Marinate vegetables: Any citrus vinaigrette or white wine vinaigrette will work as a marinade. If you marinate in mustardy barbecue sauce, keep it farther from the flame when cooking or it will burn. String 18–24 (depending on size) mushrooms on 4 skewers and coat with marinade; serve them in addition to the asparagus in a salad, with cooked rice or pasta as a side dish.

Trimming Asparagus Ends

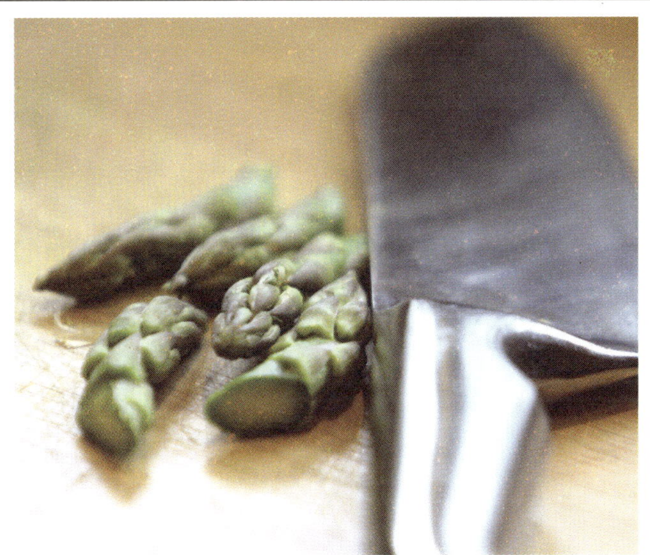

- Remove the tough, woody ends from stalks of asparagus.

- Using a potato peeler, simply start peeling where the asparagus gets thick but is still green.

- Peel thick stalks if nubby or 2.5 cm in diameter at the widest. Only peel the green part; discard the tough white or purple ends.

- Break off the end of one stalk, then line it up with the rest. Using it as a guide, cut the rest of the stems with a knife.

Green or White Asparagus?

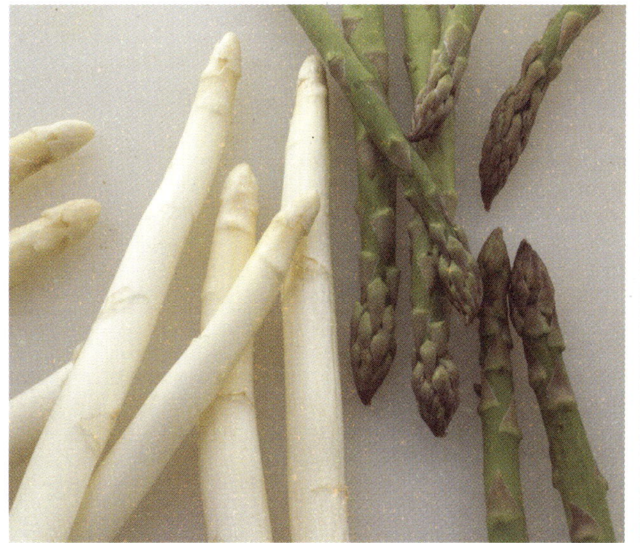

- Although white asparagus is considered a gourmet delicacy, try to get the greenest produce in the market.

- White asparagus is white because it is deprived of light; no sun touches it. Therefore, the vegetable does not make chlorophyll.

- Chlorophyll is the product of photosynthesis; plants turn light into chlorophyll, which gives them their green colour.

- There are a lot more vitamins and minerals in green asparagus than in the white, which is grown under a tent or pot.

GREEN VEGETABLES

BROCCOLI WITH GARLIC SAUCE

Broccoli is a 'power' food because it's packed with nutrients

From florets to stems, broccoli is a superfood. Use the florets for your green vegetable side dishes, salads and snacks. Use the stems for soup.

Broccoli is a member of the crucifer family of vegetables, which also includes Brussels sprouts, kale, turnip tops, cauliflower and various forms of cabbage. All these vegetables should be eaten regularly as they are full of antioxidants, which fight cancer by literally killing off the free radicals we get from other sources.

Garlic is a very healthy aromatic herb and goes very well with broccoli. Garlic in a little oil or low-fat margarine, or mixed with vinaigrette, enhances the flavours of vegetables whether they are cooked or raw. It's strongest when chopped, mildest when left whole or cut into large slices.

Ingredients

Serves 4

2 tablespoons lemon juice

2 tablespoons olive oil

2 cloves garlic, smashed and slivered

Salt and pepper to taste

450 g broccoli, separated into small florets, stems set aside

Broccoli with Garlic Sauce

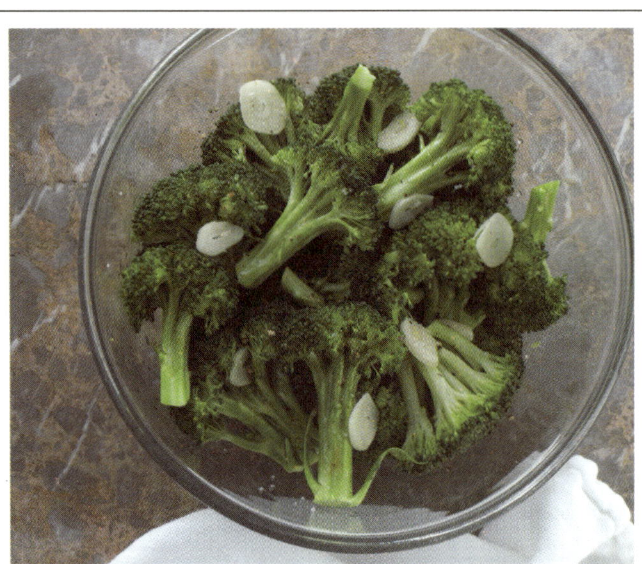

- Place the first 4 ingredients in a non-metal bowl and mix.

- Rinse the broccoli but do not dry it. Swish it around in the lemon-oil-garlic mixture.

- Cover with paper towels.

- Microwave for 2 minutes. Turn the broccoli and microwave for another 2–4 minutes, depending on desired level of tenderness.

Calories 91, **Fat** 7 g, **Carbohydrates** 5 g, **Protein** 2 g, **Fibre** 0, **Saturated Fat** 3 g, **Cholesterol** 0, **Sodium** 20 g.

Broccoli and citrus: This recipe is very quick and delicious, as well as being nutritious. Add 1 tablespoon fresh lime juice to garlic sauce, omitting the lemon juice. One teaspoon of lemon zest adds flavour. If some members of your family like broccoli to be more crisp, simply microwave some of the broccoli for 2 minutes and the rest of it for 4 minutes.

Boiling broccoli: A second method of cooking is to drop the broccoli into boiling, lightly salted water. Cook for 5 minutes, then remove from the cooking water. Refresh by plunging it into iced water, then drain. Make the sauce in a large sauté pan over medium heat. Add the broccoli to the sauce in the pan.

Preparing Broccoli Stems for Soup

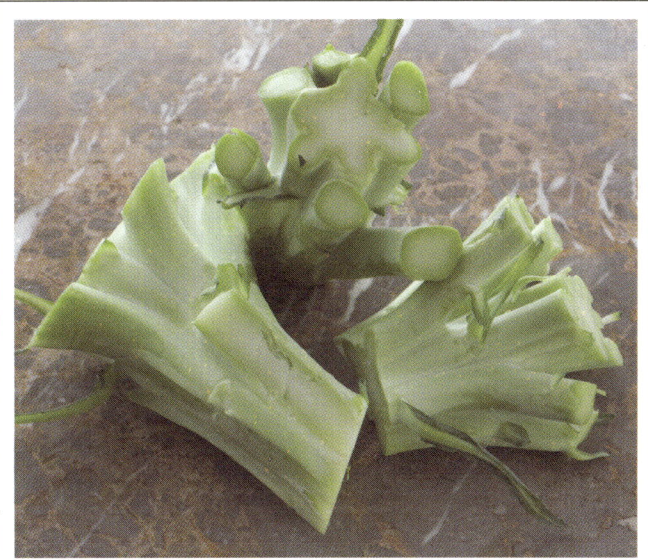

Another Broccoli-Like Vegetable

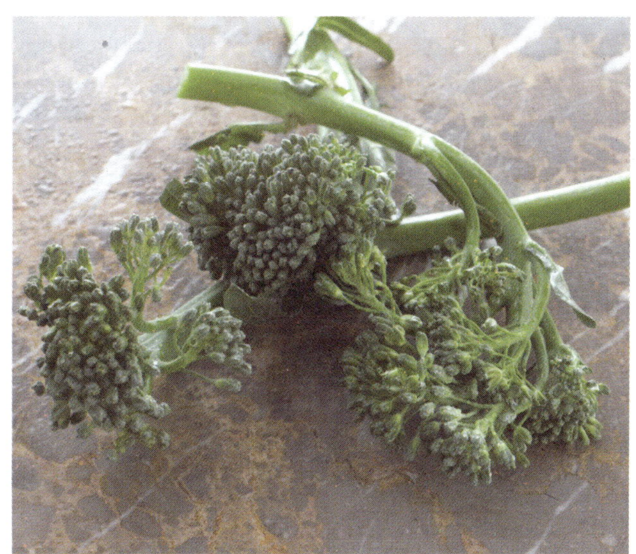

- Wash the stems. Cut $1/8$ inch off the very bottom of each stem.

- Cut the broccoli stems crosswise, into 6-mm 'coins.'

- Cook the stems in boiling salted water or light chicken stock to cover.

- Sauté 1 onion and 2 cloves garlic until soft. Add to the soup ½ teaspoon each thyme and oregano for flavour. Cool a little, then blend in batches in a food processor or blender.

- Broccolini is not, as many people think, very young broccoli. It is a cross between broccoli and a Chinese cabbage called kai-lan.

- It was developed in Japan and has become very popular worldwide because of its pleasant flavour and high nutritional content.

- Cook broccolini exactly as you would cook broccoli. It's smaller, so takes less time.

- Broccollini is tender and delicious, and high in vitamin A, calcium and iron.

GREEN VEGETABLES

TURNIP TOPS WITH PASTA

Fans of this slightly bitter vegetable claim it is positively addictive

Turnip tops, also known as broccoli rabe or rapini, are beloved by the Italians, Spanish and Portuguese. They are blanched and then sautéed in oil, butter or low-fat margarine.

Turnip tops look a lot like broccoli: unlike calabrese, you eat the stems and leaves as well as the flower buds. They have a slightly bitter or pungent flavour, which is subdued by blanching. They are very popular in Italian restaurants as a side dish, or as a main course with sausages. In Puglia they're traditionally eaten with orecchiette pasta. They're also popular on pizza, when they are precooked by blanching, mixed with two or three kinds of cheese, and baked on the crust.

This recipe can make an entire meal because it contains protein from the cheese and carbohydrates from the pasta, as well as the vegetables.

Ingredients

Serves 6

450 g turnip tops, washed and chopped into 2.5-cm pieces

450 g low-fat ricotta cheese

40 g Parmesan cheese, finely grated

1 egg, lightly beaten

$1/4$ teaspoon nutmeg

Juice of $1/2$ lemon

Freshly ground black pepper to taste

225 g whole-wheat pasta

50 ml extra-virgin olive oil

1 teaspoon dried oregano

Calories 380, **Fat** 18 g, **Carbohydrates** 35 g, **Protein** 21 g, **Fibre** 5 g, **Saturated Fat** 7 g, **Cholesterol** 31 mg, **Sodium** 275 mg.

Turnip Tops with Pasta

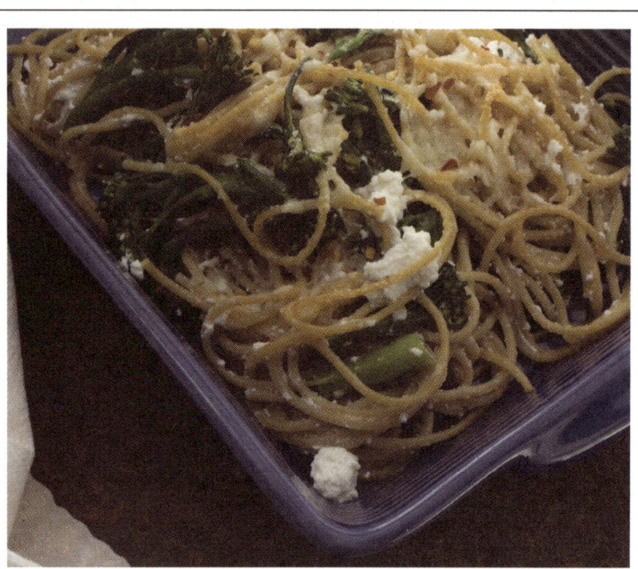

- Blanch the turnip tops for 3 minutes in boiling water; place in colander to drain.

- Mix the ricotta, Parmesan, egg, nutmeg and pepper together in a bowl. Add lemon juice. Preheat oven to 170°C.

- Cook the pasta and drain; place in a large, ovenproof serving bowl. Toss the olive oil and oregano with the pasta.

- Add the turnip tops and the cheese mixture. Mix well and bake for 20 minutes.

Always blanch turnip tops: Unless your taste buds are very well conditioned, always blanch turnip tops for a couple of minutes in boiling water to remove the bitterness. And remember, you can and should eat the leaves and stems, too. After blanching, you can cut the stems into 2.5–5-cm segments for sautéing as a side dish, mixing with other ingredients or spreading on a white pizza. If you are sautéing, do so with garlic and a drop of olive oil, then sprinkle with lemon juice. You can also use shallots instead of, or in addition to, garlic.

Blanching Vegetables

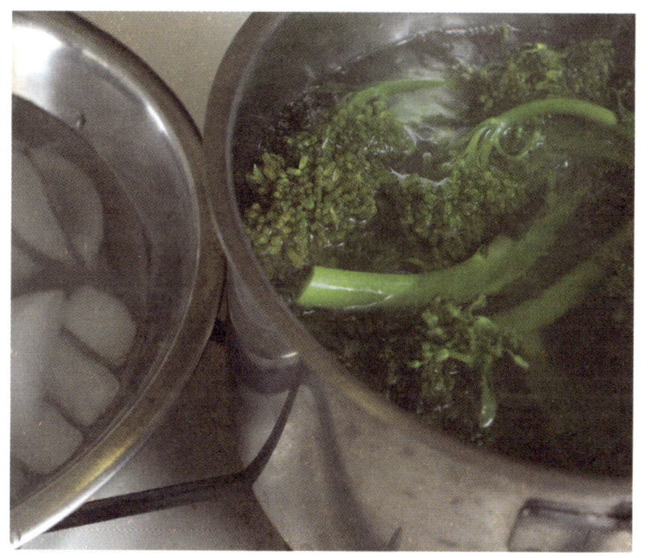

Refreshing Vegetables

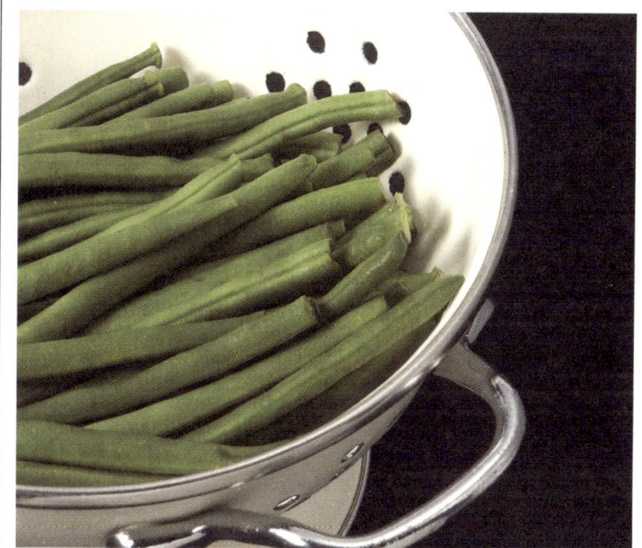

- You can blanch any green vegetable to keep it crisp-tender, then refresh it to keep it a bright green.

- Bring a large pan of water to a rolling boil. You can add a little salt, but it's not necessary.

- Immerse the vegetables in the boiling water. Return to the boil and cook for 1–5 minutes, depending on the kind of vegetable and how tender you want it.

- Drain.

- After blanching, refresh your vegetables to stop them cooking and brighten their colour. Drain, then plunge them into a bowl of iced water.

- Don't blanch and refresh spinach; it will turn limp and watery.

- Blanch and refresh green beans, asparagus, turnip tops, broccoli, broccolini and artichokes (prior to baking).

- Blanching and refreshing prior to sautéing vegetables also tenderizes them.

SAUCY GREEN BEANS

These green beans soar to new heights with a little freshly made tomato sauce

Green beans are great for mixing with other goodies. They go well with nuts, mushrooms, garlic, shallots and, in the case of this recipe, fresh cherry tomatoes made into a quick sauce.

Always blanch and refresh green beans (see technique on page 101). They will stay crisp-tender and very green. Then you can add them to a vegetable salad, dress them with a sauce, sauté them or mix them with other vegetables in dishes such as pasta bakes or frittatas.

Freshly blanched and refreshed green beans give a finer flavour to this dish than frozen ones. Since fresh green beans are available all year round, it makes good sense to use them every time.

Ingredients

Serves 6

450 g fresh cherry tomatoes, rinsed and stemmed

2 tablespoons olive oil

2 cloves garlic, smashed, peeled and sliced

2 shallots, peeled and sliced

450 g green string beans, trimmed

1 teaspoon dried rosemary or 1 tablespoon fresh rosemary

1 teaspoon dried oregano or 1 tablespoon fresh oregano

Salt and freshly ground black pepper to taste

Garnish: 2 tablespoons freshly grated Parmesan cheese

Calories 94, **Fat** 5 g, **Carbohydrates** 11 g, **Protein** 3 g, **Fibre** 4 g, **Saturated Fat** 1 g, **Cholesterol** 2 mg, **Sodium** 30 mg.

Saucy Green Beans

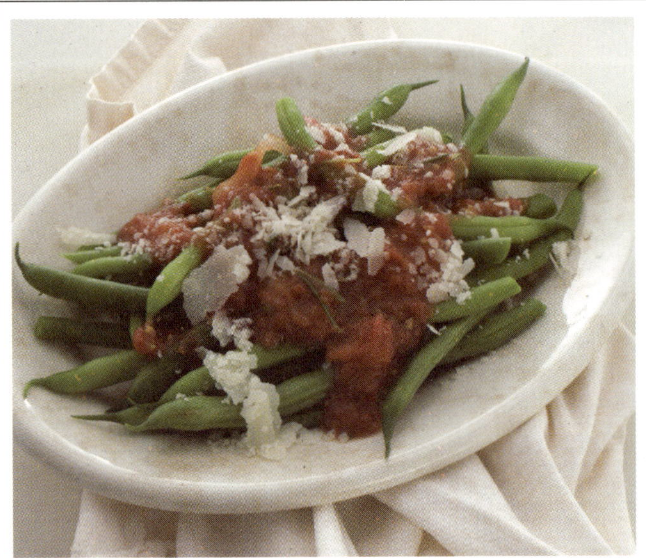

- Place half the tomatoes in a blender and purée; add the other half and purée until very fine. Set aside.

- Heat olive oil over medium heat in a large sauté pan; add garlic and shallots. Sauté, stirring to cook evenly.

- Add the tomatoes and cover; reduce heat to low.

- Blanch and refresh the beans; drain.

- Add the beans, herbs, salt and pepper to the tomato sauce. Cover and cook for 5 minutes. Sprinkle with cheese and serve.

Storing beans: Green beans store well in the refrigerator and can also be frozen for future use. If freezing, wash them first and then dry thoroughly. Line a baking sheet with baking parchment. Place the beans on the baking sheet, making sure they are not touching, and put them in the freezer for about 45 minutes. Quickly place handfuls of beans in storage bags, seal tightly, and put straight back into the freezer. Of course, there is nothing wrong with commercially frozen green beans, but they are never as crisp as the ones you freeze yourself. Also, if you have a garden full of green beans, you have the satisfaction of eating food you've grown, tended and lovingly prepared.

Why Your Sauce Turns Pink

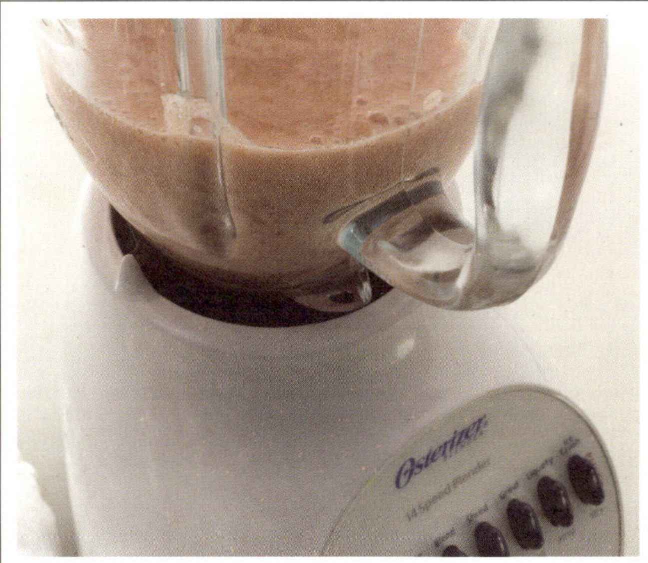

- When you purée tomatoes in a blender, they turn pink. This is because the air and water dilute the tomatoes.

- Don't worry; you won't end up with a pink tomato sauce.

- Just let it cook for a while, and it will change back to a true red. This foolproof technique can also be used for a soup base.

- Tomatoes vary in juiciness. Mix the base with 1 tablespoon tomato purée to thicken, or with 250 ml chicken or beef broth if it is too thick.

Dried vs. Fresh Herbs

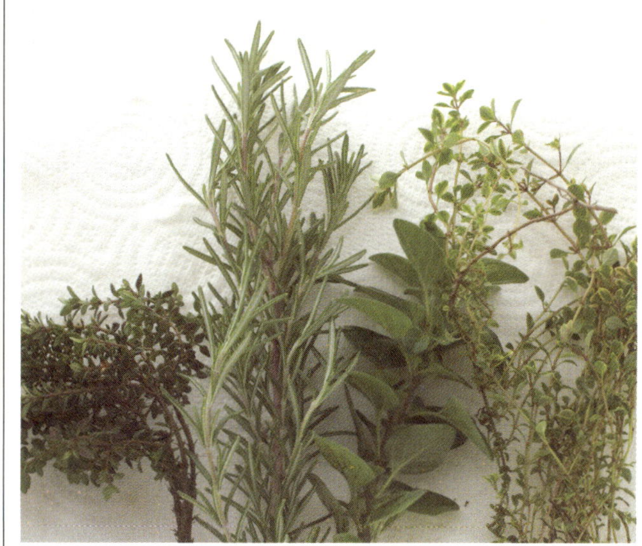

- Fresh herbs are full of moisture. Flavours are concentrated in dried herbs.

- That's why you use two or three times the amount of fresh herbs compared to dried herbs.

- Use dried herbs as soon as possible. They lose their power and aroma when stored for months on end.

- This is not so true of spices, such as nutmeg, cloves and cinnamon. They hold their flavours longer.

COURGETTE & TOMATO CASSEROLE

Here's what to do with all those courgettes from the garden

Courgettes abound in summer gardens, and those who grow them always seem to have too many. Friends with gardens will post them through your letter box, or leave them on the seat of your car or your back doorstep.

However, they are wonderful in soup and bread and as a simple vegetable side dish. This recipe has everything you need for a complete meal.

There are many ways to add extra nutrition to the dish. When you are layering the sausage and courgettes, you can add a layer of haricot beans or chickpeas. Layering with two or three different cheeses is another way to make this casserole a bit richer and more delicious.

Ingredients

Serves 6

3 tablespoons olive oil

1 teaspoon garlic powder

Salt and pepper to taste

1 tablespoon dried basil or 3 tablespoons fresh basil, shredded

2 teaspoons dried oregano or 4 teaspoons fresh oregano

1 tablespoon dried rosemary or 2 tablespoons fresh rosemary

2 medium courgettes, trimmed and thinly sliced

1 large onion, peeled and thinly sliced

4 ripe tomatoes, thinly sliced, or 250 ml tomato sauce

1 (375-g) can haricot beans, rinsed and drained

40 g seasoned dry breadcrumbs

40 g grated Parmesan cheese

Calories 304, **Fat** 12 g, **Carbohydrates** 34 g, **Protein** 16 g, **Fibre** 5 g, **Saturated Fat** 7 g, **Cholesterol** 63 mg, **Sodium** 1641 mg.

Courgette and Tomato Casserole

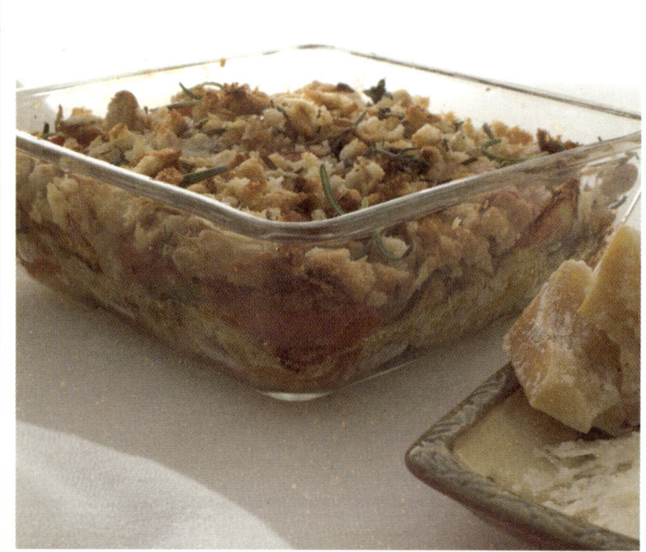

- Preheat oven to 180°C. Mix 2 tablespoons of the oil, garlic powder, salt, pepper and herbs together.

- Lightly oil a 2-litre baking dish. Layer half the courgettes, onion and tomato. Spread with beans. Top with the rest of the vegetables. Drizzle with the remaining oil and herb mixture. Sprinkle with breadcrumbs and Parmesan.

- Bake for 25 minutes, or until the casserole sizzles and the top is golden.

Fun variations: This casserole provides great flexibility. The more goodies you add, the more people it will feed. Instead of green courgettes you can use yellow ones, which look very pretty and have a buttery flavour. Parmesan cheese is essential, but you can also layer slices of mozzarella or other low-fat cheese.

Tomatoes or sauce? Use fresh tomatoes or tomato sauce, your own or bottled. Or use a can of chopped tomatoes with some extra fresh herbs. If you use canned tomatoes, use extra breadcrumbs to soak up some of the juice from the can. Commercial pasta sauces can be heavily seasoned; if you use a jar, taste it before you add any additional seasonings.

How to Layer a Casserole

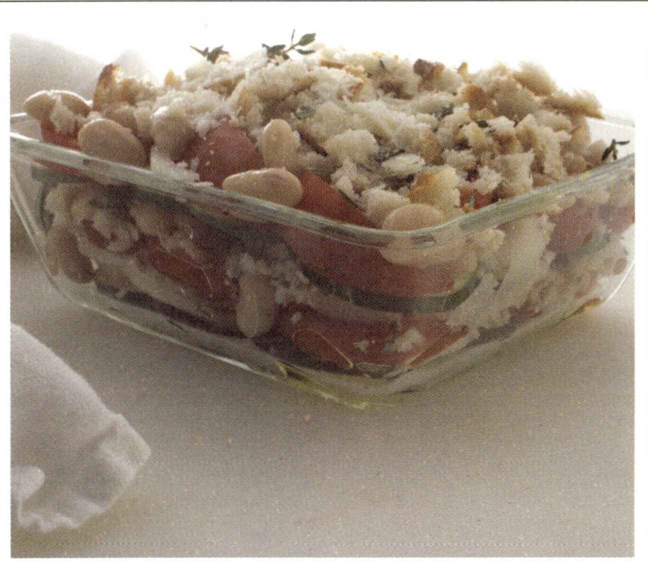

- Because the ingredients range from moist to wet, try to layer in plenty of breadcrumbs and things that go well together.

- Add beans between the layer of tomatoes and the layer of courgettes.

- The cheese can go over the tomatoes or between the layers.

Make Your Own Breadcrumbs

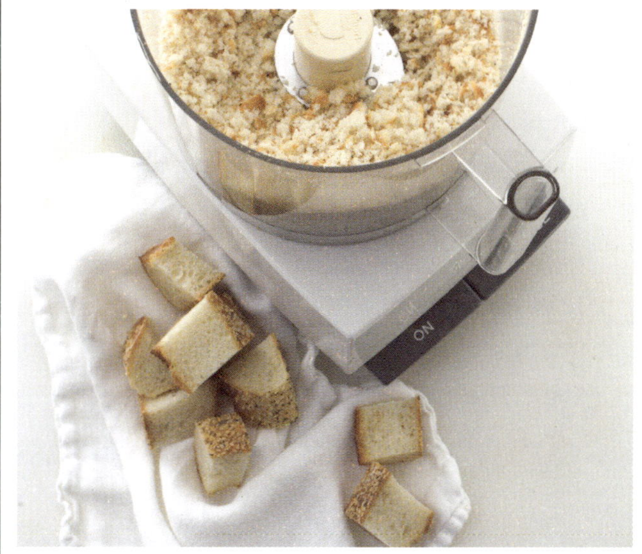

- Dry breadcrumbs are a cinch to make. Simply cut some stale French or Italian bread into chunks.

- Put the bread in a food processor or blender. Blend more for fine crumbs or less for coarse crumbs.

- You can add dried herbs, Parmesan cheese, salt and pepper to the crumbs.

- Store them in an airtight container in the refrigerator.

YELLOW WAX BEANS

Yellow wax beans, string beans and snap beans are one and the same

Yellow beans have a slightly sweet flavour. You can cook them in all the same ways that you cook green beans. They add a bright spot of colour to a dinner plate and are as good as green beans in bean salads. Yellow wax beans make an attractive presentation when paired with green herbs and/or tomatoes.

The garnishes for this recipe are fresh summer herbs and toasted walnuts. You can use pecans or almonds; however, buttery walnuts are wonderful.

You might also enjoy mixing yellow and green beans for an even more colourful side dish. This go-with-everything vegetable is a great accompaniment to any meat or poultry.

Ingredients

Serves 4

1 teaspoon low-fat margarine

40 g walnut pieces

450 g yellow wax beans, trimmed

120 ml water

1 tablespoon olive oil

6 fresh basil leaves, shredded

2 sprigs fresh rosemary, chopped

Salt and freshly ground pepper to taste

Juice of $^1/_2$ fresh lemon

Calories 70, **Fat** 4 g, **Carbohydrates** 9 g, **Protein** 2 g, **Fibre** 3 g, **Saturated Fat** 1 g, **Cholesterol** 0, **Sodium** 11 mg.

Yellow Wax Beans

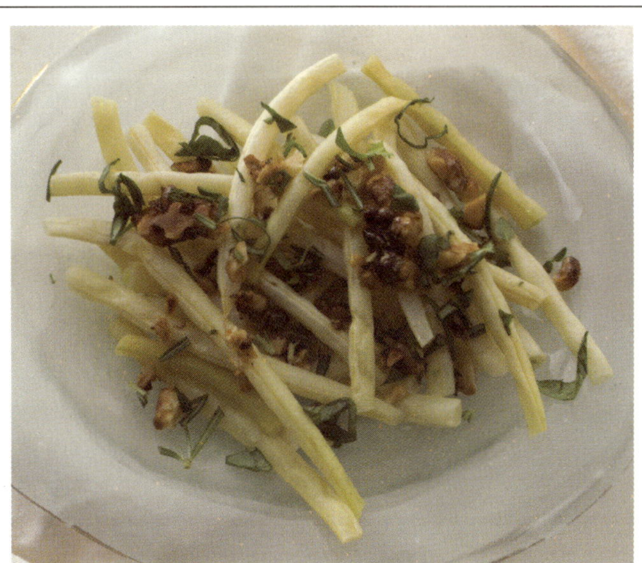

- Heat the low-fat margarine in a nonstick pan. Add walnuts and sauté for 5 minutes, shaking pan, until crisp but not burned.

- In a saucepan, steam beans in the water, covered, for 6–10 minutes.

- Drain beans and place in a serving bowl. Toss in olive oil and add herbs.

- Season with salt and pepper; sprinkle with lemon juice. Toss in sautéed walnuts.

Strictly vegetarian: You can make your vegetarian relatives and friends a delicious main course with yellow beans. The formula is simple. Steam the beans lightly and put them in an oiled ovenproof dish. Add 1 (400-g) can of black beans, rinsed and drained. (You can also use haricot beans, pinto beans or red kidney beans.) Then mix in 175 g salsa and 225 g of any good sharp Cheddar cheese or low-fat cheese. Bake for 15 minutes. While still hot, sprinkle with fresh chopped coriander or flat-leaf parsley. On the side, have plenty of fresh chopped onions. Serve the bean casserole with cornbread or thinly sliced whole-grain bread.

Cutting Beans

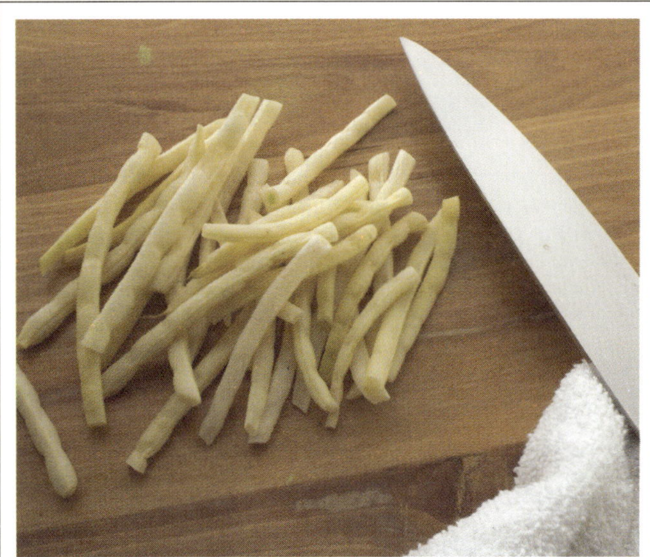

- Trim the stems from the beans. Wait until after the beans are cooked to cut off the pointed ends.

- If you cut the beans into bite-size pieces, more moisture will be depleted than if you leave them whole.

- To trim the stems, line up the beans in batches with all the ends in a row. Cut all the stems off with one swipe of the knife.

Microwaving Vegetables

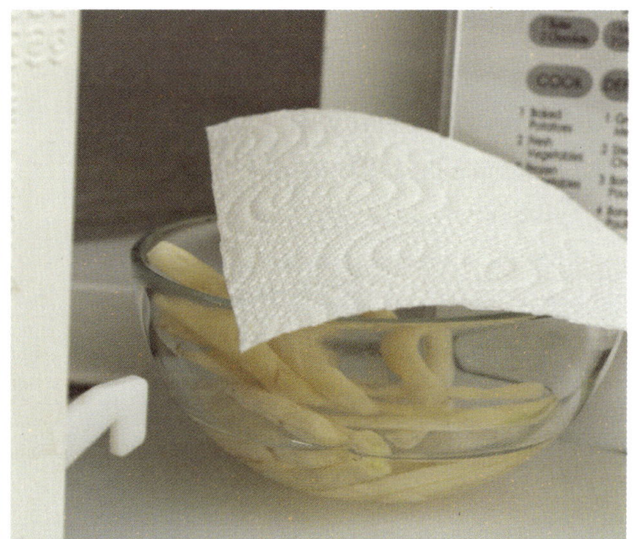

- Boiling, steaming or microwaving vegetables is the healthiest way to cook them.

- They will actually steam in the microwave. It takes less time, and you have less to clean up.

- Wash the vegetables, then put them in a glass or ceramic bowl with a little water.

- Cover with a paper towel. Microwave on high for 60 seconds; check that the beans are done and cook for longer if necessary.

PURÉED TURNIPS

Sweet and delicately flavoured, mashed young turnips can be combined with other root vegetables

Small turnips are delicate root vegetables, quite different from the big yellow and orange suedes that are available all through the winter.

Turnips are approximately 5–6 cm in diameter, and their attractive purple and white skins are easy to peel. Many really great old recipes call for these turnips to be added to soups and/or stews, and they are also wonderful mixed with other root vegetables and tubers, such as potatoes, carrots, and parsnips. In this dish the vegetables are mashed and whipped into a creamy purée topped with a scattering of crunchy pine nuts.

Ingredients

Serves 4

450 g turnips, peeled and sliced

1 carrot, peeled and cut into slices

1 baking potato, peeled and cut into chunks

1 tablespoon low-fat margarine

120 ml semi-skimmed milk

$1/2$ teaspoon nutmeg

Onion powder to taste

Freshly ground black pepper to taste

65 g pine nuts, toasted

Calories 157, **Fat** 6 g, **Carbohydrates** 23 g, **Protein** 4 g, **Fibre** 4 g, **Saturated Fat** 1 g, **Cholesterol** 1 mg, **Sodium** 77 mg.

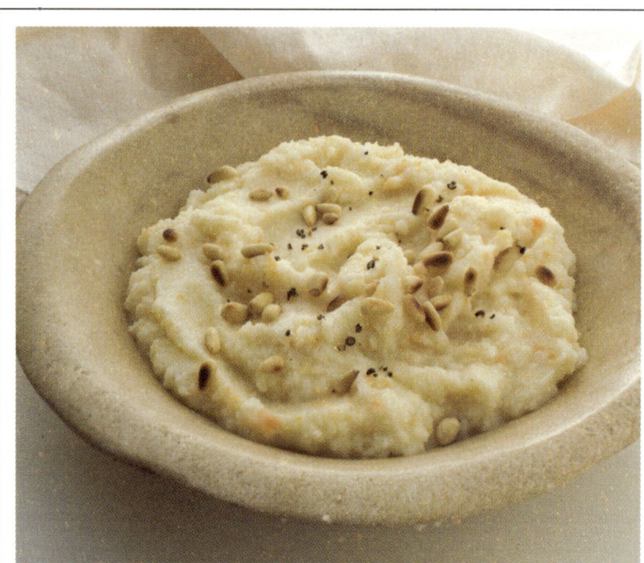

Puréed Turnips

- Place the turnips, carrot, and potato in a saucepan with 20 ml of water. Cook over medium-high heat until tender, or microwave on high for 4 minutes.

- Mash the cooked vegetables by hand or with an electric mixer.

- Beat in the margarine, milk and spices.

- Place the turnip mixture in a serving dish, and sprinkle with toasted pine nuts. Keep warm until ready to serve.

Winter vegetables: Winter vegetables are those that keep over the winter. Many of them ripen and can be picked in late September or early October, though some root vegetables can stay in the ground much longer. Winter vegetables include turnips, carrots, beetroot, parsnips, potatoes, pumpkins, winter squash, onions, garlic and a few greens, including cabbage, kale, turnip greens, Brussels sprouts, leeks and broccoli. The vitamins and minerals derived from winter vegetables help us to get through the winter without getting scurvy from a lack of vitamin C.

How to Pick a Turnip

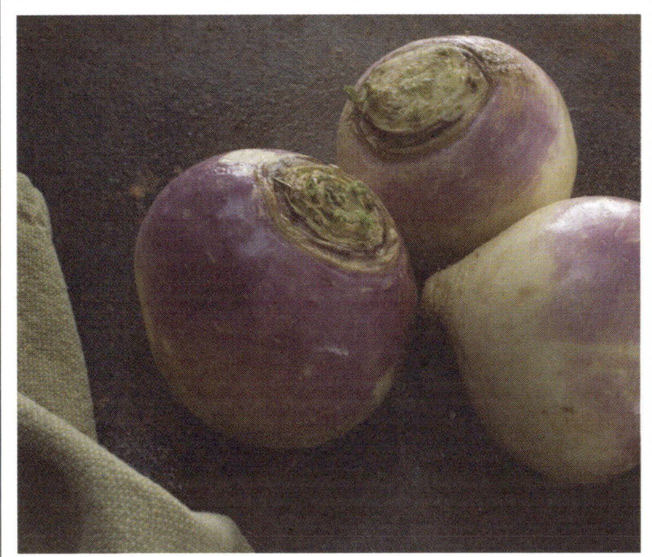

- Look for a turnip with a snowy white body and fresh mauve flush.

- Make sure the stem ends are stiff and very green.

- Squeeze the turnips to make sure they aren't wizened or soft.

- Store turnips in your refrigerator vegetable drawer for up to 3 months.

How to Peel a Turnip

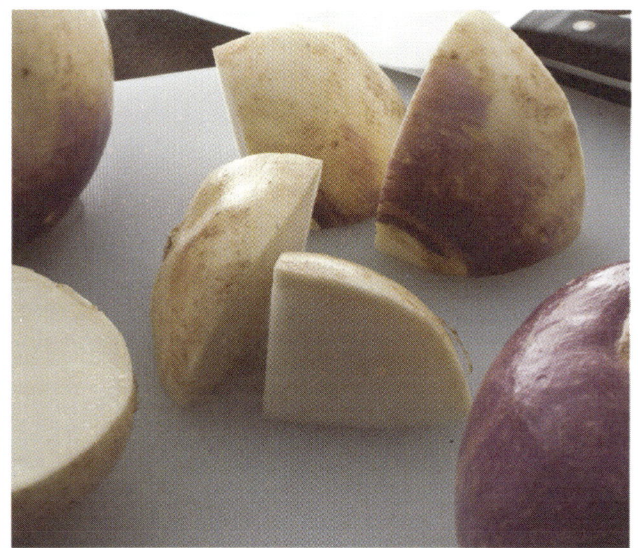

- Using a very sharp knife, remove the stem and root ends of the turnip.

- Peel off the skin.

- Cut the turnip crosswise in 8-mm rounds.

- Place in cold salted water until ready to cook.

BAKED POTATO CHIPS

Baked, not fried, these golden chips are appealing to the eye and crisp to the taste

Because they are baked and not fried, these potatoes are fat free, and no fat is added to the dish. Golden-fleshed potatoes can be used any way you would use white potatoes, but they stand up especially well to baking and oven-frying.

Look for Mediterranean varieties of potato such as Nicola and Marfona. They have a creamy texture and a buttery flavour, so they require less butter to taste good (which also makes them ideal for baking in their skins).

This recipe is equally good as a side dish for dinner or as a snack for a beer-drinking crowd watching football on TV.

Ingredients

Serves 6

3 large Nicola potatoes, peeled and cut into thin strips

3 egg whites, beaten until stiff

$1/2$ teaspoon garlic powder

$1/2$ teaspoon salt, or to taste

$1/2$ teaspoon freshly ground white pepper

50 g cornmeal

Calories 180, **Fat** 0, **Carbohydrates** 38 g, **Protein** 6 g, **Fibre** 5 g, **Saturated Fat** 0, **Cholesterol** 0, **Sodium** 233 mg.

Baked Potato Chips

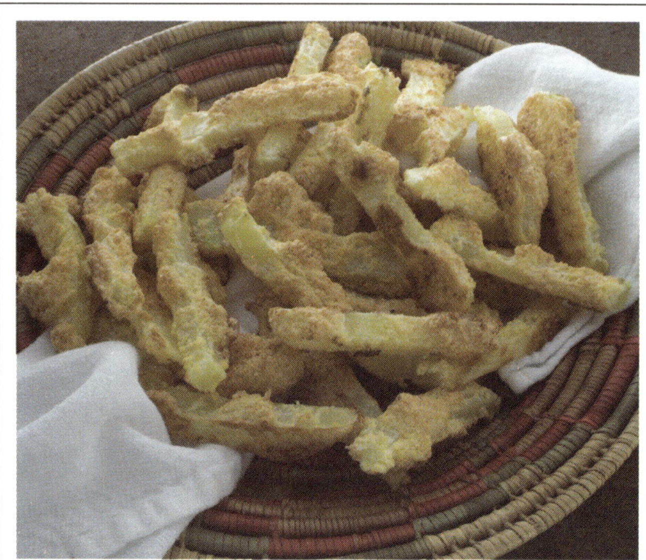

- Preheat oven to 230°C. Cover a baking sheet with aluminium foil and oil the foil lightly.

- Parboil the potatoes until crisp-tender, about 10 minutes; drain and then dry them on paper towels.

- Mix the beaten eggs with garlic powder, salt, pepper and cornmeal.

- Coat potatoes with the egg mixture and spread on the baking sheet. Bake for about 8 minutes per side or until crisp on the outside and tender inside.

Peeling Potatoes

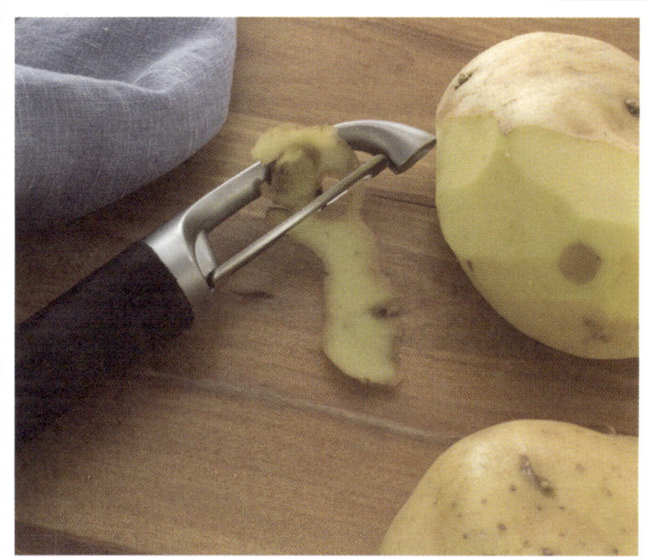

- Run your peeler from end to end when you peel these potatoes, which tend to be oval and fairly flat in shape.

- Peeling with a knife wastes a lot of potato.

- One way to peel a potato with a knife is to cut the strips first, and then carefully slice off the skin.

- The peeler should be really sharp; throw it away when it gets blunt.

Slicing: Knife or Mandoline?

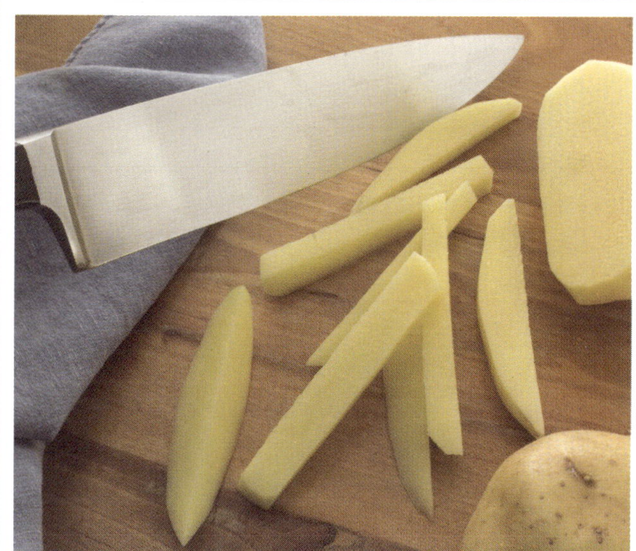

- Use a very sharp knife for making potato chips, and try to cut them evenly so that they all cook at the same time.

- If you are making potato crisps, use a mandoline set at 1–2 mm.

- If you are slicing for scalloped potatoes, use a mandoline set to cut potatoes in 3 mm slices.

- Some mandolines have handles; those are the ones to get. Otherwise, it's too easy to slice your fingers.

ACORN SQUASH WITH APPLES

A bit of sugar brings out the natural sweetness of acorn squash when roasted

When you roast acorn squash, you have the option of making it sweet or savoury, or both at the same time. The savoury aspect comes from adding herbs such as sage, rosemary and thyme. The sweetness is in the squash. A bit of reduced-sugar Splenda and some low-fat margarine is an excellent seasoning for winter squash.

There are many winter squashes, from butternut to pumpkin, to turban shapes with stripes, confetti and other interesting markings. They all taste similar, but some are sweeter. Buttercup squash is one of the sweetest. Use a sharp knife to cut any squash. A razor-sharp knife is safer to use than a blunt one, which can slip when you're cutting.

Ingredients

Serves 4

2 acorn squash, 450 g each, cut in half, seeds removed

4 tart eating apples, such as Granny Smith, peeled and coarsely chopped

$1/4$ teaspoon ground cinnamon

2 tablespoons Splenda for baking

2 tablespoons low-fat margarine

Calories 221, **Fat** 1 g, **Carbohydrates** 51 g, **Protein** 2 g, **Fibre** 7 g, **Saturated Fat** 0, **Cholesterol** 0, **Sodium** 50 mg.

Acorn Squash with Apples

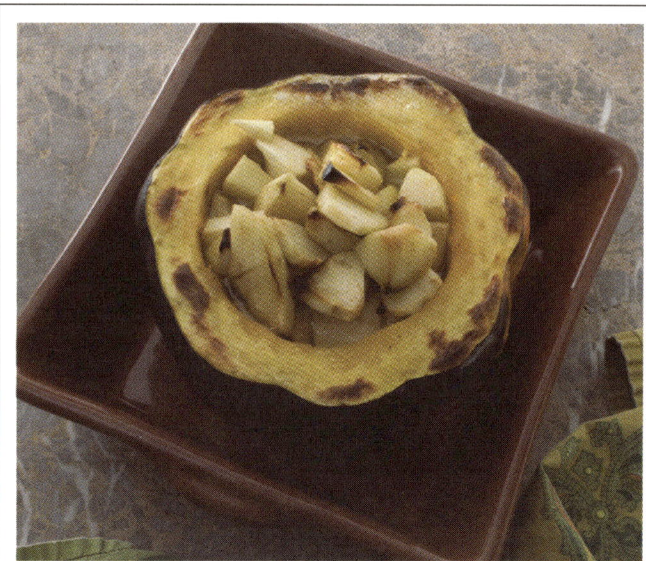

- Part-cook squash, either by roasting it in the oven (180°C for 30 minutes) or in the microwave, wrapped in paper, 8–10 minutes on high.

- In a saucepan, combine apples, cinnamon, Splenda and low-fat margarine with 2 tablespoons water.

- Preheat the oven to 180°C if it's not already hot. Place squash halves in a baking dish. Add the apple filling to the hollowed-out halves.

- Bake for 35 minutes or until both the squash and apples are soft and steaming hot.

Once the acorn squash is cut in half, scrape out all the seeds and partially bake it at 180°C or microwave for 4 minutes on high to soften it. You can then stuff the squash with any number of delicious fillings. Turkey stuffing made with cornbread is very good. Mix in some cooked sausage, sage and apples. Or try making a multigrain-bread stuffing with lots of herbs, onions and garlic.

Winter squash come in bright orange, green, beige and blended colours. With this recipe for acorn squash, it doesn't really matter whether you get the orange ones or the dark green ones. You do want to get good-sized squash because you will be cutting them in half, with one half per person per serving. If you can only get tiny squash, count on a whole one for each serving.

Cutting Squash

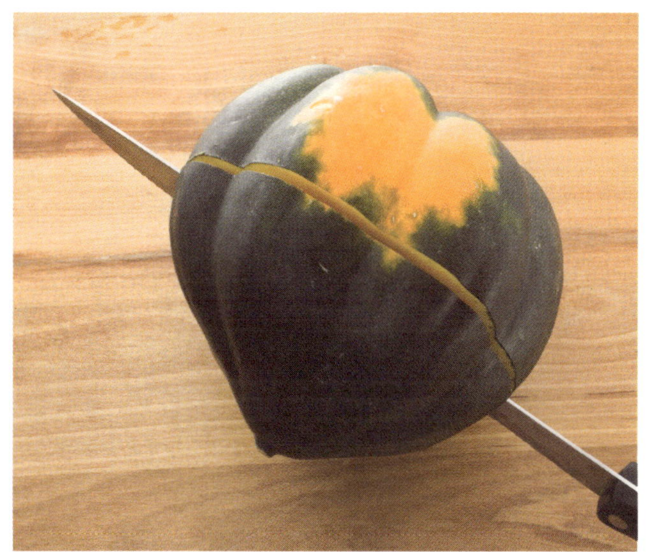

- Cutting up squash can be tiresome and frustrating.

- To eliminate stress, use two knives: a very sharp one to make the initial cut and a serrated knife to saw your way through.

- Wearing a rubber glove to hold the squash steady is also very useful.

- Remember, the sharper the knife, the better.

Roasting Seeds

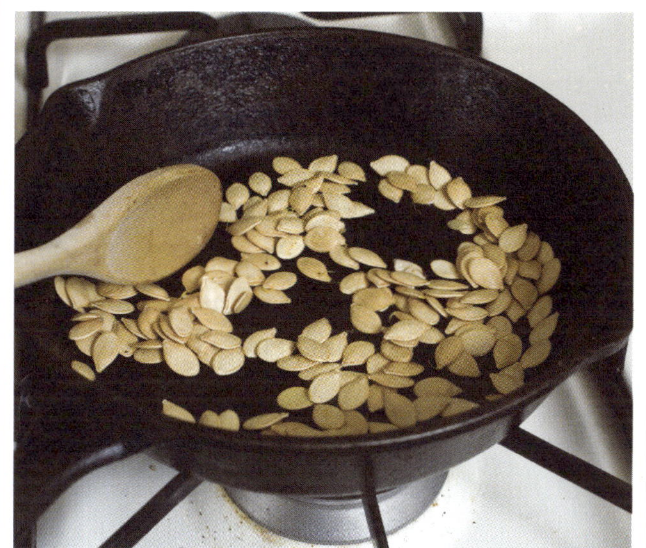

- Squash and pumpkin seeds are very much the same.

- Begin by cleaning the squash or pumpkin seeds under running water to remove fibres.

- Dry them thoroughly. Place on a baking sheet that

you've covered with aluminium foil, lightly oiled.

- Toss the seeds in melted low-fat margarine with some salt, seasoned salt or sugar, and roast in the oven for 45–50 minutes at 170°C.

CORN, SPRING ONIONS & TOMATOES

With this recipe, you can recapture the taste of late summer all year-round

If you make this dish during the summer when fresh young sweetcorn is available, it's wonderful. However, you can use frozen or canned sweetcorn during the winter and create almost the same effect. Cherry tomatoes and fresh basil are available all year round these days, but you can substitute dried basil if necessary.

Spice up the tomatoes with cayenne pepper, adjusting the heat to suit your family's taste buds. Use fresh or dried rosemary with the basil or marjoram. Sage leaves are also quite good with this, giving the dish a totally different flavour.

This colourful meal is very attractive when served in a rustic terracotta or ceramic dish.

Ingredients

Serves 4

4 young corn on the cob, shucked (if the corn is mature, it should be precooked)

115 g low-fat margarine

1 bunch spring onions, chopped

1 bunch basil leaves, rinsed and chopped, or other herbs, fresh or dried

1 teaspoon dried thyme or 1 teaspoon dried rosemary (optional)

Salt and freshly ground black pepper to taste

625 g cherry tomatoes, rinsed, halved and roasted

Calories 105, **Fat** 2 g, **Carbohydrates** 22 g, **Protein** 4 g, **Fibre** 4 g, **Saturated Fat** 1 g, **Cholesterol** 0, **Sodium** 187 mg.

Corn, Spring Onions and Tomatoes

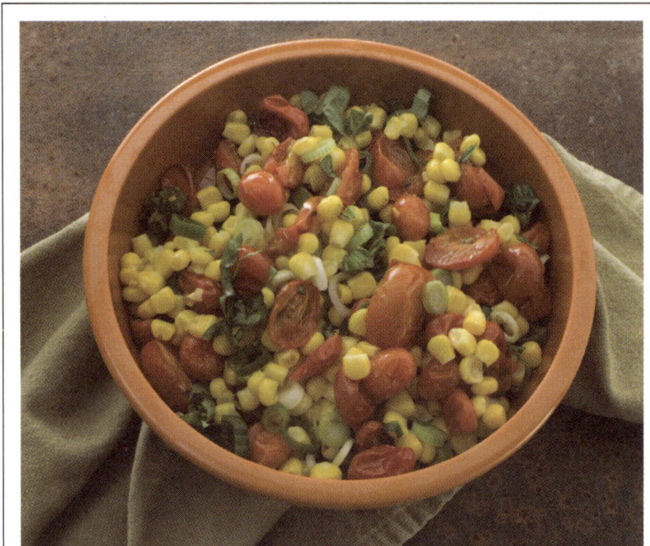

- Cut the sweetcorn from the cobs on to a sheet of greaseproof paper.

- In a large sauté pan, melt the margarine; add the sweetcorn and cook gently for 3–4 minutes. Then add spring onions, basil, herbs, salt and pepper.

- Add roasted tomatoes to the sweetcorn and butter mixture. Heat thoroughly.

- Turn into a warmed serving dish and enjoy.

Great additions and substitutions: If you add 225 g frozen edamame beans, cooked, to the corn and tomatoes, it becomes a classic combination of the American South called succotash. This will be enough for six people. You can also add 115 g fresh or frozen petits pois to this recipe, and a small jar of roasted red peppers; or chipotle chillies add a nice zing.

A main dish for vegetarians: To turn this recipe into a vegetarian main course, add 225 g cubed low-fat Cheddar cheese and 225 g frozen lima beans, cooked. Run the dish under the grill to melt the cheese. For vegans, who eat absolutely no animal products, add cubes of silken tofu and either 225 g broad beans, cooked, or 1 (400-g) can black beans, drained and rinsed, to the basic recipe.

Roasting Cherry Tomatoes

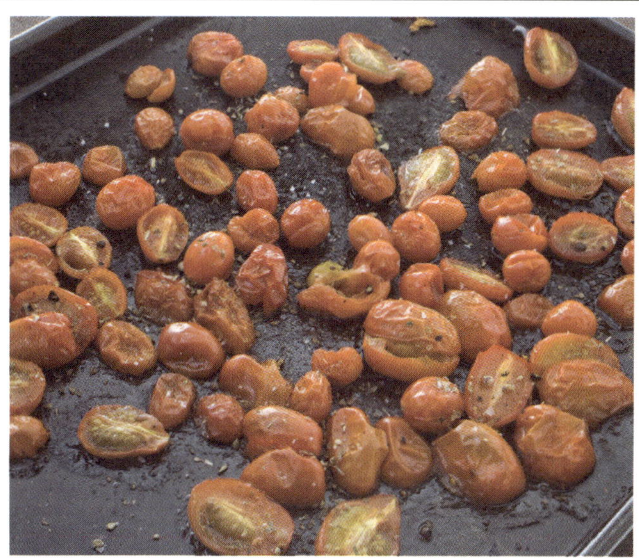

- Preheat the oven to 150°C. Oil a nonstick baking sheet or line a baking sheet with foil and oil the foil.

- Wash the tomatoes and cut in half. Arrange on the baking sheet cut side up and brush with olive oil.

- Sprinkle the tomatoes with cayenne pepper or freshly ground black pepper.

- You can also sprinkle them with dried oregano and salt if you wish. Cook for up to 1 hour, until collapsed and concentrated in flavour.

Olive Oil: Brush or Spray?

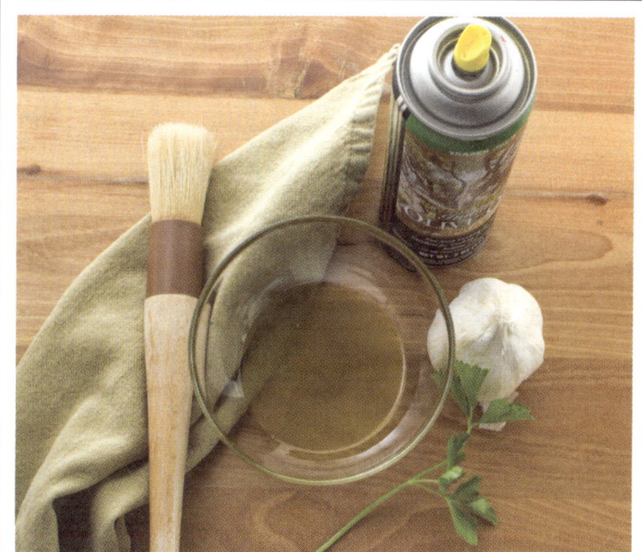

- There are good reasons for brushing and for spraying olive oil. When you spray oil, it's generalized and covers a wider area.

- You can spray olive oil on salad leaves and large vegetables.

- It's better to brush olive oil on to the cherry tomatoes on the baking sheet to get most of the oil on the tomatoes and less on the sheet.

- Pastry brushes come in several sizes. Use the smallest on the tomatoes.

ROASTED CAULIFLOWER

Even the pickiest eaters will be surprised at the taste of this unique dish

Cauliflower is exceptionally good for you. It contains zero fat, lots of vitamin C and fibre and very good carbohydrates, in addition to micronutrients that we all need.

When you roast cauliflower, the natural sugars are concentrated and caramelized, and the cauliflower becomes crisp. You have loads of flavouring options. Parmesan or pecorino cheese is very nice, and as well as salt and pepper you can use chilli powder for seasoning. This recipe provides a different and healthy alternative to plain steamed cauliflower or creamy stuff. Although a cauliflower gratin tastes very good, it also contains a lot of fat and calories. This recipe is more in line with the goals of diabetes management.

Ingredients

Serves 4

1 cauliflower

2 tablespoons olive oil

1 teaspoon salt

$^1/_2$ teaspoon cayenne pepper or chilli powder, or both

Freshly ground black pepper to taste

2 tablespoons Parmesan cheese (optional)

Calories 103, **Fat** 7 g, **Carbohydrates** 7 g, **Protein** 3 g, **Fibre** 4 g, **Saturated Fat** 2 g, **Cholesterol** 0, **Sodium** 25 mg.

Roasted Cauliflower

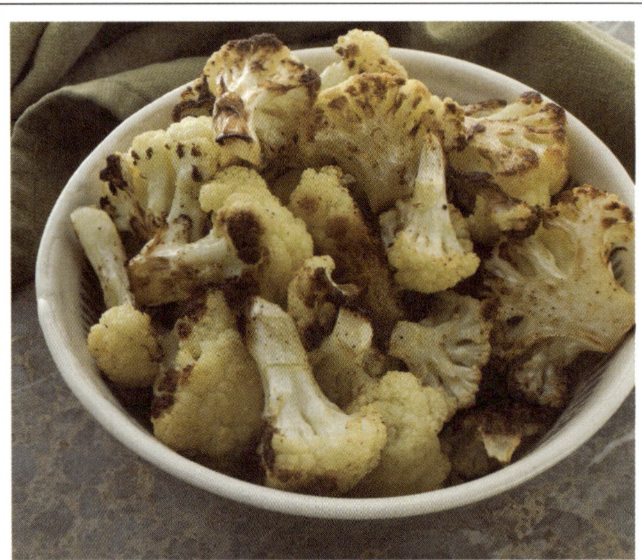

- Preheat oven to 250°C. Remove green leaves and core of cauliflower. Break into small florets, cutting off long stems. Rinse well; dry thoroughly between paper towels.

- Mix the olive oil, salt and seasonings in a large bowl.

- Toss the florets in the oil mixture.

- Place florets on a lightly oiled baking sheet. Roast for at least 30 minutes. Turn cauliflower and continue to roast until deep golden brown.

Fun variations: Experiment with adding garlic powder, onion powder, and some of the seasonings that are formulated to substitute for salt. Try crushing some caraway seeds with salt for a different and delicious flavouring. While you are at it, roast some carrots whole and serve a medley of vegetables. Try making very small florets and serving the cauliflower with cocktail sticks as a snack, which would be especially nice accompanied by a dipping sauce. Use any good-quality tomato sauce or your own fresh pasta sauce. You might try a low-calorie Russian dressing made with low-fat mayonnaise, chilli sauce and chopped spring onions, or onions and dill pickle.

Cleaning and Preparing Cauliflower

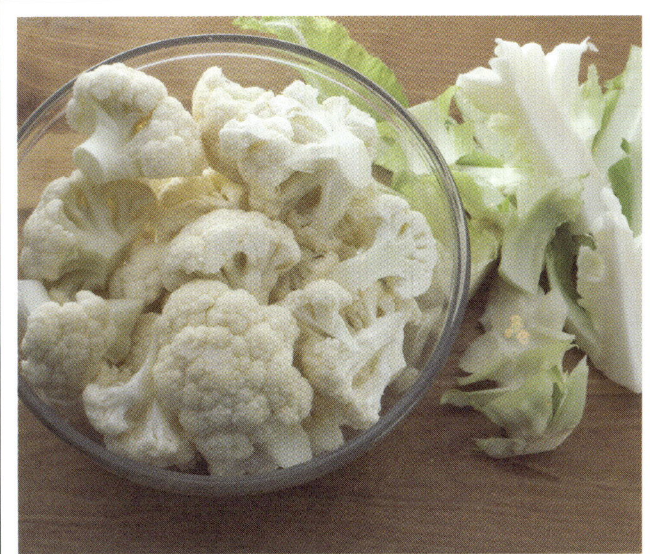

- Pull or cut off the green leaf stems and discard. Cut the cauliflower into quarters.

- Cut out the core and discard it.

- Break the quarters into florets. Make them smaller for snacks and larger for side dishes.

- Rinse the florets under cool running water. Make sure they are dry before adding seasonings and roasting.

Why Dry Cauliflower Before Roasting?

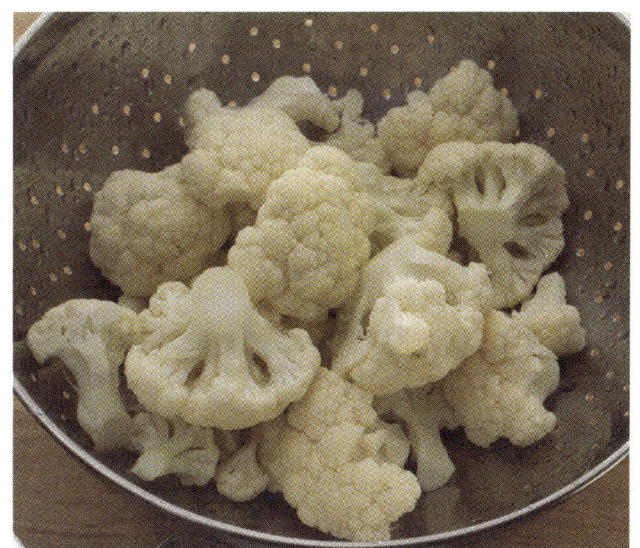

- It's important to dry cauliflower before roasting for a couple of reasons. One, it will get mushy and steam rather than roast if it's still wet.

- Two, the oil and seasonings will drip off wet cauliflower, but they will adhere well to dry cauliflower.

- If you can't get the florets dry between paper towels, leave them to air-dry for an hour or so.

- Add the olive oil and seasonings only when the cauliflower is dry and ready to go into the oven.

LENTIL & SAUSAGE CASSEROLE

A little bit of turkey sausage goes a long way in this hearty mix of vegetables and lentils

You can mix just about any meat and/or vegetable into a lentil dish, and it will be delicious. If you don't want to use turkey sausage, you can substitute pieces of chicken, pork or lamb.

This casserole is very easy to make. Lentils come in a variety of colours. Grey-green German lentils are the most prevalent and readily available. There are also delectable smaller French varieties, such as Puy lentils, as well as red, orange and yellow lentils. They are all a great source of protein and fibre, particularly for vegetarians who may not be getting other sources of protein in a meal.

Ingredients

Serves 6

1 tablespoon olive oil

450 g turkey sausage, cut into 2.5-cm pieces

2 large onions, red or white, peeled and cut into chunks

4 cloves garlic, smashed and peeled

2 carrots, peeled and cut into 2.5-cm pieces

2 parsnips, peeled and cut into 2.5-cm pieces

450 g German lentils, rinsed

750 ml chicken stock or water

Salt and black pepper to taste

Pinch of ground cloves

2 bay leaves

Calories 235, **Fat** 8 g, **Carbohydrates** 29 g, **Protein** 14 g, **Fibre** 9 g, **Saturated Fat** 3 g, **Cholesterol** 30 mg, **Sodium** 544 mg.

Lentil and Sausage Casserole

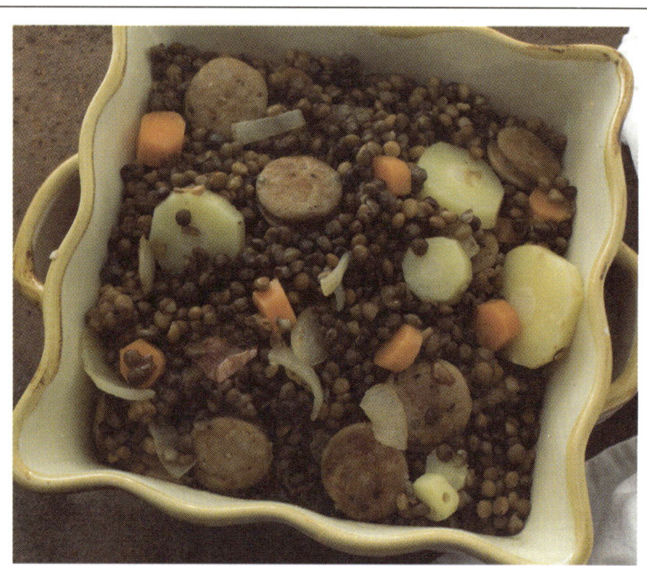

- Preheat oven to 170°C.

- On the hob, heat oil in a large, ovenproof casserole dish over medium heat. Lightly brown the sausage, onion and garlic.

- Add the rest of the ingredients. Cover and place the casserole in the oven; cook for 1 hour.

- Taste a small spoonful of lentils. If they are still tough, continue cooking. Check every 15 minutes or so until the lentils are tender.

ZOOM

One of the great things about lentils is that you don't have to soak them prior to cooking. Not only that, they also take far less time to cook than beans. However, you can use any bean you wish in this recipe, or you can substitute split peas, green or yellow. The easiest option is to use canned beans. Otherwise, if using dried beans you have to soak them for several hours or overnight and cook them for 3–4 hours. Aduki, cannellini or haricot beans are very good in casseroles, and the canned ones are always softer than those you cook yourself. If you use beans, you can omit the meat, as the beans have a great deal of excellent protein.

Rinse Your Lentils

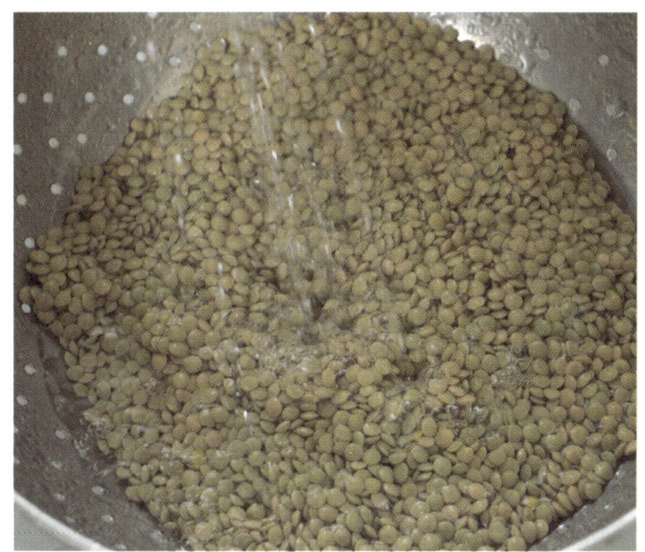

- Always rinse your lentils under cool running water.

- This will clean off any dirt and dust they may have acquired during harvesting.

- Rinsing will make any pieces of grit more visible, as they change colour when wet.

- A good rinse will also freshen the lentils up.

Storing Dried Lentils and Beans

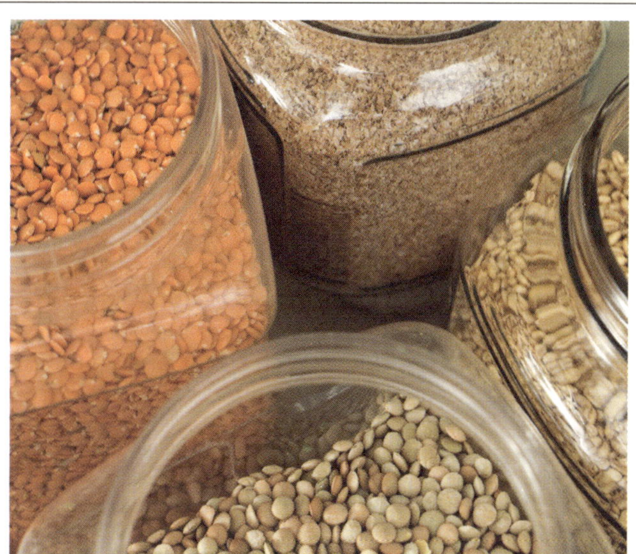

- Dried lentils and other dried beans should be stored in airtight containers; plastic is fine.

- They should not be subjected to damp, or they will get mouldy.

- Beans and lentils should not be kept loose in a bag, or they will attract insects.

- Mice love to get into bags of beans. Make sure that your containers have tight-fitting lids.

WARM LENTIL SALAD

Lentils with roasted red peppers and Chinese leaves are a study in contrasting textures and flavours

The texture of the warm lentils is soft, the cabbage is crisp. The lentils have a nutty flavour and the peppers are sweet.

Chinese leaves may be the most underused of all cabbages, yet they are among the most versatile. They are good raw or cooked, in combination with other ingredients or alone. The pale green colour and crunchy texture make them an ideal contrast with the other items in this salad. You can either roast the red peppers yourself or buy a jar of roasted peppers at the supermarket.

The garnish for this salad is very much to your own taste. Black olives, Greek or Italian, add a sharp touch, as does the recommended vinaigrette.

Ingredients

Serves 4

400 g Puy lentils, rinsed

170 ml red wine vinegar

4 tablespoons olive oil

1 teaspoon prepared mustard

1 teaspoon Worcestershire sauce

Juice of 1/2 lemon

Salt and pepper to taste

100 g roasted red pepper, diced

200 g shredded Chinese leaves, rinsed and shredded

Optional garnish: 50 g stoned and chopped black olives, 2 tablespoons capers or 1 tablespoon green peppercorns

Calories 359, **Fat** 19 g, **Carbohydrates** 33 g, **Protein** 14 g, **Fibre** 15 g, **Saturated Fat** 4 g, **Cholesterol** 0, **Sodium** 62 mg.

Warm Lentil Salad

- Over medium heat, cook the lentils in 120 ml vinegar and enough water to cover for 30 minutes.

- In a bowl, whisk together remaining 50 ml vinegar, olive oil, mustard, Worcestershire sauce and lemon juice.

- Drain the lentils and place in a large bowl; add the dressing, salt, pepper and red peppers.

- Divide the shredded Chinese leaves among serving plates. Arrange the lentils over the leaves and garnish as desired.

• • • • RECIPE VARIATION • • • •

Some good substitutes: Although Chinese leaves are recommended for this dish, you can substitute romaine or iceberg lettuce. Just be sure to use something good and crunchy with a slightly sweet taste. You can use beans instead of lentils; however, the lentils hold the flavour of the vinegar added to the cooking liquid, and they have a tangier flavour than beans with thick skins.

You can substitute chickpeas, yellow or green split peas, or use any colour lentil you wish, although the small, French grey-green ones seem to come out the best in this recipe. If you decide not to use olives for garnish, add a few capers. For a sophisticated touch, garnish with green peppercorns packed in brine.

Roasting Red Peppers

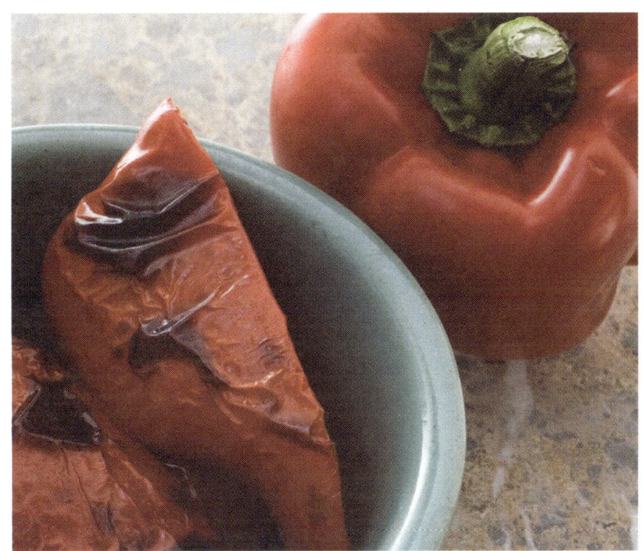

- Roasted red peppers are sensational in salads and soups, and as garnishes and hors d'oeuvres.

- If you have a gas stove, put a pepper on a long-handled metal fork and hold it over the flame, turning until evenly charred.

- Or, cut peppers in half and remove seeds and cores. Place on greased aluminium foil under a preheated gas or electric grill.

- To remove charred skin, place in a plastic bag immediately after cooking. When cooled, the skins will slip off easily.

Precooking Lentils for Salad

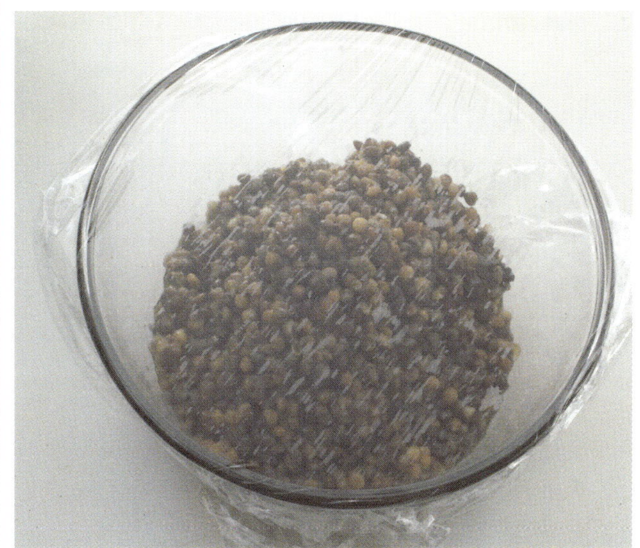

- To enhance the flavour of lentils for salads, cook them the day or night before. Then marinate them in the dressing suggested for the recipe.

- Use any vinaigrette with vinegar, or make a citrus dressing. Use plenty of flavourings, herbs and garlic.

- Make sure the lentils are well coated with dressing.

- Dress the lentils in a nonreactive bowl – glass or ceramic is best. Cover tightly and marinate overnight.

CANNELLINI BEANS & DUCK

Adding aromatic vegetables to this lovely dish makes it an ideal winter entrée

Inspired by cassoulet, a complex French casserole, this recipe is not nearly as difficult or time-consuming as the classic, and it's delicious.

If you can't get duck breasts, substitute pork tenderloin. However, duck breasts are widely available from supermarkets and butchers. Keep in mind that duck is much higher in total fat and saturated fat than other poultry. It is fine to have occasionally, though. Using canned beans is a huge time-saver. Sausage is an optional addition to this dish and adds flavour and volume. Fresh thyme is another excellent flavour that is important to this dish. Use dried thyme if you can't find the fresh herb.

Ingredients

Serves 6

1 tablespoon flour

Sprinkling of salt and pepper

2 duck breasts, about 175 g each

2 tablespoons olive oil

225 g turkey sausages (optional)

1 large sweet onion, chopped

4 cloves garlic, smashed and peeled

3 carrots, peeled and chopped

3 parsnips, peeled and chopped

3 sticks celery, cut into bite-size pieces

1 celeriac, peeled and cut into small pieces

250 ml chicken stock

250 g canned Italian plum tomatoes, drained and chopped

1 tablespoon dried or 4 teaspoons fresh rosemary or thyme

2 (375-g) cans cannellini beans, drained and rinsed

20 g fresh breadcrumbs or 2 tablespoons dried breadcrumbs

Calories 369, **Fat** 13 g, **Carbohydrates** 47 g, **Protein** 18 g, **Fibre** 14 g, **Saturated Fat** 4 g, **Cholesterol** 29 mg, **Sodium** 931 mg.

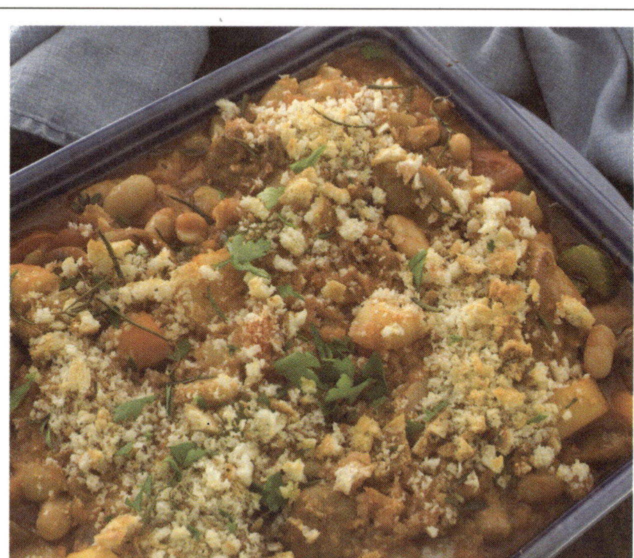

Cannellini Beans with Duck

- Preheat oven to 180°C. Sprinkle flour, salt and pepper on greaseproof paper. Roll duck in flour mixture. On hob, heat oil in large, flameproof baking dish.

- Brown duck and sausages, if using; remove. Sauté onion, garlic, carrots, parsnips, celery and celeriac.

- Add stock, tomatoes, herbs and beans. Cut sausages and duck into pieces. Return meat to casserole.

- Mix well; sprinkle with breadcrumbs. Bake for 45 minutes. Serve.

Good substitutions: If you opt to add sausages to this dish, 225 g sausages will add two to three servings. You can also substitute rosemary for thyme. Rosemary works very well with duck, chicken, pork or turkey. It is a terrific aromatic herb that also goes beautifully with lamb.

Party-size proportions: For a party, double the quantities and serve the dish buffet-style. With it, serve plenty of multigrain French or Italian bread, toasted and drizzled with a little olive oil and a sprinkling of herbs. A big green salad with lots of romaine lettuce and rocket, watercress or baby spinach also goes very well with this casserole.

Brown and De-fat Your Sausages

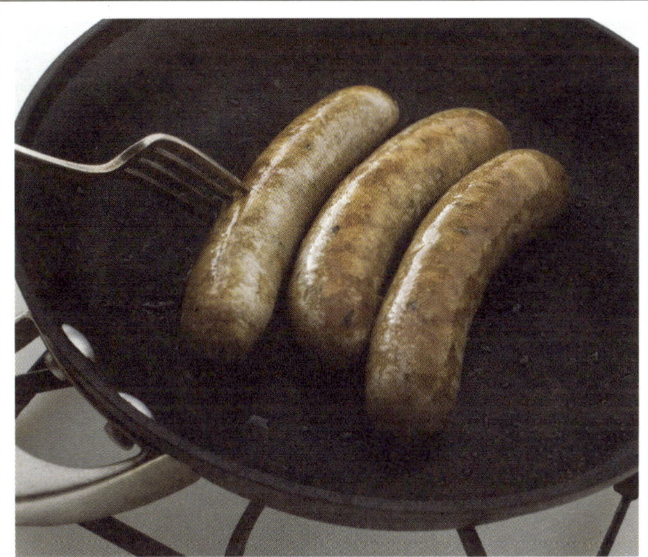

- When you brown sausages before using them in any dish, try to get most of the fat out of them.

- Of course, if you are using turkey sausage, you probably won't have a lot of fat. However, pork and beef sausages may be quite fatty.

- When heated, the fat liquefies. Thus, if you prick the sausages with a fork, the fat will run out into the pan.

- Then you can drain off the fat, leaving just enough oil for your vegetables.

Party Dishes: Bite-Size Pieces

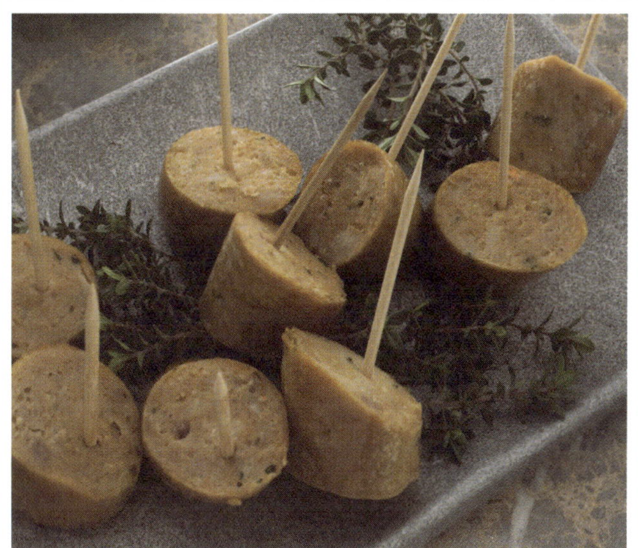

- For a buffet-style party, it's important to have all your ingredients in bite-size pieces for your guests.

- With little effort, you can cut up meat and vegetables, and tear or shred salad leaves.

- The last thing you want is guests dropping half their dinner in their laps or on the floor.

- Think ahead, and prepare your party dishes early so that you have plenty of time for chopping and cutting up the ingredients.

CANNELLINI BEANS & MEATBALLS

A dish of cannellini beans and tomato sauce serves as a great vehicle for meatballs

Tiny meatballs are an Italian favourite. They are an essential ingredient in Italian wedding soup, which also contains beans, pasta and vegetables.

Make lots of meatballs and store them in the freezer. Then, if guests pop in unexpectedly, you can use them for cocktail snacks, or add them to some pasta sauce and feed a crowd.

Using minced turkey saves lots of calories, and turkey meatballs have an excellent flavour when well seasoned. Picky eaters love these treats, and they are great for portion control. A few meatballs go a long way when served with beans and vegetables. Shredded carrots, chopped tomatoes, courgettes and peas are also good in this dish.

Ingredients

Serves 4

225 g minced turkey (used for analysis), veal or lean beef

25 g soft breadcrumbs

1 tablespoon chilli sauce

1 tablespoon milk

1 clove garlic, chopped

1 teaspoon onion powder

1 teaspoon oregano

Salt and freshly ground black pepper to taste

Pinch of cinnamon

1 egg

1 tablespoon olive oil

1 large onion, peeled and chopped

3 cloves garlic, peeled and chopped

350 ml well-seasoned tomato sauce

2 (375-g) cans cannellini beans, drained and rinsed

120 ml chicken or beef stock

Calories 383, **Fat** 5 g, **Carbohydrates** 60 g, **Protein** 27 g, **Fibre** 13 g, **Saturated Fat** 1 g, **Cholesterol** 26 mg, **Sodium** 719 mg.

Cannellini Beans and Meatballs

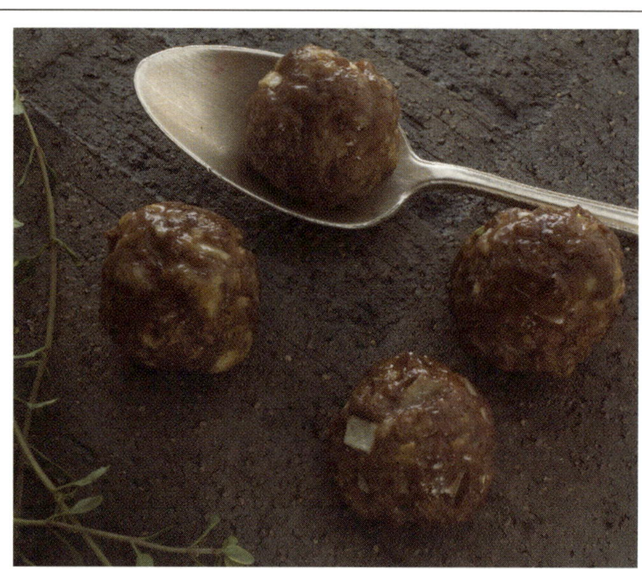

- Preheat oven to 170°C. Mix the first 10 ingredients in a bowl. Form into very small meatballs (about 2.5 cm in diameter).

- Arrange on an oiled baking sheet and bake for 25 minutes. When done, drain on paper towels.

- Heat olive oil in a large pot. Sauté onion and garlic over medium heat until softened.

- Add tomato sauce, beans, stock and meatballs. Stir gently so as not to break up meatballs but just to cover them completely with sauce.

If you are watching your budget, beans are an excellent source of nutrition and a fine way to make your money go further. They can also serve as a meat substitute, adding protein and fibre to a meal. Beans by themselves are bland in flavour and need plenty of aromatic vegetables and herbs.

• • • • • RECIPE VARIATION • • • • •

Lower-calorie meatballs: Make meatballs with minced veal or lean minced beef. Because minced turkey has less fat and fewer calories, it is preferable. Dried cannellini beans are terrific, but they must be soaked – overnight is best. If you cook beans and vegetables together, making a gravy while you prepare the meatballs, the results are delicious. The beans soak up the flavours.

Using a Melon Ball Scoop

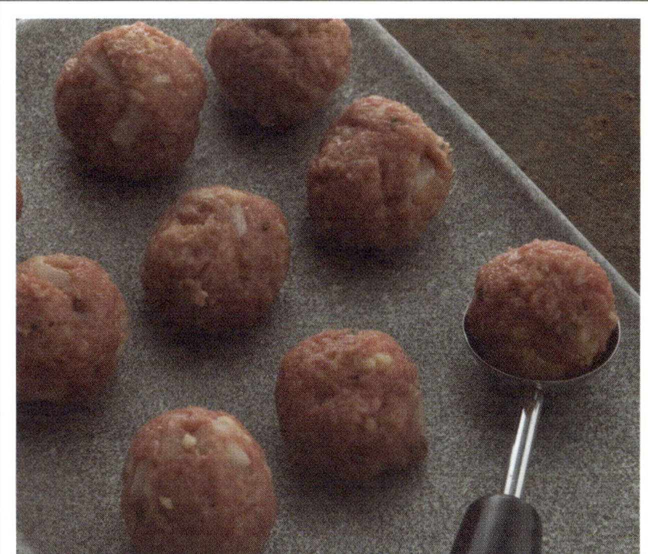

- Use a melon ball scoop to form your meatballs evenly.

- Or use a teaspoon. Just roll the balls between your palms to compress them and make them round. Elliptical meatballs, shaped like rugby balls, do not brown evenly.

- If meatballs are all the same size, they should cook evenly.

- If the meatballs are not baking evenly because your oven does not provide even heat, turn the tray and roll the meatballs over from time to time.

Adding Spices to Minced Meats

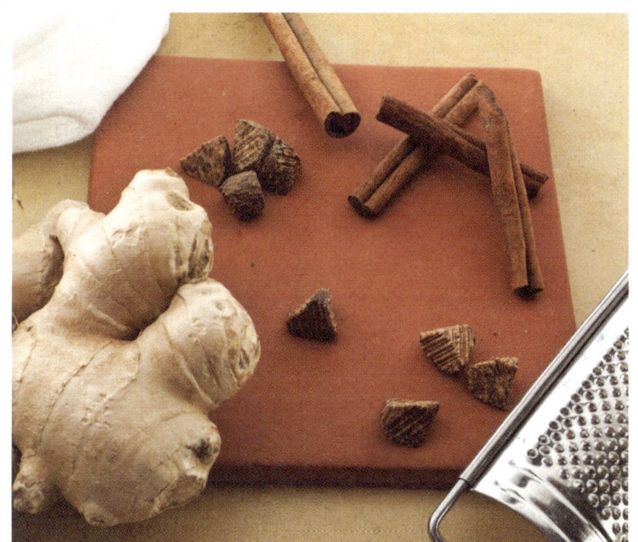

- It's an Italian tradition to put a pinch of cinnamon in meatballs and meat sauce.

- A pinch is $1/16$–$1/8$ teaspoon. You don't want to use enough to make the flavour pronounced, or even really discernible. What you want to achieve is a delightful hint of flavour.

- You can also use fresh or candied ginger in turkey, pork and beef dishes.

- When fresh ginger was unavailable, cooks would crumble gingernuts into beef stew, adding enough zip to make the stew interesting.

TURKEY CHILLI WITH BEANS

Quick to make and perfect for feeding a crowd, this chilli is high in flavour but low in fat

The longer you cook chilli, the better it gets. You can use a slow cooker and start the cooking before you go to bed at night, or early in the morning before you go to work. Just let the slow cooker do its thing.

If you don't have a slow cooker, you must be very careful to set a very low heat so that the chilli simmers and won't burn.

Burned chilli is ruined chilli – it can't be saved. Or bake the chilli in the oven, set at 120°C, for 3–6 hours.

The various seasonings make this chilli different. You will find your guests licking their lips and asking about that delicious flavour. Of course, it's many flavours married together and an unusual secret ingredient – cocoa powder.

Ingredients

Serves 10

50 ml olive or canola oil

450 g minced turkey

4 onions, peeled and coarsely chopped

4 cloves garlic, smashed and chopped

3 green peppers, cored, seeded and diced

1–2 serrano chillies, or 3 jalapeños, chopped, seeds in for extra heat

1 red pepper, roasted and peeled (from a jar is fine)

2 teaspoons cocoa powder

2 teaspoons dried thyme

2 tablespoons chilli powder, or to taste

1 teaspoon freshly ground black pepper

1 teaspoon salt

175 g low-sodium beef stock

2 (400-g) cans Italian plum tomatoes

175 ml flat beer

450 g red kidney beans, soaked overnight (used for analysis), or 4 (400-g) cans kidney beans, drained and rinsed

Calories 344, **Fat** 11 g, **Carbohydrates** 42 g, **Protein** 22 g, **Fibre** 13 g, **Saturated Fat** 3 g, **Cholesterol** 37 mg, **Sodium** 180 mg.

Turkey Chilli with Beans

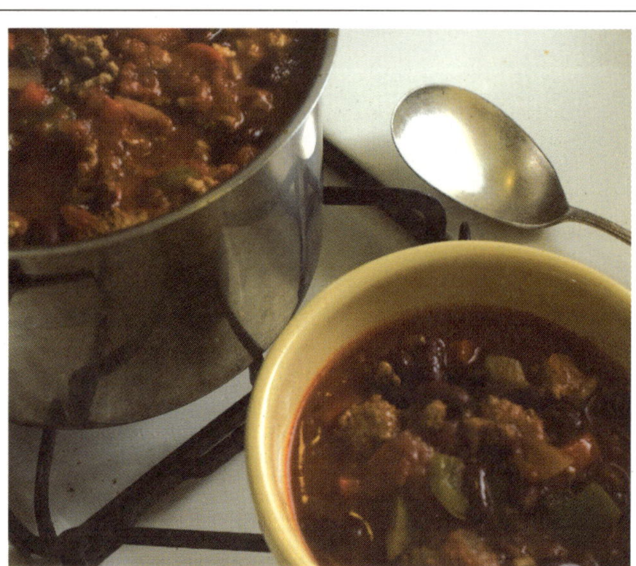

- Heat the olive oil in a large pan and lightly brown the turkey, then add the vegetables. Cook until the onions are transparent.

- Stir in the cocoa powder, thyme, chilli powder, pepper and salt; mix well.

- Add the liquids, tomatoes and beans; stir to blend.

- Pour into slow cooker and cook on low for 4–6 hours. Or bake in the oven at 120°C for at least 3–4 hours.

Seasoning chilli: Some of the flavourings in this recipe may surprise you. Cocoa, an ancient Inca flavouring, charms the palate without overwhelming the integrity of the chilli. You will also add ½ bottle of good beer – Mexican beer is great. A good chilli powder is a must, as are some fresh and canned chipotle chillies – and don't forget peppers. Add dried chilli flakes if you don't have time to prepare fresh hot chillies. For a leaner option, turkey replaces beef very nicely. Many chilli contests have been won using minced turkey. However, if you do use beef, choose lean chuck steak (more than 90 per cent lean, or fat free), coarsely minced.

Checking That Beans Are Done

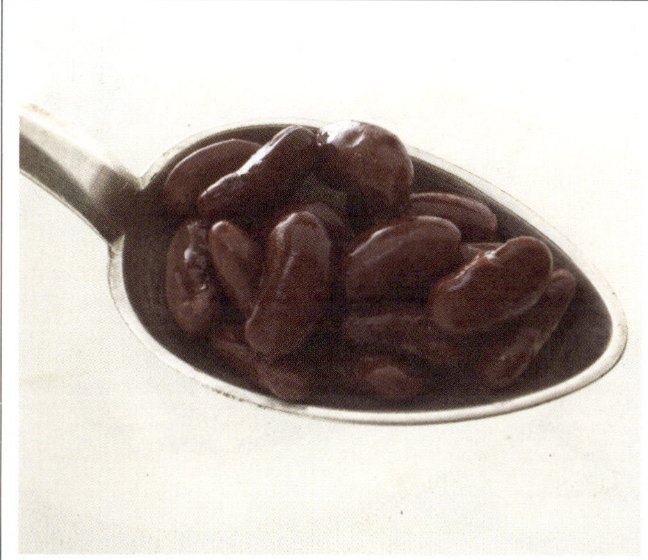

- Beans that have not cooked enough are not very good to eat. They are hard, dry and tasteless.

- If you are using dried beans, they may require 250 ml more liquid from time to time, even though you've soaked them.

- Make sure they don't dry out. Add more beer, stock or water to keep them nice and saucy.

- When you are checking that your beans are done, also check the flavouring. Adjust for salt and add spice.

Fire-Roasted Chilli

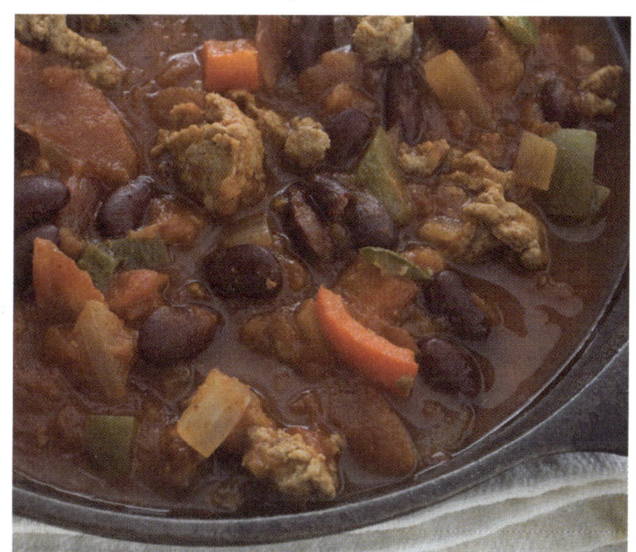

- Many chilli recipes call for roasting chilli over a wood fire.

- You can do this under your grill or over a gas flame on the hob.

- Place the final chilli ingredients in a cast-iron pan over a low, smoky fire. Cook uncovered for 3 hours. Or bake in the oven at 120°C for 3 hours.

BEANS, MACARONI & KALE

This dish shines with flavour when kale is in season

The minute you see huge bunches of fresh kale, dark green and crisp, in the supermarket or greengrocer's, buy it. Kale is a fantastic vegetable that is incredibly nutritious, as it is filled with antioxidants.

When you buy kale, there should be no limp, yellow or 'tired'-looking leaves. The whole bunch should epitomize freshness. When you get it home, remove the heavy stems all the way up to the leaves. Discard the stems. Break it up, and then run the kale under cool water to remove sand and grit.

When it is perfectly clean, drain and wrap the kale in a clean cloth or paper towels. Place in a plastic bag and refrigerate until you're ready to use it.

Ingredients

Serves 6

2 tablespoons olive oil

1 large sweet onion, chopped

2 cloves garlic, peeled and chopped

2 tablespoons tomato purée

500 ml chicken or vegetable stock

1 large bunch kale, stemmed, cleaned and torn into pieces

200 g elbow macaroni

2 (375-g) cans haricot or pinto beans, drained and rinsed

1 tablespoon dried rosemary

1 teaspoon dried oregano

Salt and pepper to taste

Garnish: 1 tablespoon grated Parmesan cheese, freshly chopped parsley

Calories 236, **Fat** 6 g, **Carbohydrates** 37 g, **Protein** 11 g, **Fibre** 5 g, **Saturated Fat** 1 g, **Cholesterol** 1 mg, **Sodium** 215 mg.

Beans, Macaroni and Kale

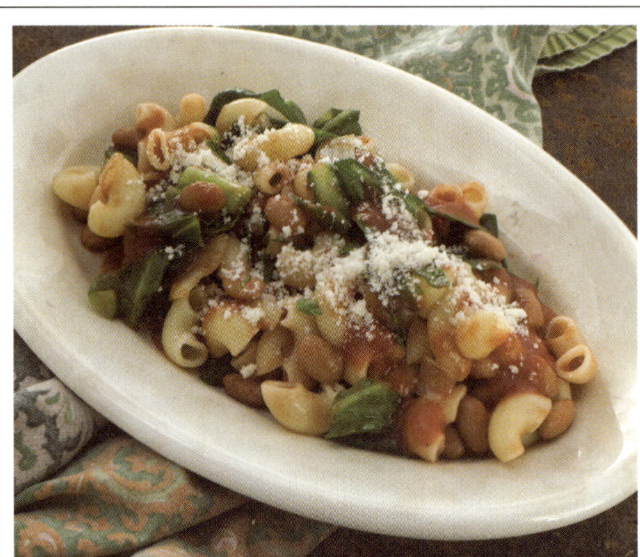

- Heat oil in a large saucepan. Add onions and garlic; sauté until soft, about 4–5 minutes.

- Stir in tomato purée and stock, then stir in kale. It will fill the pan, but it cooks down. Reduce heat, cover and simmer for 30 minutes or until kale is tender.

- While the kale cooks, boil the pasta in lightly salted water. When al dente, drain the pasta.

- Add the pasta and the remaining ingredients to the kale; cover. Simmer for 20 minutes. Serve in individual bowls, garnished with Parmesan and parsley.

Cooking Down Greens

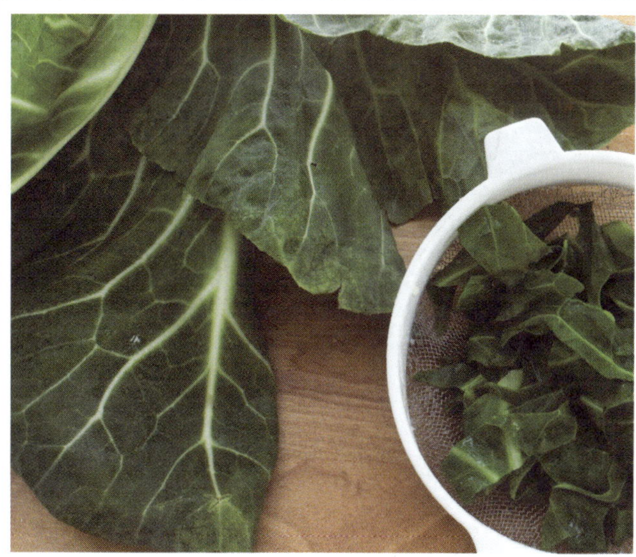

- You may think that your huge bunch of kale or turnip greens, enough to fill a 4-litre pan, will feed at least ten people.

- But once the greens are cooked, you end up with barely enough for four, as they greatly shrink and condense.

- Before you cook down the greens, you should remove the stems, which are tough and woody and often aren't good for soup.

Soaking Beans

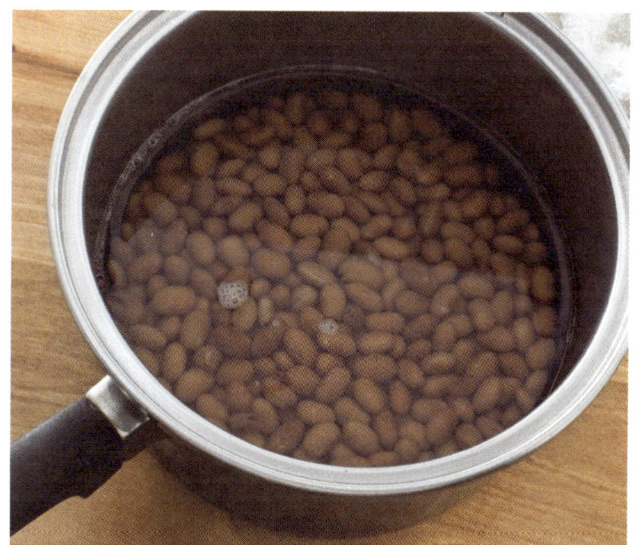

- Some beans require less soaking time than others. Lentils do not need to be soaked at all.

- Beans with stronger skins – such as haricot, kidney and pinto beans – require an overnight soak.

- Some cooks bring the beans to the boil in a pan with enough water to cover them, then turn off the heat, cover and soak for 1 hour.

- This may not work so well. You may get lots of tough bean skins, and it is sometimes better to use canned beans.

TURKEY MEATLOAF

An excellent standby for both small family get-togethers and large parties during the festive season

When you want to do something easy that's sure to please, try this recipe for a festive family meal. You can make it a couple of days in advance and refrigerate the meatloaf, or make it weeks in advance and freeze it.

The cranberries and nuts add interest, fibre and nutrients. There is vitamin C in orange juice and omega-3 fatty acids in walnuts. If you use dark turkey meat, the meatloaf will have more flavour than if you use all white meat.

Turkey meatloaf is lower in calories than beef, pork or a combination. You will find that the taste is just as good and the texture appealing if you use plenty of breadcrumbs – not dried, but fresh.

Ingredients

Serves 8

2 whole eggs

50 ml milk

50 ml orange juice

Salt and freshly ground black pepper to taste

1 teaspoon dried thyme

2 teaspoons dried rosemary, crumbled

75 g fresh breadcrumbs

500 g minced turkey

2 tablespoons low-fat margarine

175 g celery, chopped

1 small sweet onion, chopped

115 g walnut pieces, toasted

50 g dried cranberries

Calories 286, **Fat** 14 g, **Carbohydrates** 21 g, **Protein** 20 g, **Fibre** 2 g, **Saturated Fat** 4 g, **Cholesterol** 116 mg, **Sodium** 338 mg.

Turkey Meatloaf

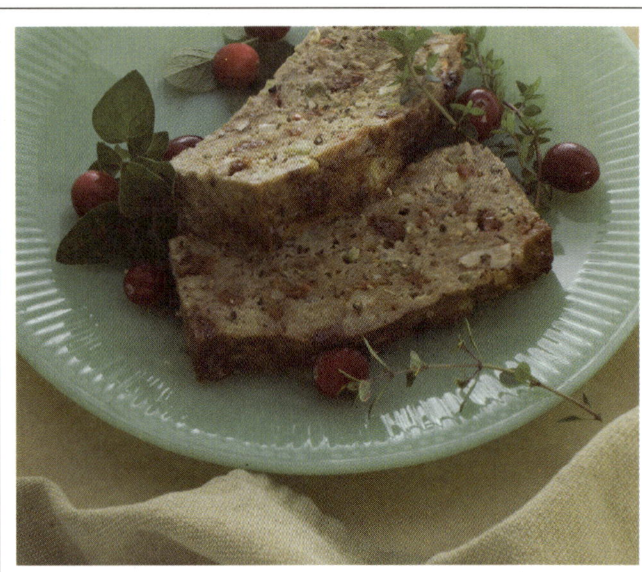

- Preheat oven to 180°C. Whisk together eggs, milk, orange juice, salt, pepper and herbs in a large mixing bowl. Add breadcrumbs and turkey, mixing well.

- Melt margarine in a frying pan; add celery and onion. Sauté until soft, about 5 minutes.

- Add celery and onion mixture to meat, with walnuts and cranberries. Mix well. Oil a 10 x 20-cm loaf tin. Pour meat mixture into tin, spreading evenly.

- Bake in bain marie for 90 minutes. Cool slightly before turning out and cutting into slices.

Fun variations: Turn this into a springtime recipe with a sprinkling of chopped basil and chives and the addition of frozen petits pois, thawed. Give your meatloaf a south of the border tang by adding 120 ml salsa and a couple of hot chillies, finely chopped, and use cornbread crumbs in place of regular breadcrumbs. Top this spicy loaf with a dollop of low-fat or fat-free sour cream. A little chopped chorizo and roasted red peppers add Spanish flavour, especially if you garnish the finished dish with chopped olives. For an Italian touch, use oregano, basil and extra garlic to season the loaf. Add 120 ml of a good Italian marinara sauce to the recipe; 40 g Parmesan cheese enhances the Italian flavourings even more. To lighten the loaf, use 2 well-beaten egg whites.

Fluffing the Mixture

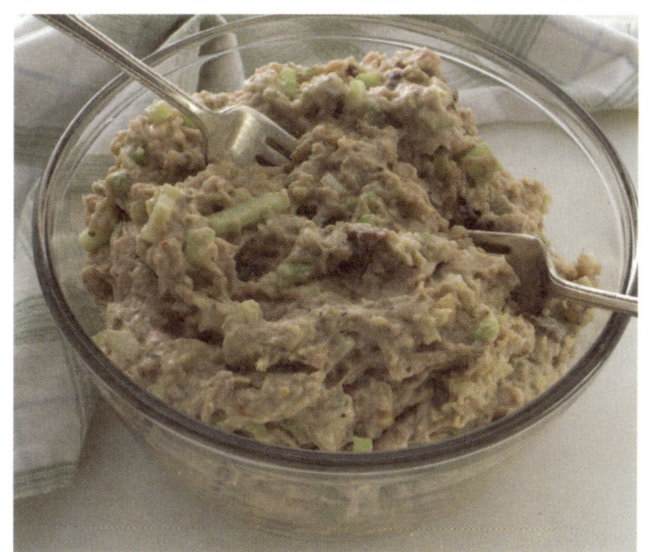

Steaming Meat Loaf in a Bain Marie

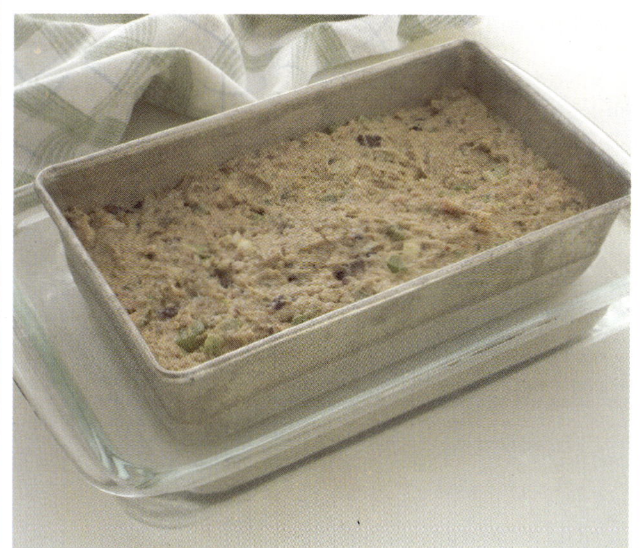

- There are many ways to incorporate ingredients, such as mixing, folding, blending and fluffing.

- To fluff, place most of the ingredients in a large bowl; the bigger, the better.

- Using two forks, bring the ingredients from the outside of the bowl towards the centre. Work your way around the outside of the bowl.

- Add the rest of the ingredients and continue to fluff them up. The result is juicy, not heavily compressed and superdense, meatloaf.

- This technique makes an extremely tender, juicy meatloaf. A bain marie is basically a hot-water bath in the oven.

- Fill a large baking dish a quarter full with hot water and place in the oven at 180°C.

- Put the loaf tin containing the meatloaf into the larger dish, and cook according to directions.

- If you need to add water for more steam during cooking, add it hot from a kettle, taking care not to get water on the meatloaf.

BEEF STEW WITH ARTICHOKES

Elevate a basic stew to new heights with the addition of artichokes, canned or frozen

When you add a can or pack of artichokes to a beef, veal or chicken stew, you will have something very different and most elegant.

Artichokes take the 'basic' out of basic beef stew. And if you don't want to use canned unmarinated artichokes, use frozen baby artichoke hearts, defrosted and cut in half. There is a chemical in the artichoke that changes the flavours to something sweetly different.

Artichokes have phytochemicals and vitamins E and C. They are high in fibre and low in calories. They are only fattening when dipped in butter, mayonnaise or an olive oil and lemon mixture. Eat them plain or with lemon juice.

Ingredients

Serves 6

25 g plain flour

$^1/_2$ teaspoon salt

$^1/_4$ teaspoon freshly ground black pepper

900 g lean stewing beef, cut into cubes

1 tablespoon olive oil

2 onions, peeled and coarsely chopped

2 cloves garlic, peeled and coarsely chopped

120 ml beef stock

120 ml red wine

Zest and juice of $^1/_2$ fresh lemon

1 (350-g) can artichokes, drained and halved, or frozen baby artichoke hearts, thawed and halved

Extra black pepper to taste

Optional: Rice or noodles to accompany (not in nutritional analysis)

Calories 338, **Fat** 11 g, **Carbohydrates** 13 g, **Protein** 42 g, **Fibre** 3 g, **Saturated Fat** 4 g, **Cholesterol** 82 mg, **Sodium** 490 mg.

Beef Stew with Artichokes

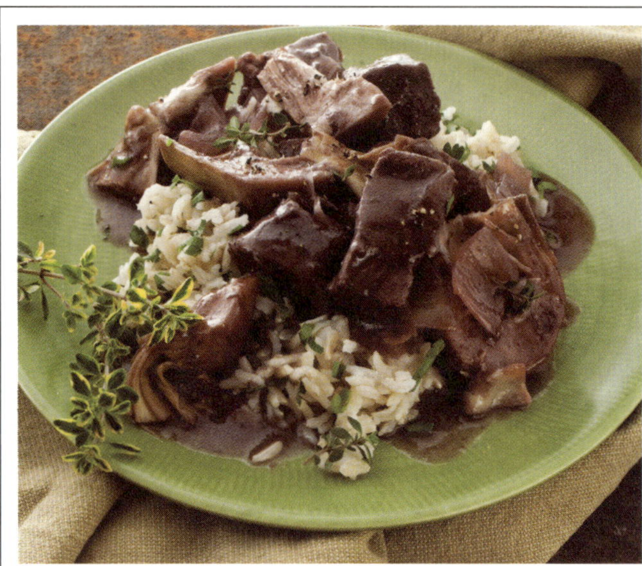

- Mix flour, salt and pepper on a piece of greaseproof paper. Roll beef in flour mixture and set aside.

- Heat oil in a large pan. Add beef and sauté over medium heat. Reduce heat; move meat to side of pan. Add onions and garlic; cook until soft, about 5 minutes.

- Add remaining ingredients; cover and reduce heat. Simmer until meat is tender, about 2–3 hours. Check occasionally, adding more water, wine or stock if the stew becomes too dry.

- Serve with noodles or brown rice.

Hungarian-style goulash: This basic recipe can quickly become Hungarian-style goulash. When you start the stew, add 250 ml tomato sauce or 250 g drained plum tomatoes. Add 3 bay leaves and a few drops of Worcestershire sauce. Sprinkle with 1 teaspoon caraway seeds and 1 tablespoon sweet paprika; mix in 450 g chopped baby carrots. Just before serving the goulash, add 250 ml low-fat sour cream and mix into the gravy, or top each serving with its own dollop of sour cream. If you've made a double quantity for serving later, it's best to add the sour cream individually to each serving. Stew kept in the refrigerator or freezer is much better off without cream, which can separate in the stew over time.

Remove Bay Leaves Before Serving

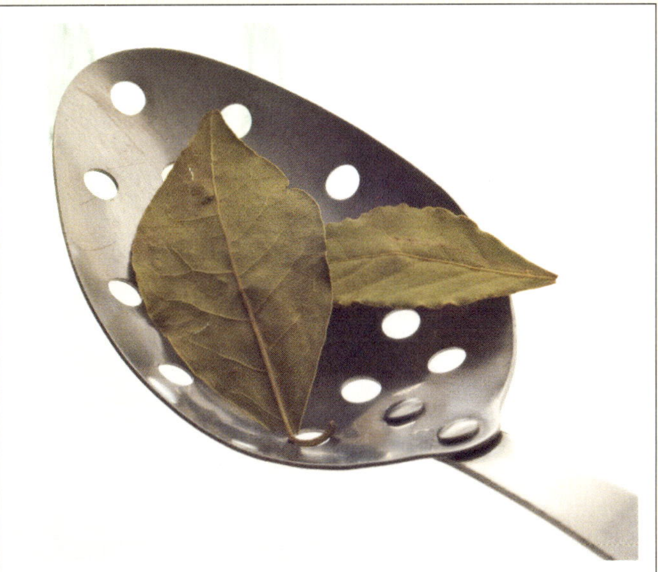

- Bay leaves add a lot of flavour to soups and stews; however, they also pose some dangers.

- Bay leaves are hard and indigestible. They also have sharp edges and can actually cut the oesophagus and stomach lining.

- Cooks working with fresh leaves must be sure to remove them before serving soups and stews. Or warn guests to remove them before eating.

Meat for Stews

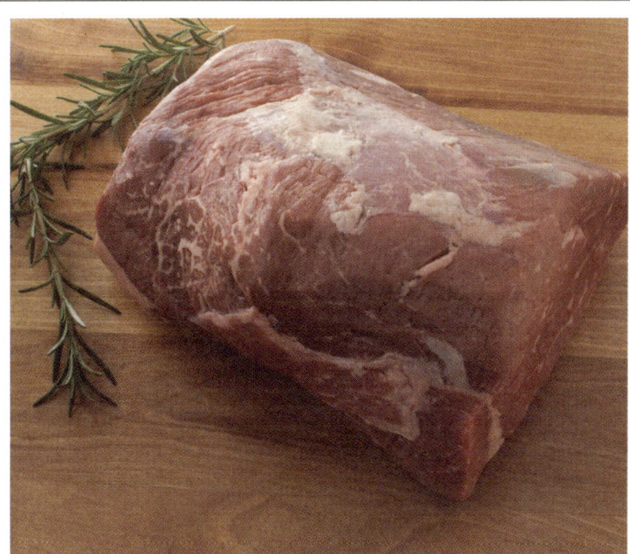

- Because of the long cooking time, you can use very inexpensive cuts of meat to make stews and soups.

- Chuck steak is flavourful, and once it is cut up and stewed, it will be tender.

- Beef skirt is also very good in stews.

- Many cuts are available for stews and soups. Different regions have different names for them. When in doubt, ask your butcher.

THAI CHICKEN STIR-FRY

Spicy Thai food excels in fresh and sparkling flavour contrasts

Thai food can be very spicy – hot is the true adjective. Although this recipe has some heat, it is adjustable for those who have sensitive palates.

Chicken breast fillets are available fresh and frozen. A big bag of them, stored in the freezer, is a boon for the cook in a rush. Tender chicken makes it easy to prepare a healthy, low-carbohydrate, low-calorie meal in no time.

A bit of coconut milk adds creamy sweetness and richness to the sauce, but use only a tiny amount, as in this recipe. Note that the milk adds saturated fat, so you may want to omit it. Red or green chilli paste is available at Asian markets and in most supermarkets, as is sesame seed oil. Fish sauce is a staple of Thai cuisine, but if you don't have any you can use Worcestershire sauce for added flavour.

Ingredients

Serves 6

25 g plain flour

¹/₂ teaspoon salt

675 g chicken breast fillets, cut crosswise into thin strips

2 tablespoons groundnut oil

1 teaspoon sesame seed oil

4 spring onions, chopped

175 g Chinese leaves, shredded

1 teaspoon cornflour

75 g unsweetened coconut milk

75 ml chicken stock

1 teaspoon green or red Thai chilli paste

Salt to taste

2 tablespoons chopped coriander or parsley

Garnish: 25 g unsalted roasted peanuts

Calories 280, **Fat** 14g , **Carbohydrates** 9 g, **Protein** 30 g, **Fibre** 1 g, **Saturated Fat** 5 g, **Cholesterol** 73 mg, **Sodium** 294 mg.

Thai Chicken Stir-Fry

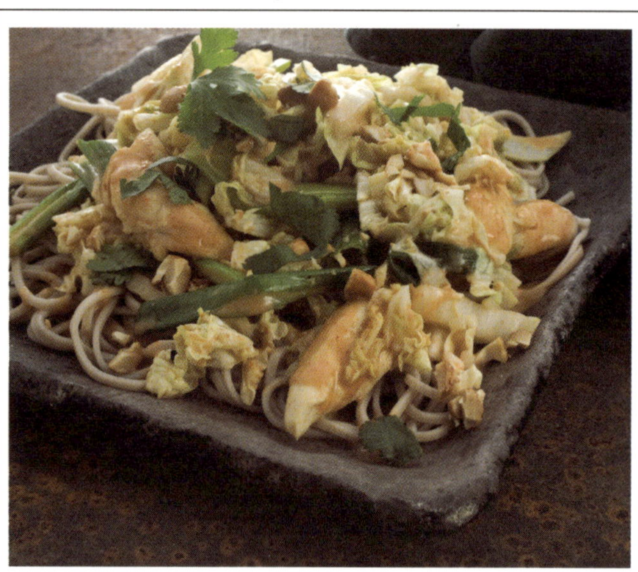

- Spread flour and salt on greaseproof paper; dredge chicken strips in flour. Heat 1 tablespoon groundnut oil and the sesame oil in a wok or sauté pan. Stir-fry chicken strips on medium-high heat, turning until golden brown on both sides. Remove cooked chicken and set aside.

- Add second tablespoon of oil; sauté spring onions and cabbage until crisp-tender, 3 minutes. Place in a bowl. Whisk cornflour, coconut milk, chicken stock and chilli paste in small bowl; blend into oil left in pan. Fold chicken and vegetables into sauce. Add coriander; sprinkle with peanuts.

Improving upon tradition: Traditionally, this recipe would be served with white rice. However, if you are trying to avoid refined and processed carbohydrates in white rice, use brown rice. Oriental noodles are delightful, especially 'glass' or 'cellophane' bean-thread noodles. An occasional lapse into true Oriental noodles is not fattening, as the noodles do not include eggs. Try using whole-grain instead of white noodles. You can always substitute parsley for coriander. Peanuts and sauces made with peanut butter are also staples of Thai cooking.

The Beauties of Stir-Frying

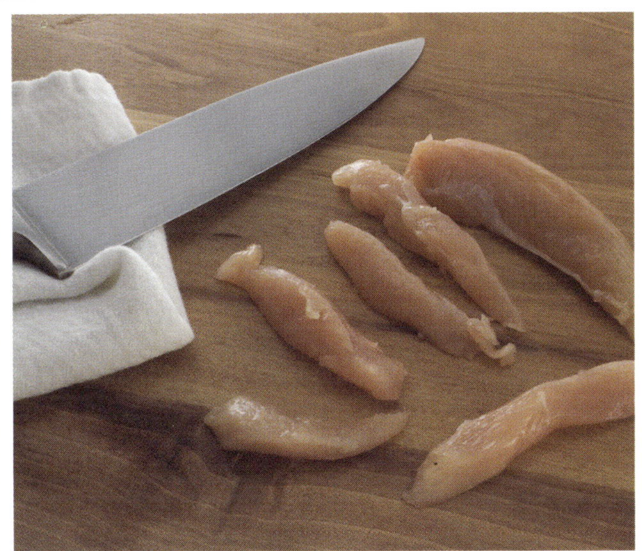

- Food is cut into small, thin strips, so that it cooks very quickly when stir-frying.

- Very sharp knives are crucial to creating a successful stir-fry. It's important that all the pieces of meat are almost exactly the same size for even cooking.

- The last thing you want with a stir-fry is to have some of the meat rare and other pieces well done.

- Chicken should never be served rare because it can carry salmonella, a very harmful form of bacteria.

Shredding Cabbage in a Food Processor

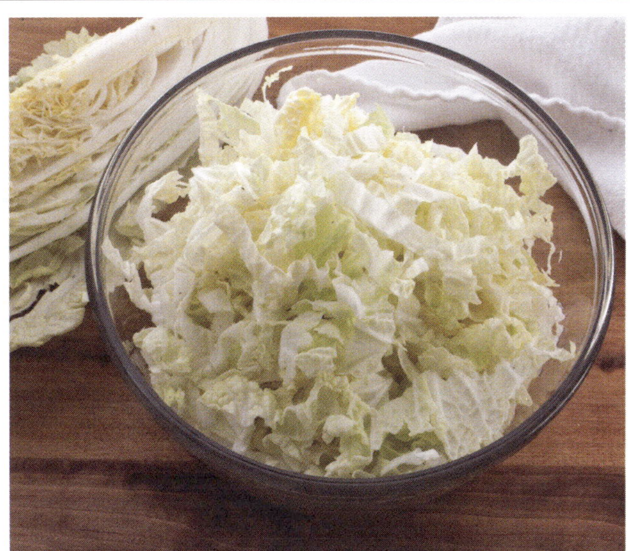

- It's easy to shred cabbage in a food processor. Remove the core and outside leaves. Cut the cabbage lengthwise so that it fits into the tube of the processor.

- Attach the shredding blade. Push the cabbage through with the pusher that comes with the machine.

- Food processors make very short work of shredding cabbage, courgettes, carrots, and just about anything else.

- Using a knife requires a lot more skill and time. Box graters also work well, but be careful of your fingertips.

PISTACHIO-PEPPER STEAK
Porterhouse steak is terrific served plain, but it's even better with a great crust

Adding a black pepper crust to a steak (steak au poivre) is a traditional French method for preparing filet mignon. It takes advantage of all the flavours that are sealed in by the pepper crust, plus there's a lot of flavour in the pepper itself.

For this recipe, get roasted pistachios that are not salted, if possible. They are available, but you may have to hunt for them. If you can't find pistachios, go for roasted hazelnuts or cashews.

You can add a drop of brandy to the sauce. Coarse salt crusts on meat or fish are popular with some chefs – they make an igloo out of the salt, and then scrape it off after cooking.

Ingredients

Serves 6

150 ml shelled pistachio nuts, coarsely chopped

1 tablespoon black pepper, coarsely ground

$^1/_2$ teaspoon salt

4 porterhouse steaks, well trimmed, about 175 g each

1 tablespoon canola or olive oil

Calories 343, **Fat** 22 g, **Carbohydrates** 4 g, **Protein** 31 g, **Fibre** 2 g, **Saturated Fat** 7 g, **Cholesterol** 70 mg, **Sodium** 267 mg.

Pistachio-Pepper Steak

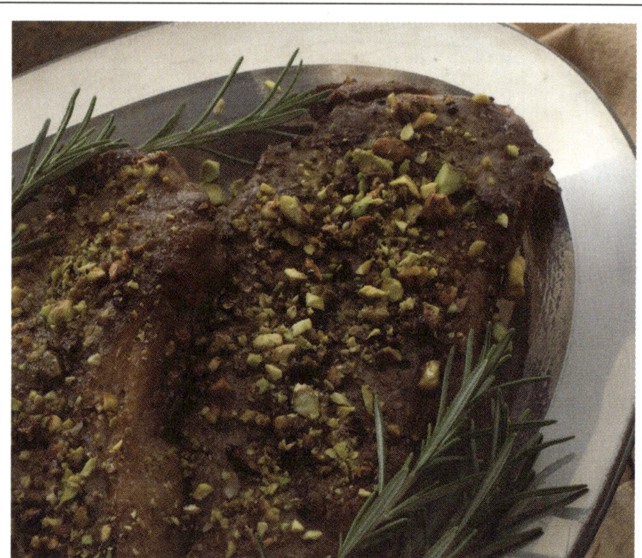

- Evenly spread the nuts, pepper and salt on a piece of greaseproof paper.

- One at a time, place the steaks on the paper, and press the nut mixture into both sides of each steak.

- Heat a sauté pan over medium-high heat. Add the oil. Sauté the steaks for 1 minute.

- Turn and reduce heat. Cook over medium-low heat, covered, until done to your liking. Leave steaks to rest for 5 minutes, covered, before serving.

Make it easy and healthy: The best way to prepare this wonderful steak is in a sauté pan on top of the stove. Of course, you can put it under the grill or on the barbecue, but sautéing both browns the nuts and seals in the flavours. Sautéing is also a very healthy technique when you use canola or olive oil – no butter, please. However, the nuts do produce a buttery flavour when browned with the steak. The nice thing about porterhouse steak is that you can cut off every bit of visible fat, and it will still be delicious. Also, the steak is so tender that you won't need to marinate it or pound it to break down the fibres.

When Is Steak Done?

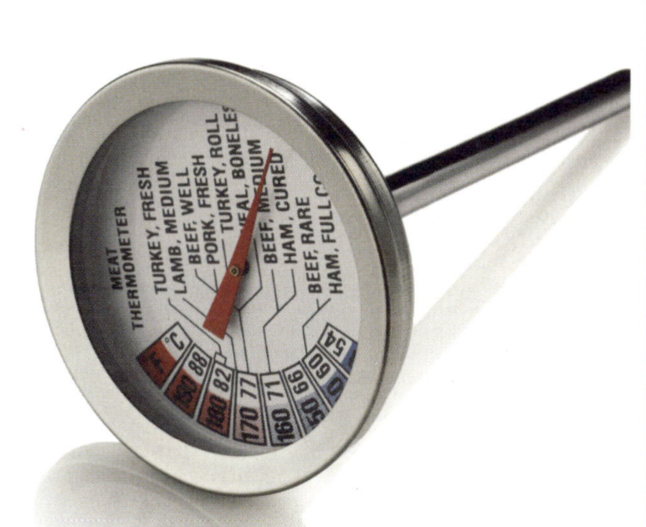

- There are two ways to know if your meat is done.

- First, you can carefully time steaks and roasts. However, because oven temperatures vary greatly, timing can be unreliable.

- Second, you can use a meat thermometer to measure the temperature. The thermometer will give a reading that will let you know the meat is done.

- A rare steak should be about 57°C; medium, 63°C; and well done, 65°C. Remember, it continues to cook while resting.

Why Let Meat Rest?

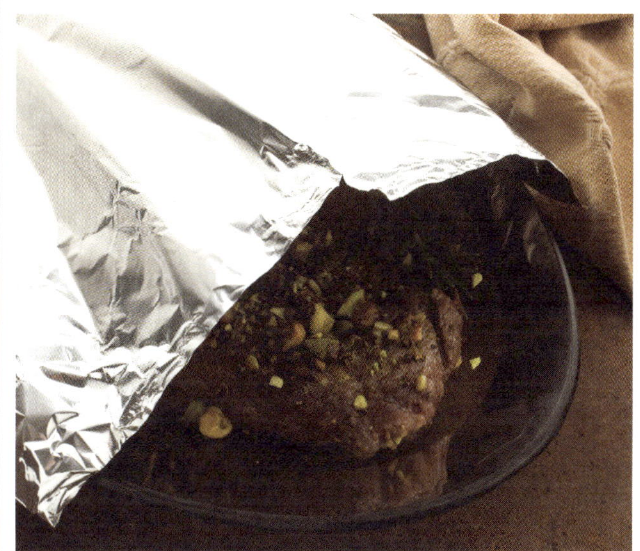

- There are two good reasons for letting a piece of cooked meat rest before cutting into it.

- The first is to let it finish cooking evenly, especially in the centre. The second is to make sure the juices do not run out on to the carving dish rather than going back into the meat.

- This principle applies to steaks, roast turkey, chicken, lamb, beef and pork.

GRILLED ASIAN CHICKEN THIGHS

These are great snacks for picnics, buffets and barbecues

Your crowd may be a bit tired of spicy chicken wings. Try using small thighs, either bone-in or boneless, for a welcome, tasty change. Bone-in is easier to eat outdoors.

Thighs are richer in flavour than wings or breast meat. And, as dark meat, they are slightly higher in calories. They also tend to be far less expensive than breasts, so you get a lot of food for your money.

A nice side dish with this recipe is fresh orange and shaved fennel salad. Or a salad of haricot beans with red onions and Chinese vegetables (bean sprouts, water chestnuts and mangetout peas) goes really well.

Ingredients

Serves 8

For the chicken:

1 tablespoon Chinese five-spice powder

200 g granulated Splenda

1 tablespoon wasabi powder, or to taste

$1/2$ teaspoon salt

Zest of $1/2$ lemon

24 chicken thighs, bone-in, skinless

For the sauce:

250 ml freshly squeezed orange juice

1 tablespoon sugar-free orange marmalade

50 ml light low-sodium soy sauce

1 tablespoon grated fresh ginger

Calories 304, **Fat** 8 g, **Carbohydrates** 14 g, **Protein** 41 g, **Fibre** 0, **Saturated Fat** 2 g, **Cholesterol** 172 mg, **Sodium** 449 mg.

Grilled Asian Chicken Thighs

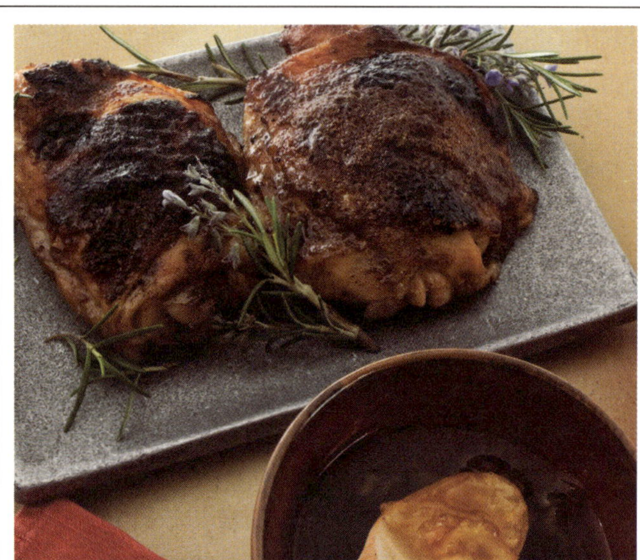

- Place seasonings and lemon zest in a bowl; mix well. Add thighs and toss to coat. Work rub under skin of each thigh. Marinate 2 hours or overnight in fridge.

- Prepare barbecue. Place thighs over medium-high heat for 3 minutes; turn and brown 3 minutes more.

- When brown on all sides, move thighs away from direct heat to a cooler part of the rack and close the lid.

- Cook through without burning the thighs, about 7 minutes off to the side.

- Mix sauce ingredients in a bowl; use for dipping.

Spice rubs and barbecue combinations: You can easily make this recipe for chicken thighs with a Cajun spice rub, or any dry barbecue rub that appeals to you. However, most rubs are high in carbohydrates, so it's best to make your own rubs using Splenda. Rubs can also be very high in sodium. A delicious dipping sauce is essential; you can always use salsa, melted cheese and pepper sauce or, as in this recipe, an Asian/citrus combination. If you use boneless, skinless thighs, you'll find that the spices work themselves into the meat more thoroughly. If using bone-in and skin-on meat, try to work some of the rub under the skin.

Bone-in vs. Boneless Thighs

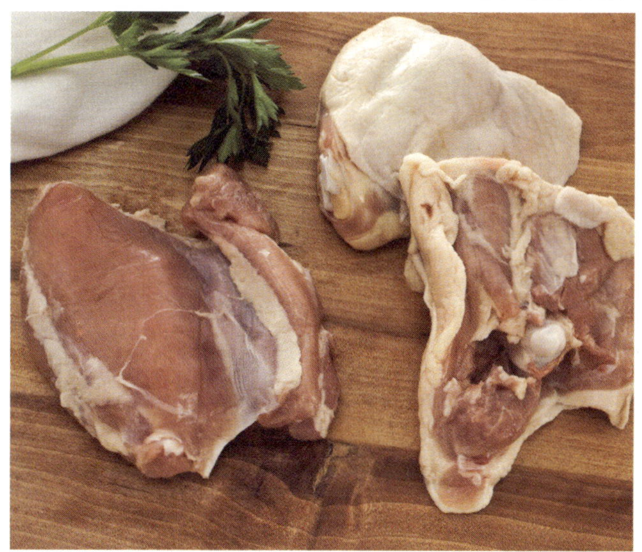

- When using skinless and boneless chicken thighs, you have to be careful not to dry them out. And they are much more difficult to eat with your hands than those with bones you can hold on to.

- Thighs with the bone in and skin on take longer to cook, and the skin has more calories.

- Be careful not to burn off the rub, especially when cooking boneless and skinless thighs.

- Cut one piece open to make sure it is done all the way through.

Charcoal vs. Gas

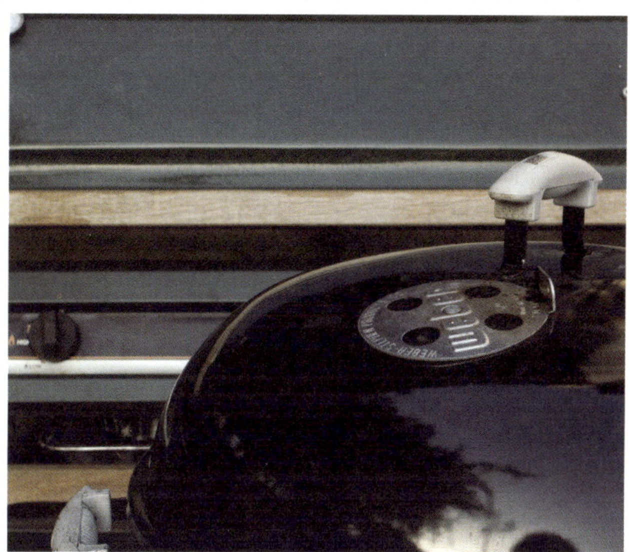

- The flame of a gas barbecue is easier to control. Some models even 'flash' cook the food at extremely high temperatures.

- A charcoal grill takes longer to bring to the proper temperature. You must let the flames die down and wait until the coals are white.

- Be sure to bank coals to one side so that you can move browned foods away from the direct heat.

- Adding herbs or wood chips enhances flavours. A bed of fennel fronds on the rack is a great addition.

BRAISED VEAL SHANKS

This traditional Italian dish can be a satisfying family dinner or a cosy meal for friends

Braised veal shanks (*osso bucco*) is a dish for 'weekend warriors' in the kitchen, as it takes a fair amount of cooking time.

Veal shanks are thick and have a large marrow bone in the middle. They should have no fat whatsoever on them. You need a big piece – allow about 225 g per person – because of the bone.

Veal shanks are excellent when served with mashed potatoes, brown rice or white beans. Pasta, such as orzo, is a traditional Italian accompaniment. Vegetables also go well. You will have lots of sauce when you braise veal shanks. The marrow is wonderful when spread on a thin slice of toasted multigrain bread.

Ingredients

Serves 6

2 tablespoons olive oil

6 slices veal shank, about 1.4 kg total weight

Salt and freshly ground black pepper to taste

2 medium onions, peeled and chopped

3 cloves garlic, smashed, peeled and coarsely chopped

120 ml low-sodium chicken stock

160 g whole Italian plum tomatoes, drained and chopped

120 ml dry white wine

2 carrots, peeled and chopped

1 tablespoon dried rosemary

1 teaspoon dried oregano

1 teaspoon dried basil

Garnish: freshly chopped flat-leaf parsley

Calories 337, **Fat** 11 g, **Carbohydrates** 7 g, **Protein** 47 g, **Fibre** 1 g, **Saturated Fat** 2 g, **Cholesterol** 79 mg, **Sodium** 392.

Braised Veal Shanks

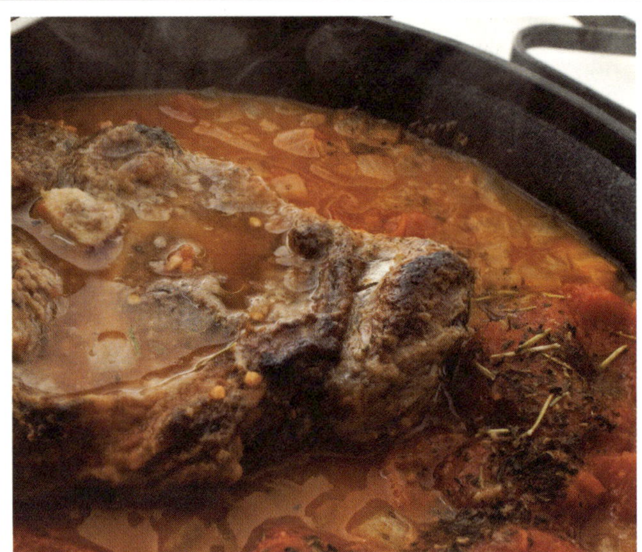

- Heat olive oil over medium-high heat in a Dutch oven or stew pan large enough to hold all the pieces of meat without crowding.

- Sprinkle veal shanks with salt and pepper; brown them in oil. Remove from pan. Sauté onions and garlic in the pan.

- Add remaining ingredients minus the fresh parsley. Return the shanks to the pan. Cover and reduce heat to simmer.

- Cook for 2–3 hours, or until meat is tender and sauce is reduced and thickened. Sprinkle with parsley before serving.

Sauces and accompaniments: Veal shanks are delicious in a brown gravy spiked with lemon, and they are also great with mushrooms in a brown sauce. Green olives will make a very good addition; they acquire a rich flavour when cooked. Rosemary, basil and oregano, together or individually, are fine complements. A dish of fennel braised with low-fat margarine and orange slices goes well with this.

Salad options: Serve a side salad to add contrast to the veal shanks. If you do not braise fennel as a hot vegetable, you might consider using it shaved, with fresh orange slices and a citrus or white wine vinaigrette. Beetroot salad with mixed leaves and a little goats' cheese is also very popular for winter meals.

Braising Meat

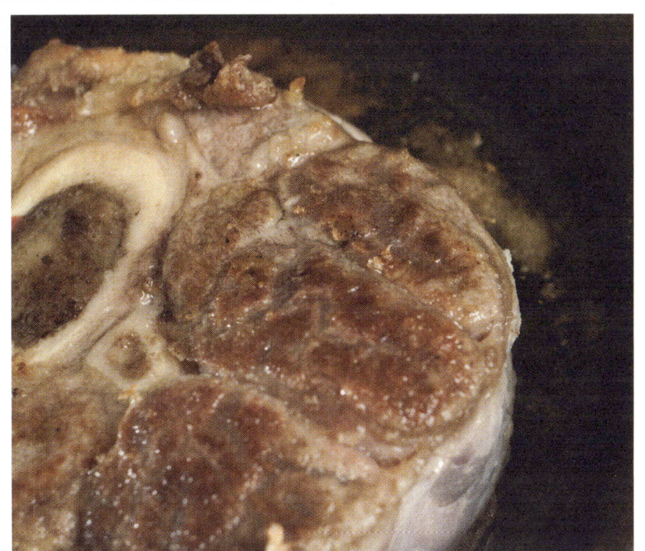

Making Gravy and Sauce from Pan Juices

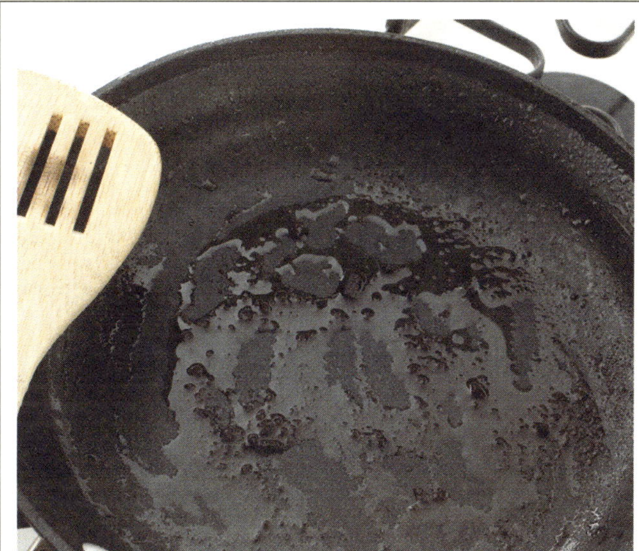

- Braising is a great tenderizer of 'muscle' meat. The shank, being part of the leg, is a hard-working muscle.

- Beef shanks make great soup. Lamb shanks are excellent when braised.

- To braise, brown meat, add aromatic vegetables and liquids; reduce heat and cover. Most braising is done on top of the stove, but you can put a casserole dish in the oven for 2–4 hours, depending on the cut.

- Braising requires very slow cooking until meat is very tender. The cooking liquid becomes sauce or gravy.

- When you braise meat, you should end up with a nice amount of rich juices.

- If you have too much liquid boil it down to reduce the volume and enrich it.

- Make sure all the brown bits on the bottom of the pan dissolve into the sauce.

- If you don't have enough liquid, add chicken, beef or vegetable stock and some wine.

- For instant thickening, make a paste with equal amounts soft butter or low-fat margarine and flour. Drop in a little at a time, stirring constantly.

GRILLED HALIBUT WTIH WATERCRESS

Mild and firm with a clean sea flavour, halibut is one of the finest fishes available

Halibut is a huge deep-sea fish. It lives only in clean salt water, and its availability has been declining over the last 20 years because of overfishing.

   Halibut doesn't need much in the way of dressing. Too much spicing, dressing, saucing and/or seasoning masks its natural fresh flavour. Salt, pepper, lemon and a watercress sauce are all you need. Don't overload it with garlic or onions. Bold flavours ruin it. Although firm-fleshed, halibut has a delicate flavour. Flavoured breadcrumbs moistened with olive oil are good on any fish, but with halibut, less is more. Olive oil, used in moderation, is recommended fat that doesn't raise cholesterol. Butter is good melted on fish, and is OK for occasional use.

Ingredients

Serves 4

1 tablespoon lemon juice

20 g chopped watercress

120 ml low-fat sour cream

4 halibut fillets, about 150 g each, skin on

1 tablespoon olive oil

Salt and pepper to taste

Garnish: sprigs of watercress

Calories 186, **Fat** 7 g, **Carbohydrates** 0, **Protein** 21 g, **Fibre** 0, **Saturated Fat** 3 g, **Cholesterol** 46 mg, **Sodium** 199 mg.

Grilled Halibut with Watercress

- Mix the first three ingredients together to make sauce; set aside. Preheat grill; place rack about 12.5 cm away from heat.

- Oil a baking sheet and arrange fish on it, skin side down. Drizzle with olive oil and sprinkle with salt and pepper.

- Grill fish until it starts to brown and flakes. If it is very thick, switch on the oven at 180°C and let it cook through until it flakes.

- Serve fish with sauce on the side or drizzled on top. Garnish with sprigs of fresh watercress.

Grill a thick fillet of fish: A good firm fish like halibut can be cooked over charcoal or on a gas barbecue – it won't fall apart. The easiest way to cook it is to run the fish under the grill. If it is a very thick cut, you will need to turn on your oven to cook it through. Cod is the preferred fish for deep-frying, as in fish and chips. However, a boneless fillet of halibut is fine for frying in a light batter. Fresh or dried dill, lemon juice and low-fat sour cream make a delicious sauce for fish. Simply combine 1 teaspoon dried dill with 120 ml sour cream and 1 tablespoon freshly squeezed lemon juice.

Checking Fish Fillets for Bones

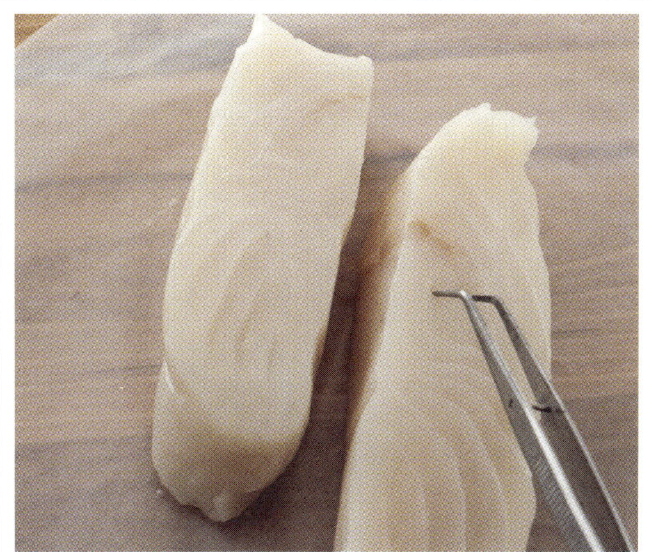

Fillets vs. Steaks

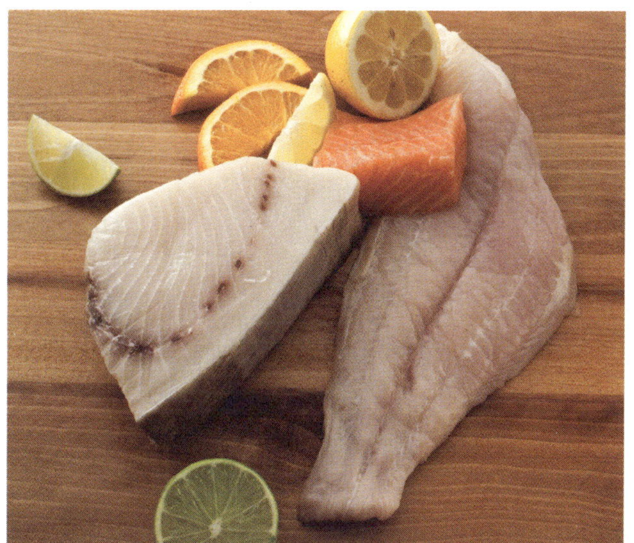

- Fish steaks may have bones in them; salmon steaks, for example, include a section of backbone.

- Fish fillets should be boneless, but may sometimes have small 'pin' bones.

- You can find these bones by running your finger over the raw fillet, back and forth against the grain.

- Should you find a bone, pull it out with tweezers.

- Mid-sized fish such as salmon, cod and halibut are often cut into steaks, which are cut across the grain of the flesh.

- Alternatively, the sides of the fish may be taken off the bone as fillets. Flat fish such as sole are either filleted or served whole.

- Fillets tend to be thicker at the end near the head than at the tail end. So move your grill pan around to ensure even cooking.

CORNMEAL-CRUSTED BAKED FISH

If you love the crispy crust on fried fish but not the fat calories, try this recipe

There are so many ways to coat a fish; this is a very good method that is sure to please the family.

You can add this crunchy cornmeal crust to fillets of any white fish, such as cod, haddock, hake or whiting. The mixture of spices and seasonings sets off the flavour of the fish beautifully. Add some Cajun spice to the fillets if your family wants a true Southern touch. Or you can rub them with an Asian spice mix, which will give you a completely different taste experience.

Generally, it's better to make your own coating. Store-bought coating mixes are loaded with salt and/or sugar, which we can all do without.

Ingredients

Serves 4

1 whole egg and 1 egg white

50 g cornmeal

50 g plain flour

1 teaspoon baking powder

1 teaspoon salt

1 teaspoon sweet paprika

$1/2$ teaspoon thyme

$1/2$ teaspoon garlic powder

$1/2$ teaspoon ground cumin

1 teaspoon cayenne pepper, or to taste

1 teaspoon freshly ground black pepper, or to taste

4 white fish fillets, about 150–175 g each

2 tablespoons olive oil, sprayed

Garnish: 4 lemon wedges and fresh parsley

Calories 256, **Fat** 8 g, **Carbohydrates** 21 g, **Protein** 21 g, **Fibre** 2 g, **Saturated Fat** 2 g, **Cholesterol** 78 mg, **Sodium** 774 mg.

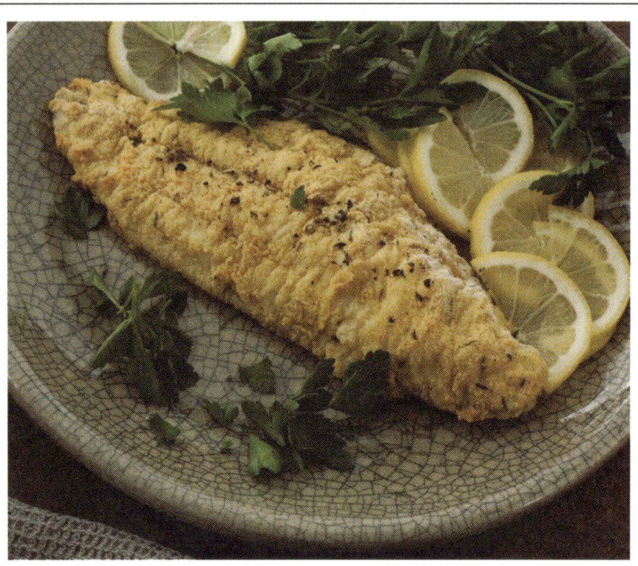

Cornmeal-Crusted Baked Fish

- Preheat oven to 180°C. Whisk egg and white in a shallow bowl; set aside. Mix all the dry ingredients on a piece of greaseproof paper.

- Dip fish fillets in the eggs and then roll in cornmeal mixture. Press dry ingredients into the flesh, and make sure they stick.

- Arrange fillets on an oiled baking dish. Lightly spray olive oil on the fish.

- Bake for 25–30 minutes until golden brown and crisp. Garnish with lemon wedges and parsley. Serve with your favourite sauce.

About fish: Fish is good for you, and it's advisable to eat at least two portions a week, one of which should be an oily fish such as mackerel, trout or salmon. White fish such as cod and haddock are rightly popular because they are delicious, but fish populations throughout the world's oceans have become seriously depleted by overfishing and in many areas are in danger of dropping to the critical point where they could die out altogether. It's important for all of us to buy fish responsibly, as far as possible making sure that we are not contributing to the problem. Buy from a reputable fishmonger or supermarket, and look for fish that carries the blue Marine Stewardship Council (MSC) logo, which guarantees that the fish comes from a sustainable source. Don't just buy the fish you know, but explore less familiar, and less threatened, species recommended by your fishmonger, so that you can eat fish with a clear conscience.

Checking Fish for Freshness

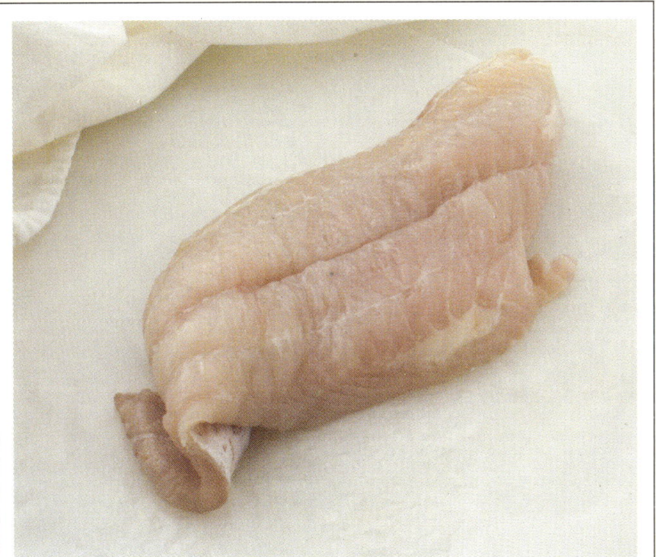

- When you buy fish, look for a nice colour and a firm texture.

- Always smell fish before you buy it.

- Any decent fishmonger or supermarket fish department should be happy to put the fish on a piece of paper and let you give it a good sniff. It should smell fresh, even milky, or like the sea on a clear morning.

- When you get fish home, check freshness; make sure the flesh springs back when pressed with a fingertip. Smell it, too. If it doesn't pass the tests, take it back.

Using Citrus Zest with Fish

- Try using orange or lemon zest in your next coating for baked fish.

- Lime zest can get very bitter when cooked, so use it only for fresh dishes. Lime juice, however, cooks very well and maintains a tart taste without bitterness.

- A mixture of orange and lemon zest is great when added to breadcrumbs for coating fish.

- Grapefruit zest is less common; however, it can be quite good on a fish that will stand up to strong flavours.

CASHEW-CRUSTED SALMON FILLETS

The baked avocado with lime dressing in this recipe adds great flavour contrast

Using nuts with fish is a fairly new idea but one that's worth exploring. You will find that as the nuts brown on the fish, they develop a buttery flavour that is absolutely delicious. In this dish, it doesn't compete with the salmon at all but does make it taste even sweeter.

The contrast with baked avocado and lime juice is stunningly good. Try using other juices, such as Seville orange juice or grapefruit juice, as a substitute for the lime juice in your dressing. Other nuts, such as pine nuts, can also be used as a crust on salmon. Macadamia nuts add as many calories as a pork chop to the meal, so try to avoid them. To cut back on the fat, eliminate either oil or avocado.

Ingredients

Serves 4

Juice of 1 lime

3 tablespoons olive oil

1/4 teaspoon salt

1/4 teaspoon Splenda

Tabasco sauce, a few drops or to taste

2 avocados, halved and stoned

4 salmon fillets, about 175 g each

50 g whole cashews, ground coarsely in the food processor

Garnish: 4–8 lime wedges

Calories 538, **Fat** 39 g, **Carbohydrates** 13 g, **Protein** 34 g, **Fibre** 7 g, **Saturated Fat** 8 g, **Cholesterol** 87 mg, **Sodium** 241 mg.

Cashew-Crusted Salmon Fillets

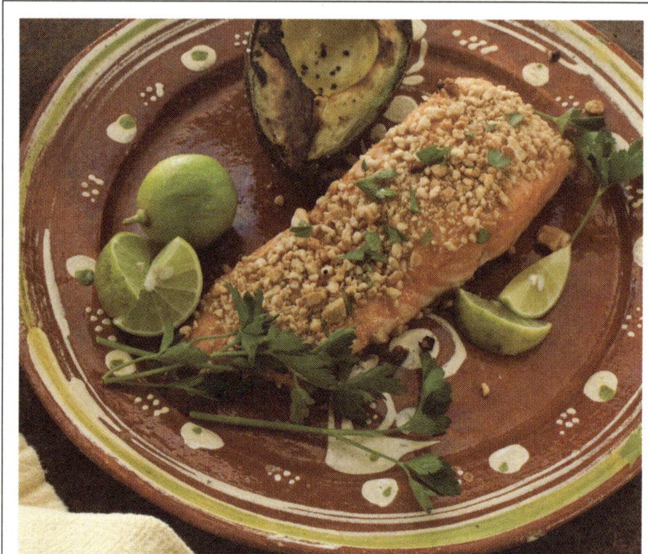

- Preheat oven to 180°C. Using a fork, whisk lime juice, oil, salt, Splenda and Tabasco sauce in a cup. Spread mixture on avocado halves and fish fillets.

- Spread the ground nuts evenly on the fish fillets and press into the flesh.

- Arrange avocado halves and fish, skin side down, on an oiled baking tray.

- Bake for 20 minutes, or until avocado is softened, nuts are brown, and fish is done. Serve with lime wedges on the side.

Kid-friendly ideas: Children can be fussy eaters. To appeal to them, try substituting peanuts for cashews. In any case, be sure that the nuts are raw and not roasted, or they will get too brown and lose their delicate taste. You may well find that children who won't eat fish will try it when it looks more like a chicken breast or their favourite nut bar.

Give your kids a great reason for eating fish. Cook small salmon fillets with fun toppings, such as 1 tablespoon of chopped tomato; a couple of olives, chopped; or chopped pieces of a peeled orange.

Grinding Nuts

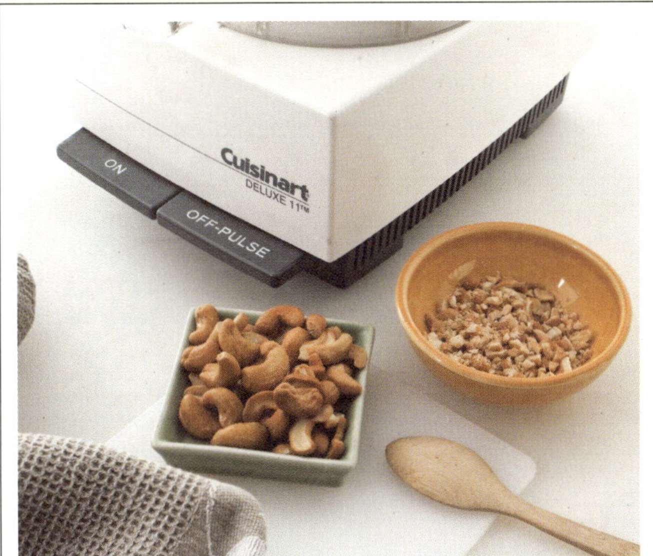

- To grind nuts coarsely, pulse them in a food processor, pausing to scrape down the sides of the bowl.

- Or grind nuts coarsely by placing them on grease-proof paper, covering them with another piece and pounding them with a cast-iron pan or meat mallet.

- For finely ground nuts, pulse in a food processor for a few seconds, then whirl the nuts on high.

- Don't use a blender. You will end up with unground nuts on the top and a paste at the bottom.

Flavouring Ground Nuts

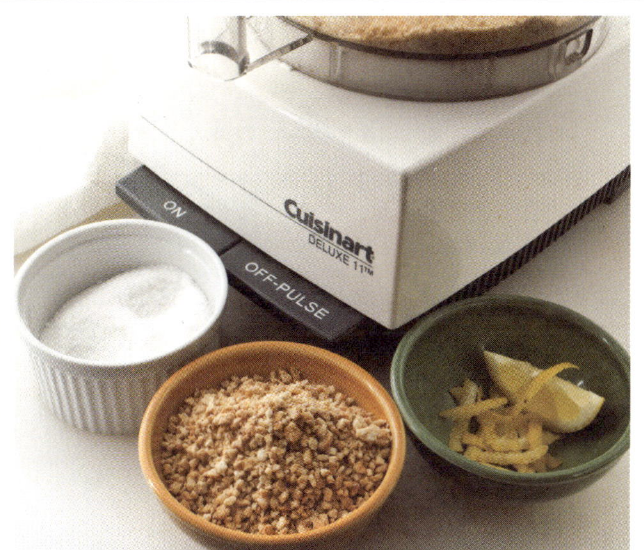

- Whether you're preparing fish, chicken breasts or pork cutlets, ground nuts make a great crust.

- Always buy raw, unsalted unroasted nuts. Then, you can add seasonings to the nutty crust that will not interfere with your recipes.

- While grinding and seasoning nuts, control your salt and sugar intake by using salt substitute and Splenda.

- Try adding dried herbs such as thyme or rosemary. Add some lemon, orange or grapefruit zest to nuts while you are grinding them.

147

SPICY BARBECUED SHARK SKEWERS

Charcoal-grilled shark is delightful when marinated or dressed in chilli-citrus sauce

Shark is tender, sweet and versatile. The only thing that will ruin a piece of shark is overcooking.

Shark is a lot like firm-fleshed swordfish, but a bit softer and milder. Making a marinade of chilli sauce, orange juice and Worcestershire sauce will enhance the fish. Barbecuing some orange slices along with the shark is sublime.

If you are using skewers, marinate the fish so that it has time to absorb the flavours. A slight charring is fine, but do not burn shark or any other fish.

Add orange sections to the shark on the skewers. Or add vegetables, such as chunks of courgette, cherry tomatoes or chunks of sweet red onion.

Ingredients

Serves 4

2 tablespoons light (low-sodium) soy sauce

Juice of $^1/_2$ Seville orange or regular orange juice (used for analysis)

1 teaspoon Splenda

1 tablespoon low-sodium tomato purée

$^1/_4$ teaspoon ground cloves

Pinch of ground cinnamon

$^1/_2$ teaspoon garlic powder

Freshly ground black pepper to taste

500 g fresh boneless shark steak, cut into 4-cm cubes

8 wooden or metal skewers (if wood, soak for at least 30 minutes)

Calories 185, **Fat** 3 g, **Carbohydrates** 7 g, **Protein** 31 g, **Fibre** 1 g, **Saturated Fat** 1 g, **Cholesterol** 46 mg, **Sodium** 292 mg.

Spicy Barbecued Shark Skewers

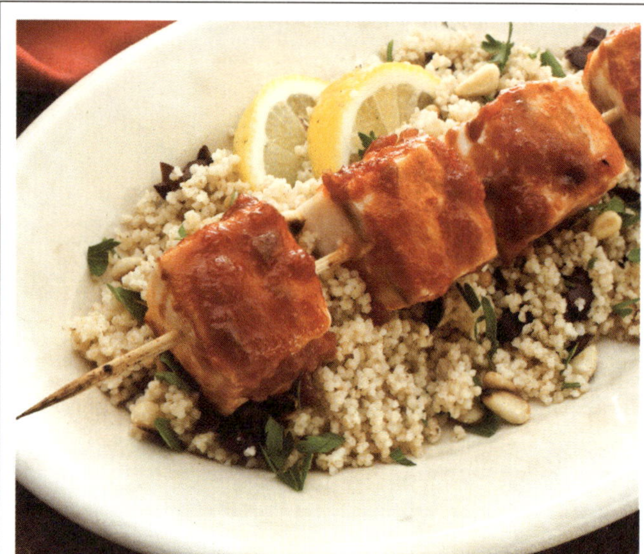

- In a large mixing bowl, whisk the first eight ingredients together.

- Add shark cubes, turning to coat. Cover and refrigerate for 1–2 hours, turning occasionally to coat evenly.

- Preheat barbecue or grill to medium-high, about 190°C.

- Place shark cubes on skewers and grill until nicely brown.

- Cook for about 3 minutes per side. Do not overcook or the shark will dry out. It's better to undercook than overcook.

Shark appetizers: Shark on skewers is a great hors d'oeuvre. Skewer shark pieces and coat with mango salsa or an Asian dipping sauce. Allow about 115 g per person. Cut into 2.5-cm cubes and thread on wooden skewers. (Soak wooden skewers before using.) Use ½ mango, mixed with 1 teaspoon chopped fresh ginger and 1 teaspoon lime juice. Grill for 2 minutes each side.

Mediterranean shark skewers: Give your shark skewers a Mediterranean flavour with a marinade of 2 teaspoons olive oil, the juice of 1 lemon and 1 teaspoon oregano for every 500 g of cubed shark meat. Marinate for 30 minutes, then thread on skewers and grill for 2 minutes each side.

Skewers: Wooden or Metal?

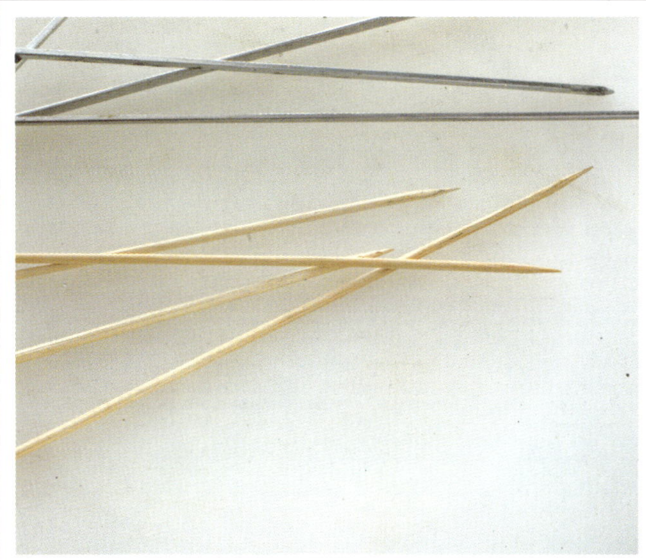

- Wooden skewers are great for grilling; however, they must first be soaked in water to prevent them from catching fire.

- As an alternative, try using rosemary stems, which give food a herbal flavour. Or use skewers made from cedar or ash wood.

- Metal skewers are reusable. They often have medallions or miniature handles on one end, like small swords.

- Metal skewers are easily cleaned with a scouring pad. Be sure to get stainless steel if you buy metal skewers.

Shark Snacks for the Cocktail Tray

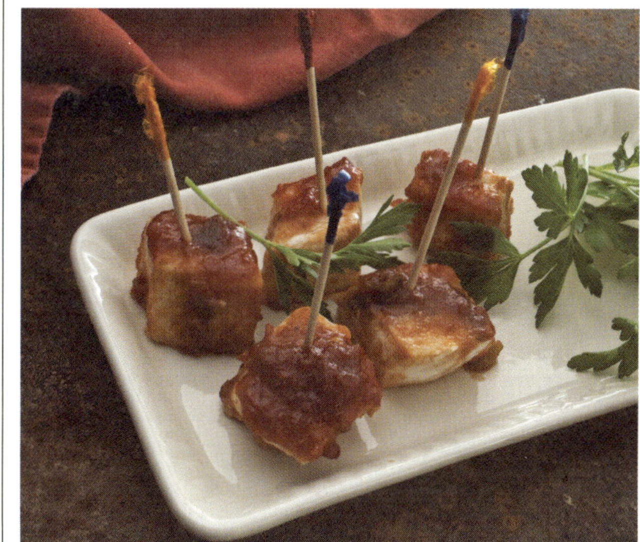

- By cutting the shark into smaller pieces, you can grill them very quickly.

- Lightly oil the grill pan, arrange the pieces of shark on it, then run it under a preheated grill. Turn the shark, and remove after a few more seconds of cooking.

- Once it's cooked, spear the shark pieces with cocktail sticks and arrange on a serving dish. Leave to cool slightly before serving.

- You can garnish the platter with lemon wedges.

FISH

GRILLED COD WITH TOMATOES

Cod is one of the most versatile of fish and is notably used in traditional fish and chips

Cod is a fine, white ocean-going fish that is extremely popular on both sides of the Atlantic.

Cod may be fried, as in fish and chips. It can also be baked, grilled, poached for fish chowder, or minced as the base for fish cakes – a staple of the frozen food department and truly delectable when homemade.

This recipe calls for grilling the fish, accompanied by cherry tomatoes. Cod is so low in fat that it needs the addition of a little olive oil or margarine to keep it moist while cooking.

Dried salt cod is called *baccalà* by the Italians and *bacalao* by the Spanish. It requires two days of soaking in fresh water and is very good.

Ingredients

Serves 4

4 cod steaks (150 g each)

Juice of 1/2 lemon

16 cherry tomatoes, cut in halves

1 tablespoon fresh dill

Salt and pepper to taste

2 tablespoons panko breadcrumbs

1 tablespoon olive oil

Calories 184, **Fat** 5 g, **Carbohydrates** 8 g, **Protein** 26 g, **Fibre** 1 g, **Saturated Fat** 1 g, **Cholesterol** 60 mg, **Sodium** 203 mg.

Grilled Cod with Tomatoes

- Preheat grill to 225°C. Oil a flameproof gratin dish.

- Arrange fish in dish. Sprinkle with lemon juice, and arrange tomato halves around fish.

- Sprinkle with dill, salt, pepper and panko breadcrumbs.

- Grill for 4–5 minutes, or until the fish is sizzling and the breadcrumbs are browned.

- Switch to oven heat at 150°C and leave fish for 3–4 more minutes to finish cooking.

Fun variations: For a wonderful variation, use mild salsa instead of fresh tomatoes. Coriander, popular in Mexican cooking, and dill, a staple of Scandinavian cooking, are strong herbs worth a try. Both can be terrific with fish, but use a light touch at first.

For a crunchy crust: Coat fish with lemon juice, spread thinly with low-fat mayonnaise, and sprinkle with 25 g panko breadcrumbs. This will give the fish a great crunchy crust and add only a few calories.

About Panko Breadcrumbs

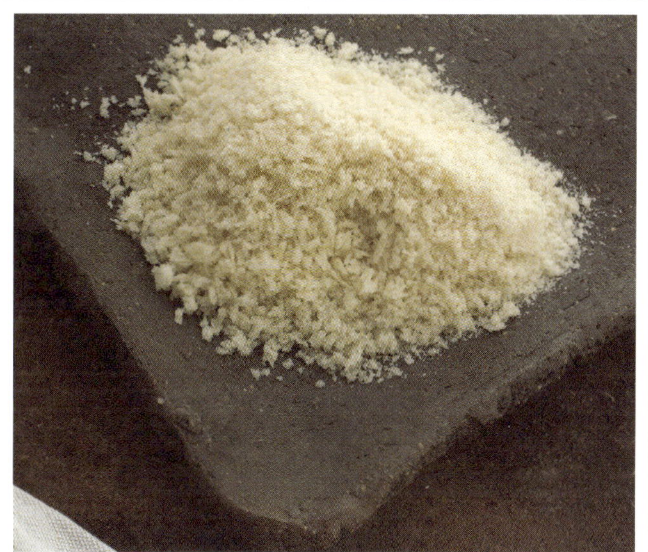

Homemade Breadcrumbs

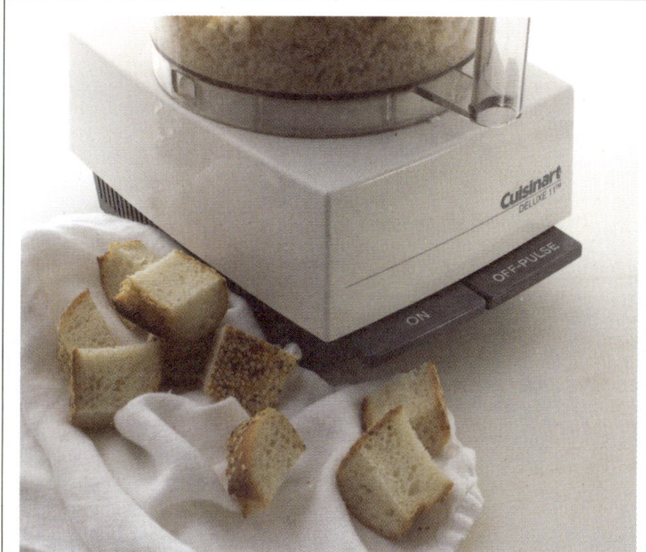

- Panko breadcrumbs are popular in Southeast Asian cooking. *Panko* means 'breadcrumbs' in Japanese.

- These breadcrumbs are made from a light white crustless bread.

- They are delightfully crisp when used in frying and baking all kinds of meat, fish and vegetables.

- You can buy panko breadcrumbs at Asian markets and in some large supermarkets.

- Fresh breadcrumbs are made with soft bread, which toasts nicely when used as a coating or crust.

- Toast and stale bread can also be used to make breadcrumbs. Cut bread into large cubes and whirl them in a food processor.

- For seasoned breadcrumbs, add garlic powder, dried oregano or any other dried herb, salt, ground black or white pepper and/or dried citrus zest.

151

GRANDMA'S FILLETS OF SOLE

Fillet of sole is a sweet and delicate fish that's wonderful when roasted

This sautéed fillet of sole is topped with 'Grandma's crust', a combination of breadcrumbs, mushrooms and lemon zest.

The fish is served with plenty of fresh rocket. Because sole is so delicate, it's important not to overwhelm it with strong herbs, spices or aromatic vegetables, such as garlic. If you do that, the subtle flavour is lost.

Sole (either lemon or Dover) is also good grilled and served plain, dressed simply with lemon and parsley. If you plan to roast the fish for a group, buy fillets or each person or roast the fish whole, and garnish it with lots of goodies. Ask your fishmonger how best to prepare the whole fish for cooking.

Ingredients

Serves 4

4 150-g sole fillets

1 tablespoon olive oil

1 tablespoon lemon juice

1 teaspoon each fresh lemon zest and fresh orange zest

Salt and freshly ground pepper to taste

40 g fine dry breadcrumbs

Garnish: sprigs of fresh parsley

Calories 188, **Fat** 5 g, **Carbohydrates** 10 g, **Protein** 26 g, **Fibre** 1 g, **Saturated Fat** 2 g, **Cholesterol** 59 mg, **Sodium** 368 mg.

Grandma's Fillets of Sole

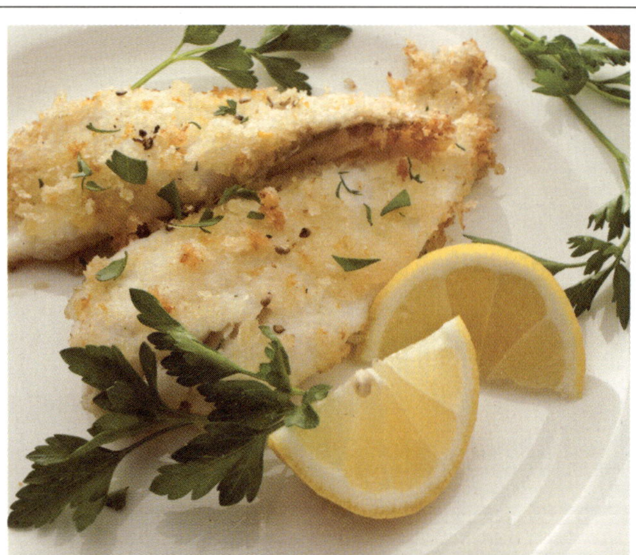

- Set sole fillets on a piece of greaseproof paper.

- Heat oil in a large nonstick pan over medium heat. Add olive oil. Sprinkle fish with lemon juice.

- Mix the zest, salt, pepper and breadcrumbs together. Spread on the sole.

- Sauté the sole for 3–4 minutes per side, until golden brown but not falling apart.

When Is the Fish Done?

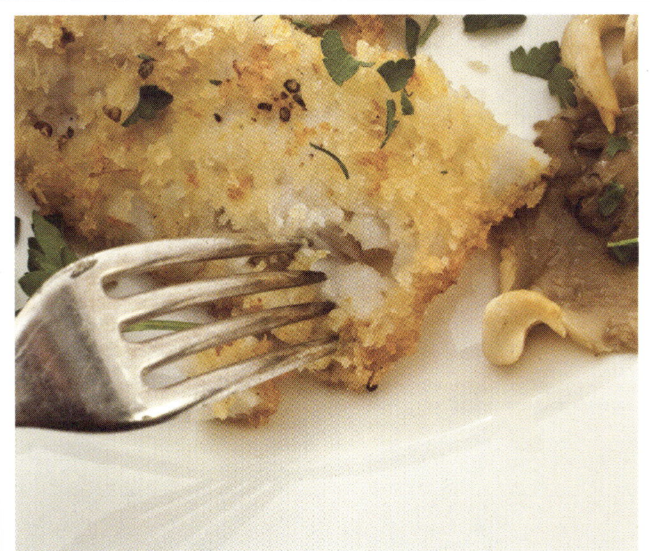

- Cookbooks used to say that fish is done when it flakes when separated with a fork.

- Today, chefs and cooks prefer not to overcook fish. Overcooking dries it out and can even make it tough.

- This method of cooking fish quickly at high heat is a good one. If the fish is very thick, it's better to brown it under the grill and then bake it.

- Learn to listen to the fish and what to look for; listen for the sizzle, and look for a delicate browning on top. Your fish will be perfectly done.

Pan-Frying Fish

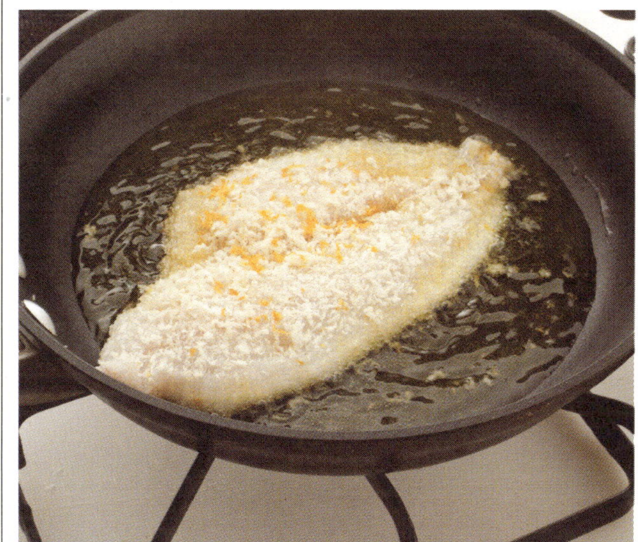

- When sautéing fish, you can make a sauce with fresh tomatoes, mushrooms, spinach, or almost anything you enjoy.

- When the fish has been turned, cook for another 2 minutes then place on a warmed plate, and cover.

- Add 115 g fresh spinach, or a chopped onion to the pan and cook until softened.

- If necessary, stir in 25 ml dry white wine or 1 teaspoon extra olive oil. Keep stirring, and then add to the fish.

MUSSELS IN WHITE WINE SAUCE

Low in calories and cholesterol, mussels are an easy-to-make delicacy

This dish is simple to prepare and a true classic. It makes a wonderful sauce that is excellent when mopped up with crusty toasted chunks of multigrain bread or served with pasta.

Mussels are a terrific source of protein. Most mussels in the market are farm raised and do not need scrubbing, but they do usually have 'beards', which are easy to pull off.

The beards enable the mussels to cling to rocks or posts when they are in the sea. They grow well along rocky shores and in bays, inlets and areas where the water is clean and frequently changing.

Mussels are very low in calories and very low in fat.

Ingredients

Serves 4

1.5 kg fresh live mussels

2 tablespoons olive oil

2–3 cloves garlic, peeled and chopped

1 shallot, peeled and chopped

Small bunch fresh flat-leaf parsley, washed and chopped

Freshly ground black pepper to taste

150 ml dry white wine

Calories 251, **Fat** 13 g, **Carbohydrates** 4 g, **Protein** 31 g, **Fibre** 0, **Saturated Fat** 2 g, **Cholesterol** 83 mg, **Sodium** 734 mg.

Mussels in White Wine Sauce

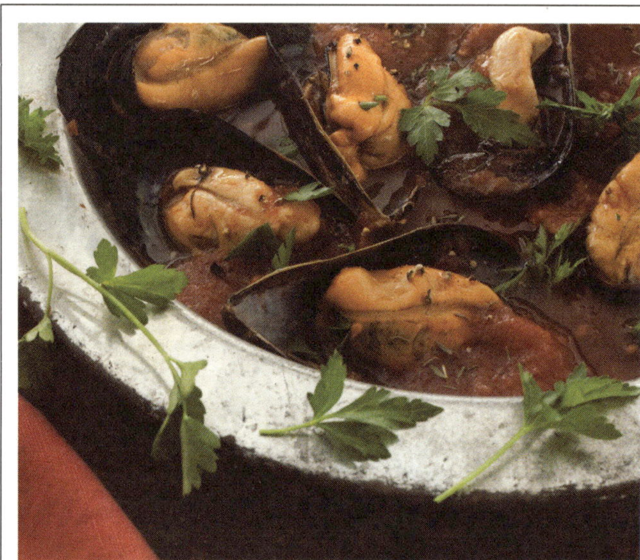

- Check mussels for cleanliness and liveliness. Rinse in cold water and remove beards. Set aside.

- Warm oil in a large pan over medium-high heat.

- Sauté garlic and shallot for about 4 minutes, until softened. Add remaining ingredients. Add mussels; cover pan and cook over high heat until the mussels have opened.

- As mussels open, transfer them to a large bowl. A nice touch is to remove the top shell of each. Cook down the sauce, reducing it by half, and pour over mussels.

Mussels are versatile, and a great dish to serve on any occasion. They are wonderful with 50 ml cream added to this basic recipe, or can be cooked in any marinara sauce. They mix well with garlic, and do more than well when cooked with shallots. Herbs are also outstanding with mussels. You can't go wrong by steaming mussels and serving them with a bit of melted low-fat margarine and lemon. Or try them just in their own stock with a touch of lemon juice. When cooked, mussels release a lot of juice, which is delicious and greatly enhances the flavour of fish soups, stews and pies. Never add salt to mussels, as they have quite a bit of salt in their systems.

Checking that Mussels Are Alive

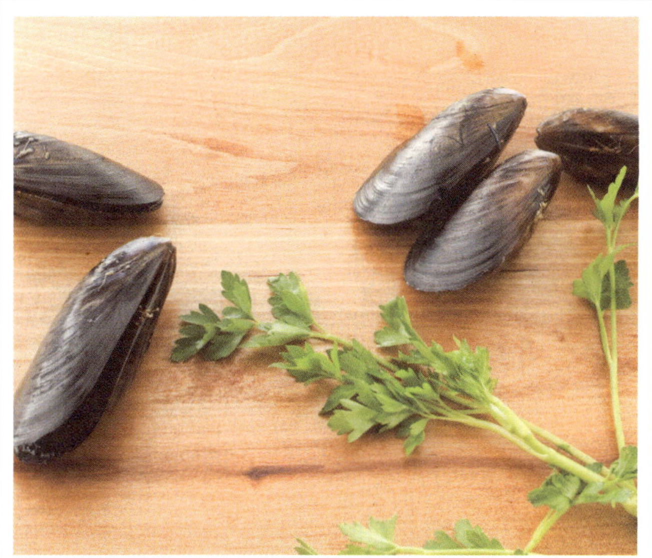

- Never, ever, cook a dead mussel. Live mussels open and close on their own. If you tap an open mussel against a closed one, it should close.

- Listen for a sharp click, not a hollow sound, when tapping mussels together. Give them all a chance to close.

- Discard any mussel that does not close; after cooking, discard any that does not open. Discard any cracked mussels.

Safe Seafood

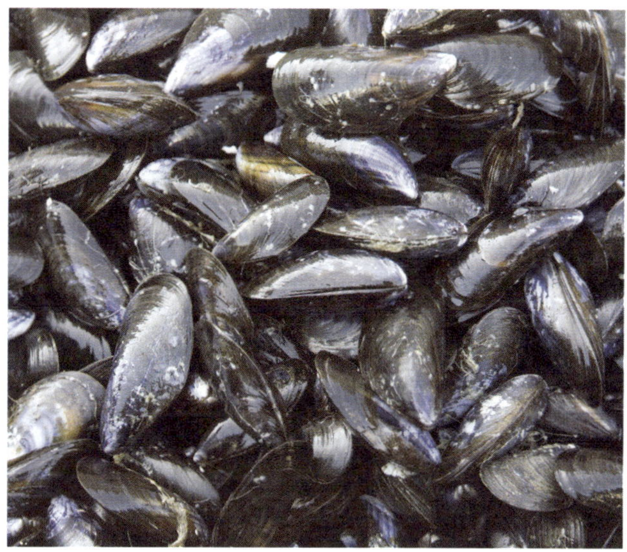

- Shipments of fresh raw fish and other seafood should be tagged to show the area of origin – in the case of mussels, where they were harvested.

- Any reputable seafood seller should be happy to show you the area of origin. If not, go elsewhere.

- If you live on the coast, you can probably bypass the retailers and go straight to the source.

- Find out the date of collection. And remember, if a mussel doesn't close prior to cooking or doesn't open when cooked, discard it. Be safe.

BREADED SCALLOPS & PRAWNS

This recipe calls for baking scallops and prawns rather than sautéing them

This recipe can be finished at the last minute with a little lee-way. Most dishes of this kind are sautéed over very high heat. This one is baked, which gives you a little more time between cooking and serving.

Scallops and prawns together are a natural combination, although scallops are molluscs and prawns are crustaceans.

Frozen raw prawns are fine, but if you can get fresh-caught prawns, the dish will sparkle.

Two types of scallop are generally available in Britain, large king scallops and the smaller, slightly cheaper queen scallops. Hand-dived fresh scallops are the best and the most environmentally friendly.

Ingredients

Serves 4

75 g fresh breadcrumbs

3 cloves garlic, peeled and chopped

1 1/2 teaspoons dried oregano

2 teaspoons sweet Hungarian paprika

Salt and freshly ground pepper to taste

50 ml olive oil

Juice and zest of 1/2 lemon

225 g raw prawns, peeled and cleaned

450 g scallops, rinsed

Garnish: sprigs of flat-leaf parsley and lemon wedges

Calories 451, **Fat** 18 g, **Carbohydrates** 34 g, **Protein** 34 g, **Fibre** 3 g, **Saturated Fat** 3 g, **Cholesterol** 131 mg, **Sodium** 566 mg.

Breaded Scallops and Prawns

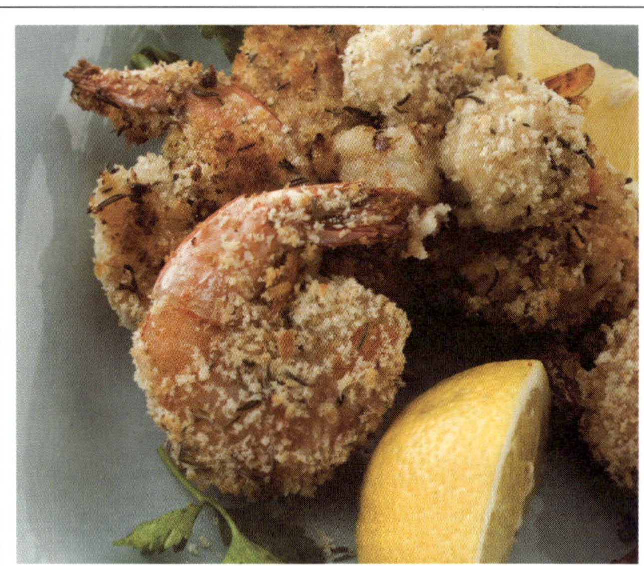

- Preheat oven to 200°C.

- Mix the first seven ingredients together, in the order listed, in a bowl large enough to hold the prawns and scallops. Toss the seafood into the mixture and coat well.

- Oil a baking tray and turn seafood on to it.

- Bake until the crumbs are lightly browned and the prawns are pink. Sprinkle with sprigs of fresh parsley, and serve with fresh lemon wedges.

The fresher, the better: As long as you use fresh or frozen raw seafood, not precooked, you'll get great results. If the seafood is precooked and you then cook it some more, it will become rubbery. If you decide to use clams, allow 6–8 per person. Simply open them and add them, raw, to the mixture described in this recipe.

• • • • • RECIPE VARIATION • • • • •

Fun variations: Use 50 ml grapefruit juice instead of lemon juice. Or substitute tomato juice for its lower acid content. Add 150 g cup chopped tomatoes. Add 100 g per person white crabmeat. Or use lobster claws and prawns (lobster meat should be parboiled). Add 25 g per person to the weight if you buy prawns in shells.

Rinse and Dry Seafood

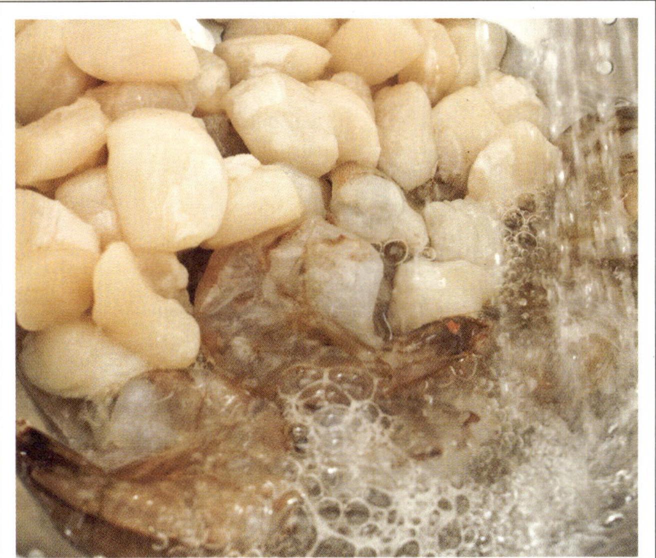

- The reason for rinsing seafood is to remove any sticky matter before cooking.

- After rinsing, dry the seafood on paper towels.

- It is important to dry the seafood if you will be baking it with crumbs so that the crumbs won't get soggy when coating the seafood.

- If you are sautéing, the water will cause your oil to snap and hiss, making it difficult to cook the seafood properly.

Moistening Food with Oil or Wine

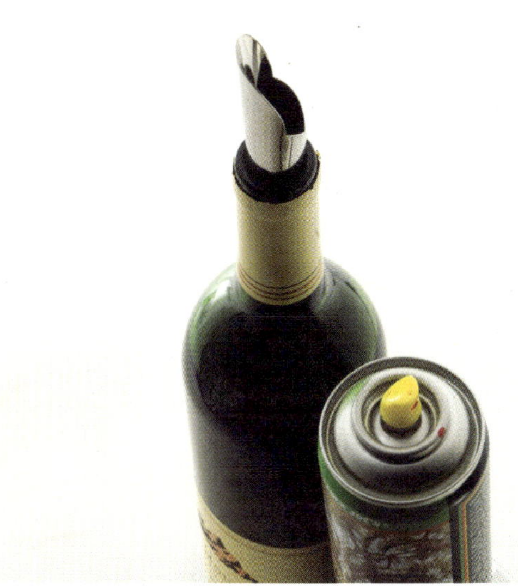

- Because breadcrumbs vary greatly, you may need to moisten yours while baking.

- Prawns and scallops also vary in their moisture content.

- Spraying on some extra oil or wine slows the cooking process.

SEARED KING SCALLOPS

King scallops are huge and rather expensive but definitely worth it

The sauce that accompanies these scallops has solid Caribbean influences. Although the sauce itself is not strongly flavoured, it is distinctive. The sweetness of the sauce comes from the natural flavour of coconut milk. The spikiness of lime juice, hot pepper and ginger combine for a piquant touch.

It's advisable always to buy hand-dived scallops for the best quality and because dredging for scallops destroys the sea bed.

Scallops have two large shells, one flat and one curved, which make excellent and attractive containers in which to serve sea-food dishes. They last for a long time and can be cleaned easily if you oil them before use.

Try this dish with couscous or brown rice. Balance your carbs and proteins, however, if you do so.

Ingredients

Serves 4

For the sauce:

250 ml unsweetened coconut milk

1 teaspoon freshly grated ginger

1 teaspoon cayenne pepper, or to taste

1 teaspoon sweet Hungarian paprika

1 teaspoon sesame seed oil

Juice of 1 fresh lime

Salt to taste

For the scallops:

2 tablespoons cooking oil, such as canola

450 g king scallops, rinsed and dried

Garnish: sprigs of coriander and lime wedges

Optional: couscous or brown rice to accompany

Calories 288, **Fat** 21 g, **Carbohydrates** 7 g, **Protein** 20 g, **Fibre** 0, **Saturated Fat** 12 g, **Cholesterol** 37 mg, **Sodium** 191 mg.

Seared King Scallops

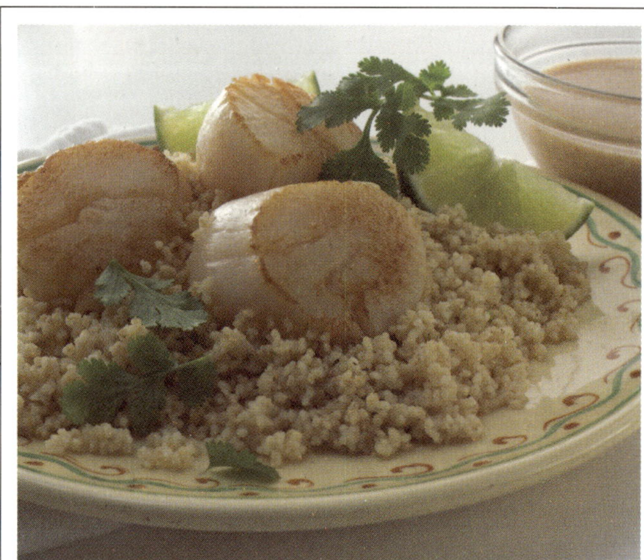

- In a saucepan, whisk all the sauce ingredients together and warm over very low heat. Keep warm.

- Prepare couscous or rice, if using. Warm plates.

- Heat cooking oil in a nonstick pan over high heat. Add scallops, and sear quickly until golden brown on each side, no more than 1 minute per side.

- Arrange scallops over couscous or rice, if using. Spoon sauce over the top of each serving and garnish.

All about scallops: Scallops are sold in two sizes: large kings and much smaller queens. They are collected either by hand (hand-dived) or machine (dredged). They are sweet and succulent, and only become tough if they are overcooked. Don't worry about cooking them through – you just want them to be hot inside and seared on the outside.

• • • • RECIPE VARIATION • • • •

With a Cajun accent: Affordable queen scallops can be used in spicy Cajun dishes. Coat 450 g scallops with a sprinkling of paprika, white pepper and allspice, then fry the scallops in 2 teaspoons olive oil for 2–3 minutes. Your favourite light cream sauce will help keep the heat under control. Serve with brown rice and a medley of vegetables on the side.

Hot Food and Cold Plates Don't Mix

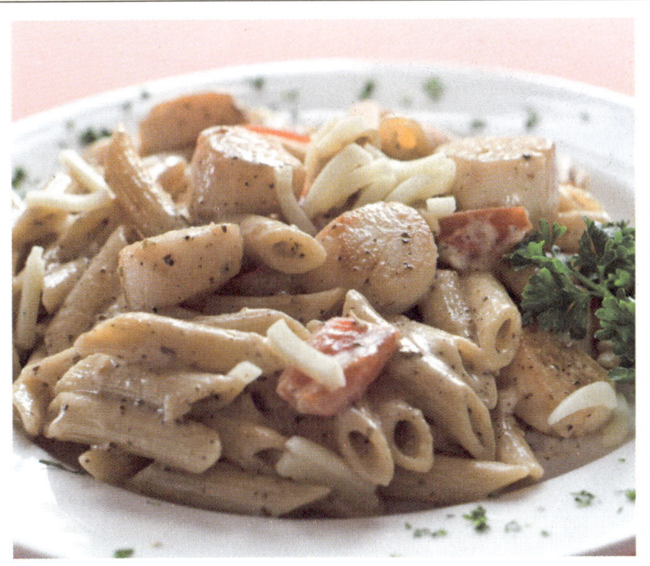

Garnishes for Caribbean-Style Dishes

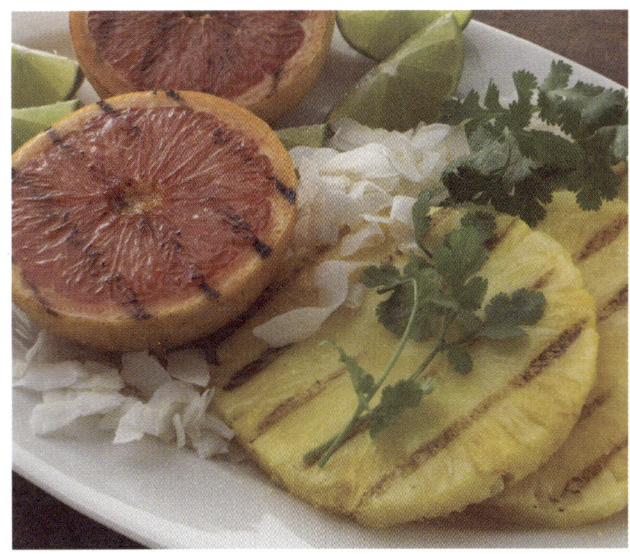

- A well-trained chef will warm plates for hot food and chill plates for cold food.

- Newer ovens have a separate warming area. If you have a double oven you can use the smaller one for warming plates.

- Hot trays are excellent for buffets when you wish to keep both the food and the plates warm.

- When serving cold salads or desserts in hot weather, put the plates in the refrigerator for a while.

- Apart from limes and coriander, there are many fun things to use as garnishes for these exotic dishes.

- Small chunks of grilled pineapple, shredded fresh coconut, and grilled coconut chips are all wonderful.

- Try serving a grilled grapefruit half with each portion. Avocados, sliced and sprinkled with lime juice, are also very colourful and tasty.

- Note that these garnishes are not in the analysis of this dish, and they add carbohydrates and fat.

SAUTÉED SOFT-SHELL CRABS

A seasonal speciality of the American Atlantic coast, soft-shell crabs are becoming popular around the world

Fresh soft-shell crabs are a great delicacy, available at times when crabs are shedding their old shells and before their new, larger shells harden. A crab needs to be eaten within 4 days of moulting to have a completely soft, edible shell. The species eaten varies around the world. Chesapeake Bay is famous for its soft-shelled blue crabs, which are also eaten around the Gulf of Mexico. The Asian mangrove crab is also eaten in this form, and good quality soft-shell crabs imported from Thailand are available frozen in Britain.

Sautéed soft-shell crabs require just the tiniest bit of flour, not a lot of breading. Olive oil mixed with canola or groundnut oil is the cooking medium of choice, not butter.

Ingredients

Serves 4

8 large (7.5–10 cm across) or 12 small (7.5 cm across) soft-shell crabs

Juice of $^1/_2$ fresh lemon

Salt and cayenne pepper to taste

25 g plain flour

50 ml mixture of olive and canola oil

50 g slivered raw almonds

Garnish: lemon halves

Calories 368, **Fat** 22 g, **Carbohydrates** 10 g, **Protein** 32 g, **Fibre** 2 g, **Saturated Fat** 3 g, **Cholesterol** 97 mg, **Sodium** 560 mg.

Sautéed Soft-Shell Crabs

- Rinse crabs in cold water and dry with paper towels. Sprinkle with lemon juice.

- Sprinkle crabs on both sides with salt and cayenne pepper; dust with flour.

- In a large frying pan, heat oil to the smoking stage.

- Add crabs and brown quickly on both sides. Drain on paper towels.

- In the same pan, sauté almonds until light golden. Place crabs on warm plates and sprinkle with almonds. Garnish with lemon wedges.

More about crabs: As with any seafood, make sure the crabs you buy smell fresh. The soft shell comes about after the hard shell is sloughed off and before a new, larger one is formed. The shells of soft-shell crabs should be tender and edible. As they start to harden they reach a stage when they are described as 'papershells', when the shells start to be crunchy and are less appetizing. Once the crab has acquired its new, hard shell its flavour and your cooking technique are different. European brown crabs are available all year round, and are sold either live or cooked. You can buy dressed fresh crab ready to eat from supermarkets and fishmongers.

A Soft-Shell Crab Sauce

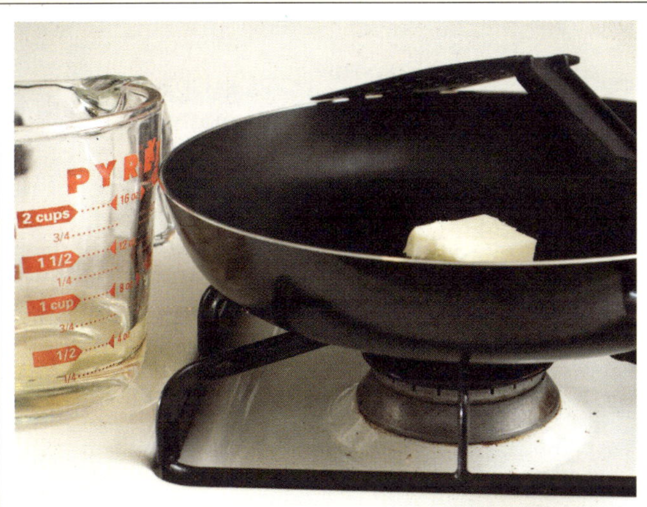

- This sauce will add flavour and interest to your soft-shell crabs.

- While the crabs are draining, remove the sautéed almonds to a bowl. Stir 120 ml dry white wine, such as Chardonnay, into the pan.

- Bring to the boil. Add a pat of unsalted butter to the pan.

- Return the nuts to the sauté pan, and pour over the crabs.

Tartar Sauce for Crabs

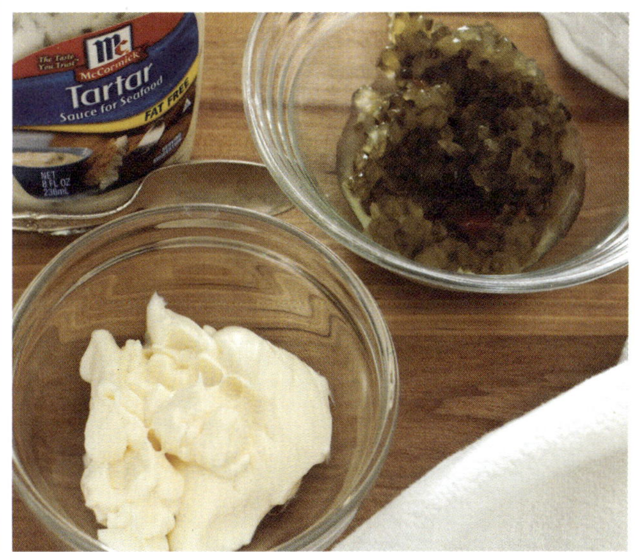

- Tartar sauce is the perfect accompaniment to most fish and other seafood.

- Bottled tartar sauce contains a lot of sugar and salt. It is easy to make your own healthier version.

- Simply mix 1 tablespoon sweet green relish (hot dog relish) with 120 ml low-fat mayonnaise.

- Mix in 2 tablespoons lemon juice and a dash of cayenne pepper, and your sauce is ready.

MIXED SEAFOOD BARBECUE

Say hello to spring or farewell to summer with this seafood feast

This recipe is especially great to serve for your first barbecue party in the spring or the last one in the autumn.

You can make a series of dipping sauces for a mixed seafood platter. Change the mixture according to the occasion, mood or even the weather. Cooking seafood on a metal platter or baking tray on the barbecue adds a wonderful smoky flavour that is enhanced with wood chips.

Plan on using 225 g of shellfish per person. Remember, shells are heavy.

To cut back on the calories, try eating the seafood with just a bit of lemon juice or an olive oil and garlic mixture.

Ingredients

Serves 4

For the basting sauce:

250 ml homemade chili sauce, sugar-free or low-sugar

Juice of $^1/_2$ lemon

2 strips orange peel

50 ml cooking oil

For the seafood:

24 clams, cleaned and checked for liveliness

24 mussels, cleaned and checked for liveliness (see page 155)

2 live lobsters, cut into sections: remove claws and knuckles, and cut tails in 5-cm chunks crosswise; or 900 g crabs or crab claws, cut into 5-cm chunks

450 g jumbo prawns, in shells

Calories 276, **Fat** 9 g, **Carbohydrates** 7 g, **Protein** 43 g, **Fibre** 1 g, **Saturated Fat** 1 g, **Cholesterol** 165 mg, **Sodium** 1295 mg.

Mixed Seafood Barbecue

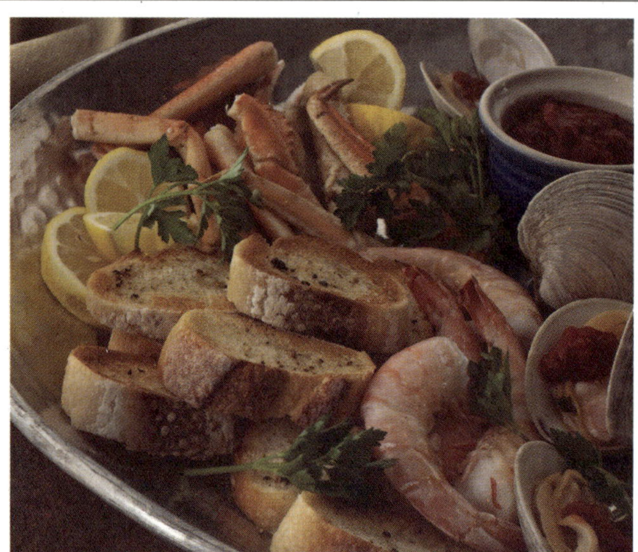

- Heat barbecue or set grill on high. Mix sauce ingredients in a bowl. Wash all the seafood and pat dry.

- Place seafood on a metal pan to be cooked in stages in the order listed at left.

- Start barbecuing or grilling clams and mussels; when they start to open, add lobster or crab, and, if using live lobster, cook until it turns red. When everything is almost done, add prawns. Cook until prawns turn pink.

- As seafood opens, brush with sauce. Let guests peel their own prawns.

This recipe calls for a variety of seafood, cooked in stages. You put the prawns on last, as they cook faster than the rest. You can use any crabmeat: brown crabs or spider crabs aren't usually considered for barbecuing, but it gives the meat a delicious flavour. When lobsters are plentiful and not overly expensive, they make an excellent addition to this mixed platter. Unshelled prawns, the bigger the better, are fine. Or use langoustine or crayfish. Clams and mussels in their shells will pop open when the heat hits them. You could also consider adding scallops threaded on skewers, or squid, which need only a brief searing.

Cooking Scallops and Prawns

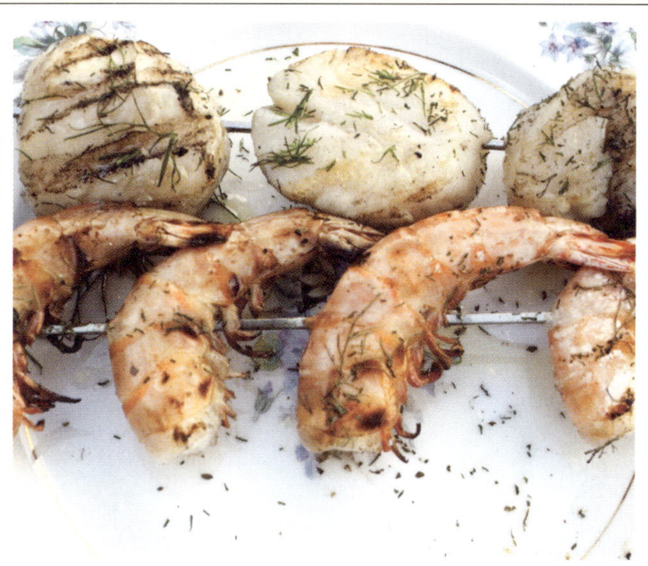

Saucing Seafood

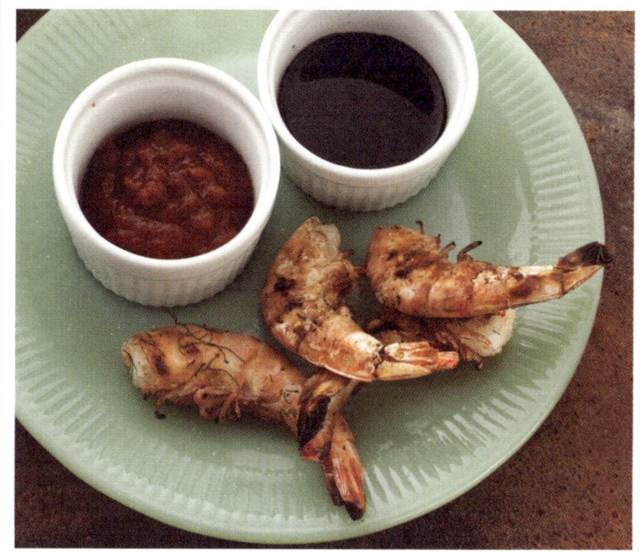

- Always put prawns and scallops on the barbecue or under the grill last.

- They will cook fast; uncooked prawns often need only about 30 seconds per side. They will turn light pink in colour and coil into the shape of a C.

- Start grilling or barbecuing clams, then add mussels or lobster chunks.

- If you are using precooked crab, defrost it if frozen and put it on with the prawns.

- Adding sauce to seafood while on the barbecue or under the grill seals in the natural flavours.

- After you've grilled the seafood, offer your guests an Asian dipping sauce that starts with 120 ml soy sauce. Add 1 teaspoon each chopped fresh ginger, lemon juice and sesame oil.

- Classic cocktail sauce is always very good. Mix 120 ml chilli sauce with 1 teaspoon each of Worcestershire, horseradish and lemon juice.

- Any simple vinaigrette is also terrific with seafood.

BASIC POLENTA

As an appetizer or side dish, polenta is so simple, so versatile, so delicious

Polenta is cooked cornmeal, a staple of the Native American diet and a key ingredient in the cooking of Italy, from where it gets its name. It can be served soft and warm, or allowed to harden for grilling and sautéing. It's a high-fibre food that can be reheated and used again the next day. Liven up basic polenta with the addition of various ingredients. It is especially tasty when topped with tomato sauce, meat gravies, seafood or grilled vegetables.

Ready-made polenta is a bit expensive. Because it's so very simple to make, it's not necessary to buy it. If you make double quantities, you can turn half into a polenta roll and refrigerate it for a few days or freeze it for up to a month.

Ingredients

Serves 8

1 litre water

1 teaspoon salt

115 g coarse-ground cornmeal

Freshly ground black pepper to taste

Optional:

40 g grated Parmesan cheese

Small bunch parsley, rinsed and chopped

1 tablespoon dried rosemary, or 3 tablespoons fresh, chopped

Calories 55, **Fat** 1 g, **Carbohydrates** 12 g, **Protein** 43 g, **Fibre** 1 g, **Saturated Fat** 0, **Cholesterol** 0, **Sodium** 296 mg

Basic Polenta

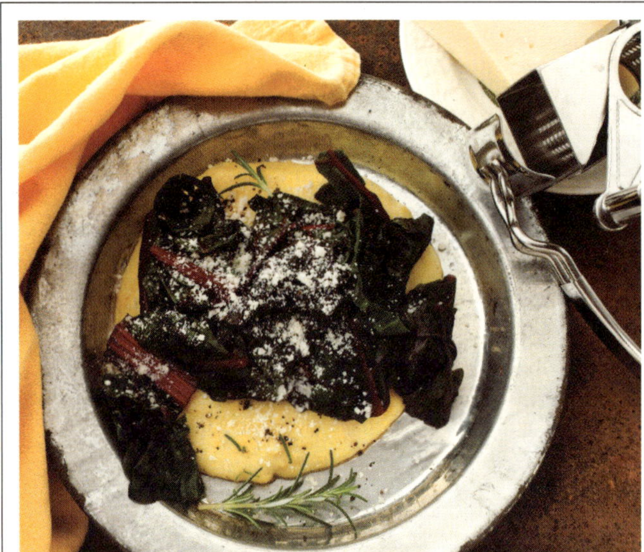

- Bring salted water to the boil in a heavy-bottomed saucepan (nonstick is best).

- Add cornmeal in a thin stream, very slowly, stirring constantly with a wooden spoon.

- Keep stirring until the polenta reaches the consistency of mashed potatoes. Add black pepper.

- If desired, add grated Parmesan cheese, herbs or whatever you desire.

Enhanced polenta: This recipe can be made richer by substituting 1 litre semi-skimmed milk for water and adding 1 tablespoon low-fat margarine. Add 40 g grated Parmesan cheese when the polenta is almost ready to serve. The cheese melts into the hot polenta for a savoury flavour. Or add 2 tablespoons extra-virgin olive oil to the hot polenta for a smooth consistency.

Adding herbs: Various herbs, fresh or dried, make excellent variations. A generous pinch or two of basil, marjoram, oregano and rosemary is recommended. You can use herbs individually or in combination. A handful of chopped fresh parsley is also a terrific addition. Remember, dried herbs are far more concentrated than fresh, so use less and taste often.

Stir Polenta Constantly

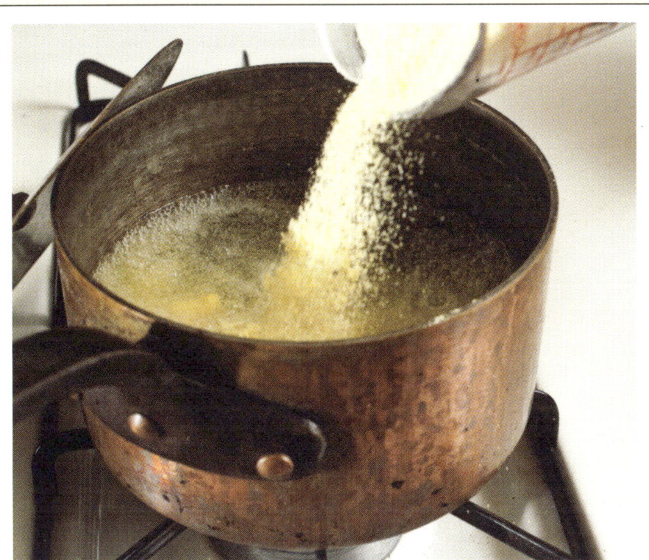

Making Polenta More Healthy

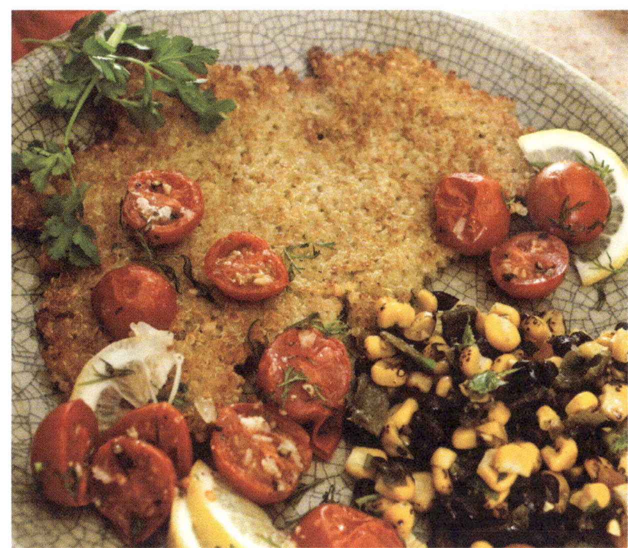

- There is a good reason for adding the cornmeal slowly and stirring it constantly.

- If you add the cornmeal all at once, you will end up with a gummy clump that cannot be saved.

- What you want is smooth, creamy polenta. Going slowly and stirring constantly will result in a lovely, smooth texture.

- For a thicker consistency, increase the cooking time by a minute or two.

- Adding vegetables to polenta will make it more attractive and nutritious by adding fibre.

- The addition of grilled or roasted chopped vegetables turns polenta into a wonderful side dish.

- Grilled and chopped cherry tomatoes are another tasty way to make your polenta healthy.

- Add the vegetables, then bake the polenta with 25 g Parmesan cheese sprinkled on top.

SAUTÉED POLENTA

Sautéed until golden brown, polenta can be fresh and fragrant or saucy and spicy

Polenta can be formed into squares or rounds for sautéing. Traditionally, it is sautéed in butter or deep fried in oil. Neither of these methods is recommended, as they load on the calories. Instead, use a skim of olive or canola oil in the pan.

Serve sautéed polenta dressed with onions and black beans for lunch. Or top polenta squares or rounds with a hearty tomato sauce, sliced black olives and a sprinkling of Parmesan cheese for a light supper.

Polenta can be spiced up with the addition of dried chilli flakes or chopped, canned chipotle chillies. Make mini polenta cakes and load salsa or guacamole on top for a fabulous party snack.

Ingredients

Serves 4

1 tablespoon olive oil

1 onion, finely chopped

2 cloves garlic, peeled and finely chopped

1 teaspoon dried oregano or other favourite herbs

40 g cooked sweetcorn (optional)

40 g finely chopped hot or sweet peppers (optional)

1 quantity cooked polenta, still warm (see recipe, page 164)

1 tablespoon canola or olive oil

Calories 108, **Fat** 5 g, **Carbohydrates** 14 g, **Protein** 4 g, **Fibre** 1 g, **Saturated Fat** 1 g, **Cholesterol** 4 mg, **Sodium** 234 mg.

Sautéed Polenta

- Place a large, nonstick pan over medium heat. Add oil, onion and garlic; stir. Cook until softened, about 4 minutes. Stir in oregano, corn and peppers. Add polenta.

- Oil a sheet of heavy-duty aluminium foil. Spread polenta on the foil and smooth evenly. Cover with cling film and refrigerate for at least 2 hours.

- Cut polenta into rounds using a biscuit cutter.

- Heat oil in a large, nonstick frying pan on medium-high heat. Sauté polenta cakes until golden brown on both sides.

Cooked polenta may be smoothed on to an oiled tray or heavy-duty aluminium foil. When hot, polenta doesn't hold its shape. As it cools, it congeals, and then you can cut it into squares or rounds with a plain cutter. Cook polenta the day before and spread it on foil, cover with plastic and refrigerate overnight. You can't make squares or patties with hot polenta – they won't hold.

Flavouring polenta: While the polenta is still hot, stir in 25 g Parmesan cheese, 1 tablespoon of your favourite dried herbs, ½ onion, chopped, 40 g cooked sweetcorn and/or chopped peppers, or whatever you plan to use as flavouring.

Sautéing Food

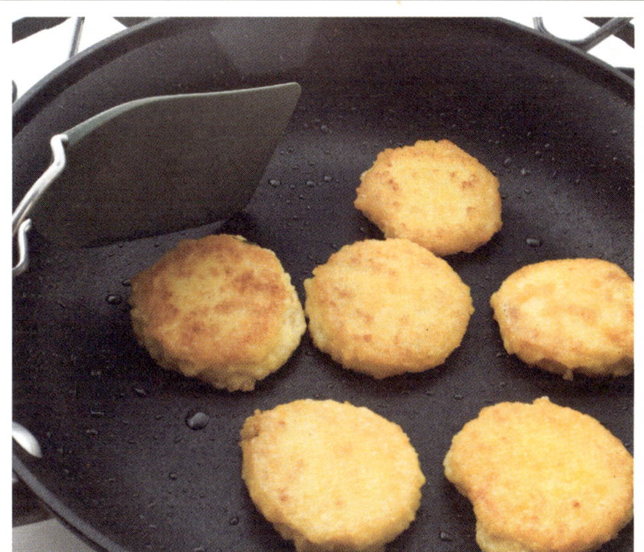

Working with Warm Polenta

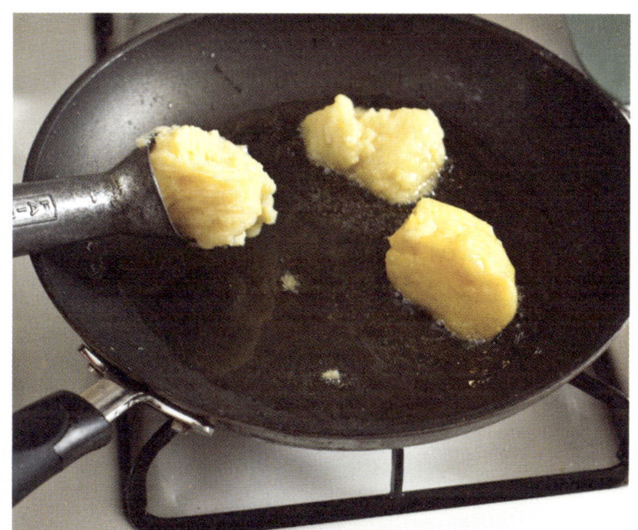

- The sauté technique is the basis of many recipes. It's a simple way to prepare highly flavourful meals.

- Sauté pans come in all sizes. Use an 18-cm pan for single-serving dishes; a 25-cm pan for double servings. Start with a tiny bit of oil over medium heat in a nonstick pan. Add food to be sautéed. Turn when either lightly browned or softened. For crisp results, heat the pan before adding oil..

- Have the food at room temperature before sautéeing.

- Allow the polenta to harden, then cut into left-over soups, such as chicken or turkey.

- If you do not have time to let the polenta cool, scoop it up with an ice-cream scoop and place it in the freezer on greaseproof paper for 10 minutes.

- If your polenta is still warm, however, it will take less time to cook.

- While it's in the pan, smooth the top down with the back of the ice-cream scoop. When it's nicely browned on one side, turn it.

QUINOA RISOTTO WITH CHICKPEAS

Quinoa is highly nutritious and works well with lots of different flavours and textures

Quinoa is grown in Bolivia, Ecuador and Peru. It is a complete food, higher in protein than any other grain. Quinoa sustained the people of the Andes for thousands of years before the Spanish arrived. It is ideally suited for cultivation in otherwise desolate mountain areas. Thinking the quinoa 'barbaric', the Spanish destroyed it, thereby condemning the natives to starvation. The crops introduced by the Spanish did not grow at high altitudes.

Fortunately, quinoa is making a comeback, and cooks love its versatility. Eat it for breakfast, lunch and dinner, as part of a main course or as a side dish. Apart from its protein content, quinoa is good for the digestive system – and it's delicious.

Ingredients

Serves 6

250 ml low-salt or salt-free vegetable or chicken stock

120 ml water

2 tablespoons olive oil

1 onion, finely chopped

1 clove garlic, peeled and chopped

175 g quinoa, rinsed and drained

1 tablespoon dried rosemary

1 teaspoon dried oregano

1 (375-g) can chickpeas, rinsed and drained

2 tablespoons red wine vinegar

Garnish (optional): chopped tomatoes, olives, capers, freshly chopped parsley

Calories 228, **Fat** 7 g, **Carbohydrates** 35 g, **Protein** 7 g, **Fibre** 5 g, **Saturated Fat** 1 g, **Cholesterol** 0, **Sodium** 278 mg.

Quinoa Risotto with Chickpeas

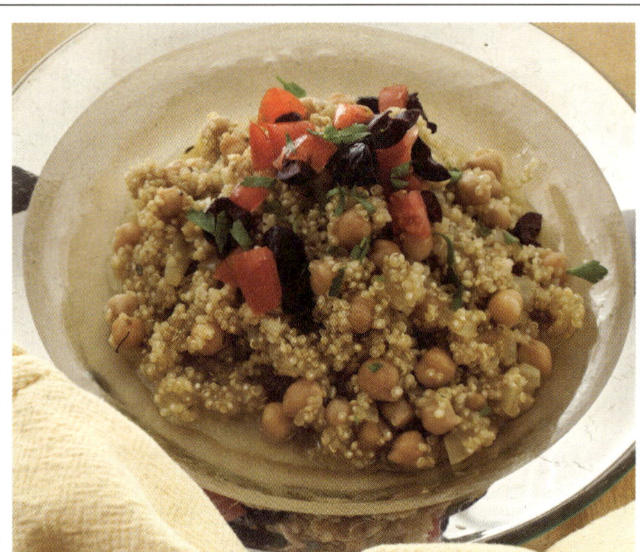

- Place stock and water in a saucepan over medium heat to warm.

- Place oil in a large pan over medium heat. Add onion, garlic and quinoa; stir to mix.

- Slowly add warm stock/water mixture to quinoa, stirring constantly. As soon as it's absorbed and the pan begins to hiss, add a bit more. When all the liquid is absorbed, stir in rosemary, oregano, chickpeas and vinegar.

- Serve warm, cool or at room temperature; garnish as desired.

Rinse Your Quinoa and Beans

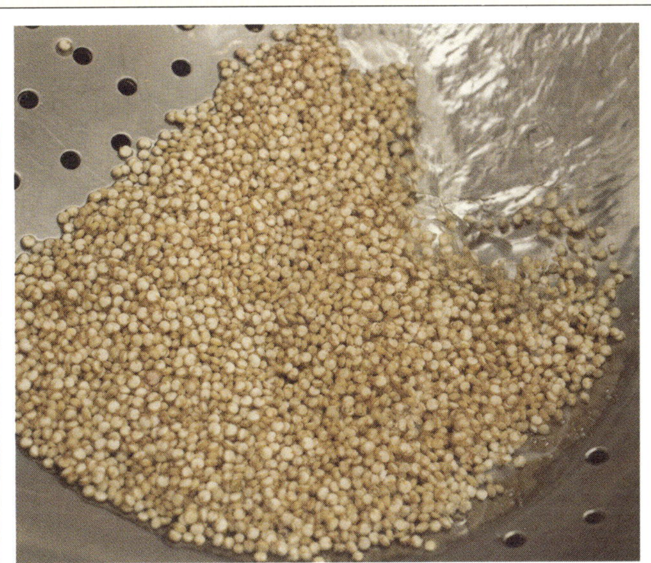

- Rinsing quinoa in a fine sieve will clean it of dirt, dust and foreign bodies, which will appear when the quinoa is wet.

- You must also rinse lentils and dried beans. Like quinoa, beans often contain pebbles and little lumps of dirt.

- A pebble can break a tooth, which is an expensive and avoidable problem.

- A lump of dirt can dissolve when liquids are added, spoiling the taste of the whole dish.

Slow Addition of Liquids

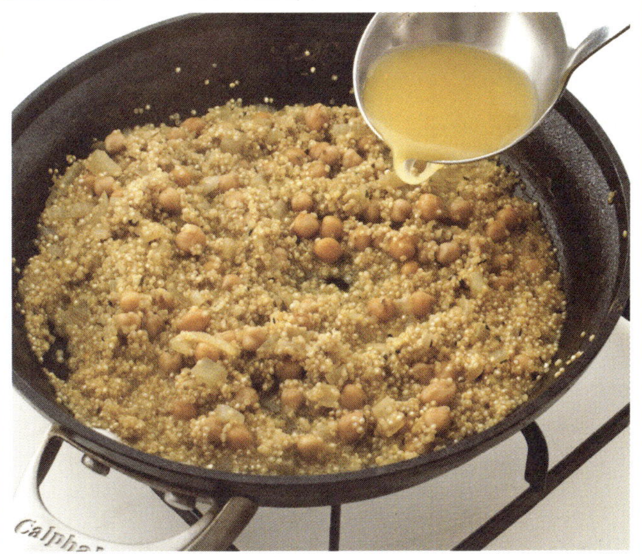

- You can boil quinoa just like rice, which some-times results in a grainy consistency.

- The texture is much nicer if you cook it like risotto. The food will tell you when to add another half-ladle of liquid – it will make slight hissing noises.

- Don't let the onions scorch. As soon as the liquid is absorbed, add another half ladle of stock.

- Watch the quinoa carefully. It takes about 20 minutes to add all the liquid, but you'll be so happy with the results.

SEASONED BROWN RICE

More nutritious than white rice, brown rice has fibre and is very versatile

Brown rice is unprocessed, unpolished, unhulled rice. To get rice to the stage where it is white, the nutritious outer hull is removed with chemicals or through a polishing process. The rice bran, the best part nutritionally, is then used to make bran muffins and bran-based cereals. Thus, brown rice has more flavour, making it far tastier than white rice.

Like white rice, brown rice lends itself to many wonderful food combinations, from the simplest recipes such as this one to the addition of meat, poultry and seafood. Leftover rice is very useful in many next-day dishes, such as salads, soups and stews. It stores very well in the refrigerator for up to a week.

Ingredients

Serves 6

2 tablespoons olive oil

2 medium sweet onions (such as Vidalia), chopped

2 tablespoons fresh rosemary leaves or
1 tablespoon dried rosemary

185 g brown rice

450 ml cups water, chicken stock or vegetable stock

Pinch of salt

Freshly ground black pepper or hot pepper sauce to taste

Calories 169, **Fat** 5 g, **Carbohydrates** 27 g, **Protein** 4 g,
Fibre 2 g, **Saturated Fat** 1 g, **Cholesterol** 0, **Sodium** 142 mg.

Seasoned Brown Rice

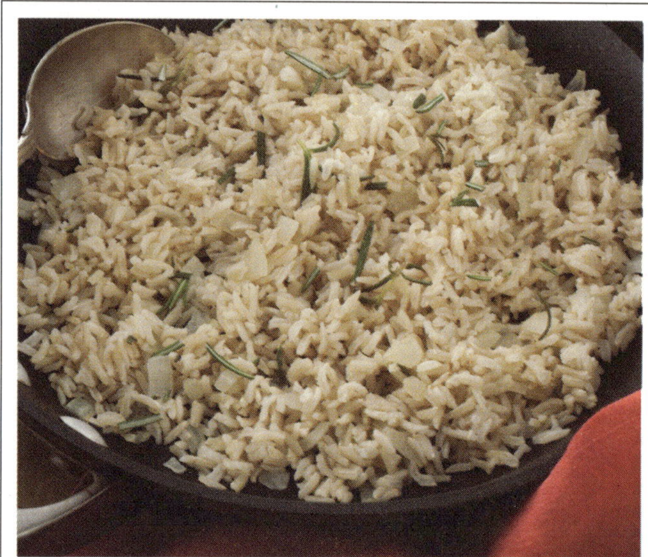

- Preheat oven to 180°C. In a large saucepan, Dutch oven or deep frying pan, heat oil over medium heat.

- Add onions and stir, cooking for about 3 minutes or until translucent. Stir in rosemary and rice, mixing to coat well. Add liquid, salt and pepper.

- Bring to the boil. Cover and place in oven for 40 minutes.

- Remove from oven. Fluff rice and re-cover. Leave to stand for 10 minutes.

Quick-cooking rice with dried fruit: Following the directions on the box, prepare 4 servings of quick-cooking brown rice. As soon as the rice is cooked, add 1 onion, chopped and sautéed; 1 apple, peeled, cored and chopped; 25 g dried cranberries; 25 g toasted walnuts; 1 stick celery, rinsed and chopped; 1 teaspoon dried thyme leaves; and 1 teaspoon fresh lemon zest. Stir to mix, and serve as a side dish.

Using the Proper Pots and Pans

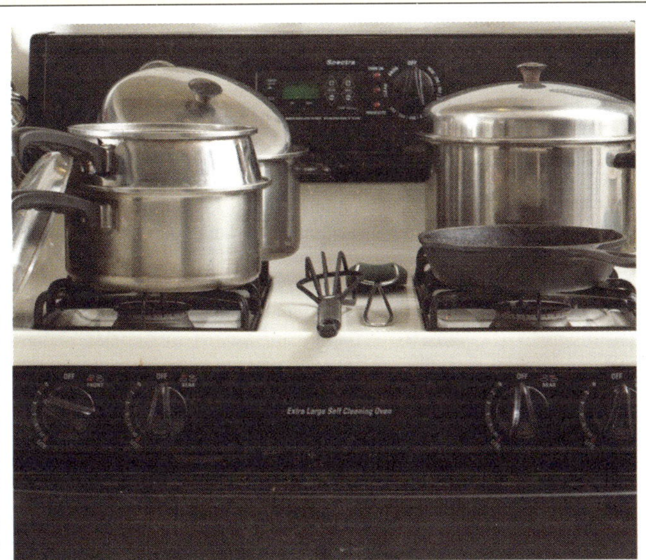

- It's best to use a heavy-bottomed, nonstick pan or Dutch oven for this recipe.

- If you use a thin metal pan, your food will stick and burn. You want slow, even heat.

- You can even use an old-fashioned, heavy-duty, deep cast-iron frying pan, if you have one with a lid.

- Be sure the lid you use fits tightly, in order to keep the steam from escaping.

Make Extra Brown Rice

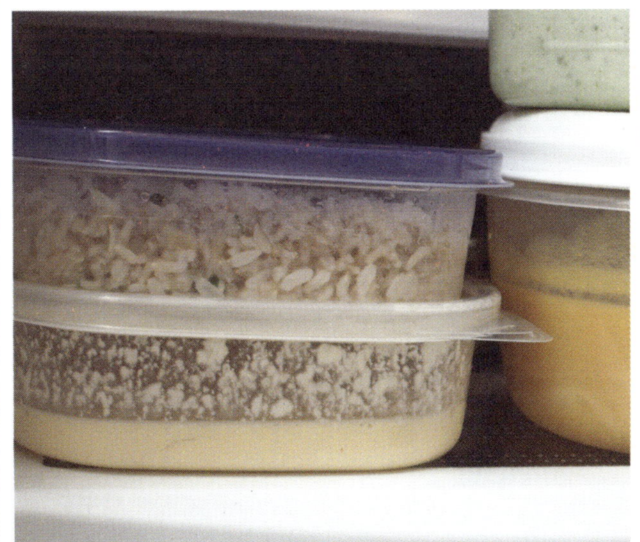

- Cook an extra quantity of brown rice. You'll then be set for tonight's dinner, with leftovers to have for lunch as the base for a salad or as part of another dinner.

- Wise family cooks always make extra quantities of staples like brown rice, whole-wheat dough, quinoa and polenta.

- If you want to lower your blood sugar or work on increasing your energy expenditure, it's important to plan ahead.

- Plan your food, exercise time and some down time.

BROWN RICE, CHICKEN & OLIVES

Brown rice is a great base for dishes with chicken, seafood, pork and aromatic vegetables

This recipe is a delightful combination of harmonious flavours. It's a surprise to find how cooking changes the taste of green olives. You will detect some of the tartness from the olives, but it will meld into the rice and chicken for a subtle overall taste. Lemon and olives are also a natural combination that makes this dish special.

You can double the quantities to serve it for a party. It has a slightly earthy, rustic flair, and it's also very good for people with diabetes because it's high in fibre and protein and low in fat. Also, rice is a carbohydrate that will be absorbed more slowly into the bloodstream, a definite plus.

Ingredients

Serves 6

120 ml olive oil

1 whole chicken, about 1.2 kg, cut into 6 serving pieces

2 tablespoons plain flour

1 teaspoon sea salt or other light salt

$^1/_2$ teaspoon ground black pepper

1 teaspoon sweet paprika

1 onion, coarsely chopped

2 cloves garlic, smashed and peeled

275 g uncooked brown rice

1 litre chicken stock or a mixture of stock and wine

50 g small green, pimiento-stuffed olives

1 tablespoon fresh rosemary

Juice of $^1/_2$ lemon

Calories 497, **Fat** 20 g, **Carbohydrates** 50 g, **Protein** 29 g, **Fibre** 3 g, **Saturated Fat** 4 g, **Cholesterol** 30 mg, **Sodium** 678 mg.

Brown Rice, Chicken and Olives

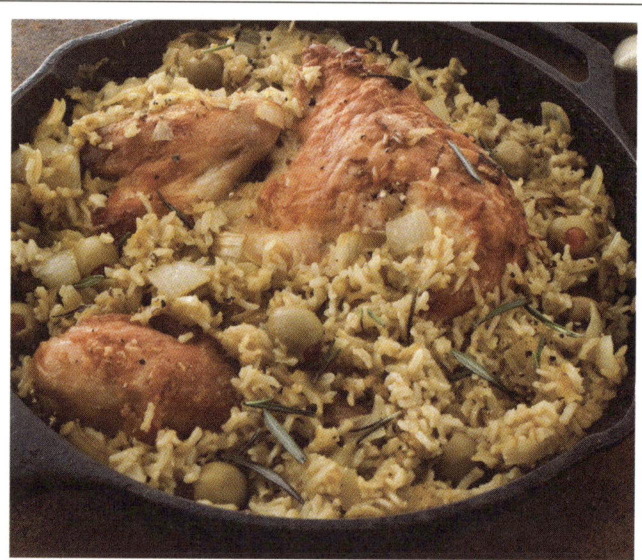

- In a large pan, heat oil over medium heat. Rinse chicken and pat dry. Mix the next four ingredients on a piece of greaseproof paper. Roll chicken in the flour mixture.

- Brown chicken in oil; remove to a plate. Sauté onions and garlic in the oil until soft, about 3 minutes.

- Add rice to sautéed onions and garlic, mixing to coat well. Add liquid, and return chicken to pan. Add olives, rosemary and lemon juice.

- Cover; bake for 50–60 minutes at 180°C. Leave to rest, uncovered, for 5 minutes before serving.

Brown rice with pears: When cooking this dish, you may want to substitute pears for olives to make a savoury/sweet dish. Stir in 2 peeled, cored and chopped pears in place of the olives. The pears, combined with a pinch of thyme or rosemary, will change the dish completely.

Brown rice with capers: Instead of olives add 1 tablespoon capers with a pinch of oregano. For grown-ups, add 1 tablespoon green peppercorns, plus your favourite herbs. Add 120 ml dry white wine to the cooking liquid. For a very sophisticated flavour, use 1 tablespoon each of capers and dry white vermouth instead of white wine.

Brown Rice on the Stove

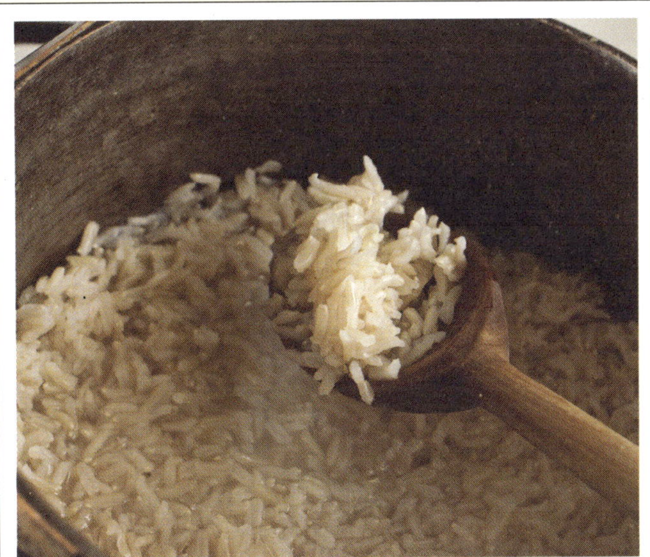

Don't Overload Rice with Liquids

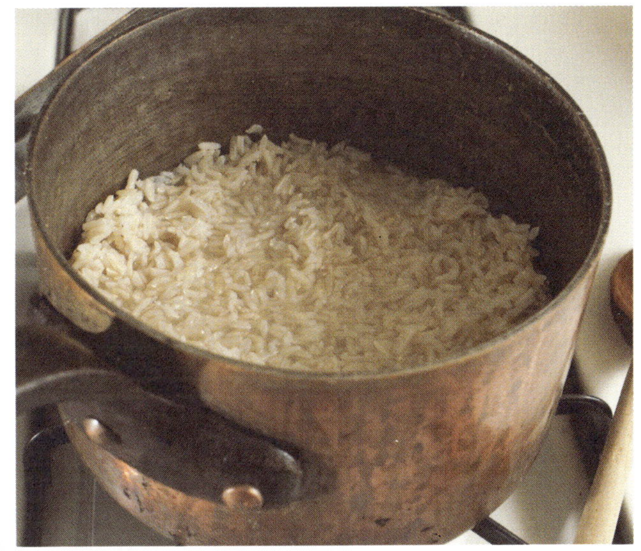

- When you boil rice on the hob, you have to watch it closely; it's easy to burn it or get a sticky mess on the bottom of the pan.

- Use a nonstick pan and stir often. If the rice gets dry, add more stock or water.

- You want the rice to be perfectly done, and brown rice is difficult to overcook.

- If you are rushed and haven't time to stand over it, use quick-cooking brown rice.

- It's better to start by following the directions on the pack.

- Depending on your elevation and the humidity, cooking time will vary, as will amounts of moisture.

- Use a fork to stir the rice often, and add additional water or stock to help keep the rice from drying out.

HIGH-FIBRE FOODS

WHOLE WHEAT WITH VEGETABLES

Whole wheat grains are a terrific source of fibre and a wonderful addition to any diet

Whole wheat grains work well in a slow cooker. Put 350 g wheat in a slow cooker in the morning with at least 1.75 litres water but no salt. Set it on low, cover it and go to work.

If the wheat grains aren't done when you get home, turn the slow cooker temperature up and add more water if necessary. Check occasionally. If they aren't done before you go to bed, turn the slow cooker temperature down and add more water, if necessary.

When the wheat is done, it will still be chewy. It makes a wonderful addition to soups, stews and salads. With herbs and a salt substitute, wheat grains make an excellent snack for munching while you work or when watching TV.

Ingredients

Serves 6

350 g whole wheat grains

2.5 litres water

2 tablespoons olive oil

2 red onions, finely chopped

2 red or green peppers, chopped

2 sticks celery, cleaned and chopped

1 fennel bulb, cut into thin slices

1 teaspoon orange zest

Salt and pepper to taste

Calories 175, **Fat** 5 g, **Carbohydrates** 27 g, **Protein** 5 g, **Fibre** 5 g, **Saturated Fat** 1 g, **Cholesterol** 0, **Sodium** 451 mg.

Whole Wheat with Vegetables

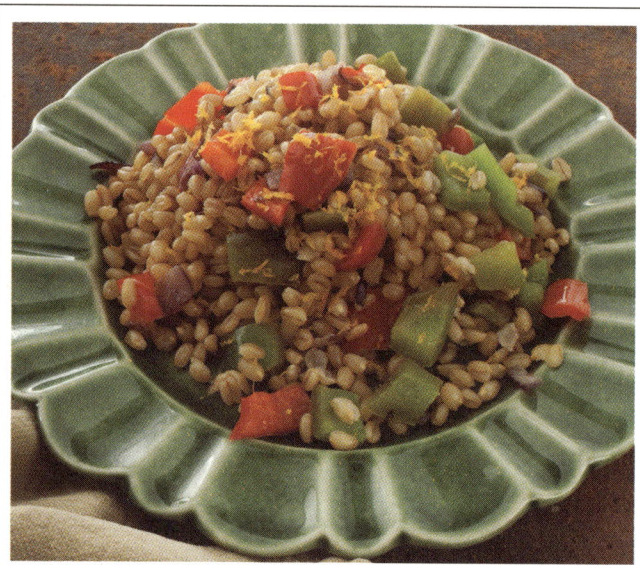

- Place wheat grains and water in a saucepan. Simmer for 2 hours.

- When wheat is done, heat 2 tablespoons olive oil in a large frying pan over medium heat. Add onion, peppers, celery, fennel and orange zest, and sauté.

- After about 4 minutes, when the vegetables are softened, remove from heat.

- Mix the cooked wheat with vegetables, and serve as a side dish.

Hearty wheat salad: If you marinate the cooked wheat in a vinaigrette, the acid in the marinade will soften the grains. Combine 175 g cooked wheat grains in a container with 75 ml red wine vinegar and 120 ml olive oil. Add 1 smashed garlic clove and a dash each of oregano, salt and pepper. Cover and refrigerate overnight. Serve with crisp leaves for a hearty salad the next day.

Wheat and vegetable soup: Add 175 g cooked whole wheat grains to 1.2 litres leftover turkey soup. Add 150 g cut-up tomatoes, 150 g sliced carrots, a sliced parsnip and a few small turnips cut into small dice. Serve with some crusty slices of toasted multigrain bread and a green salad, and dinner's ready.

Rinse Wheat

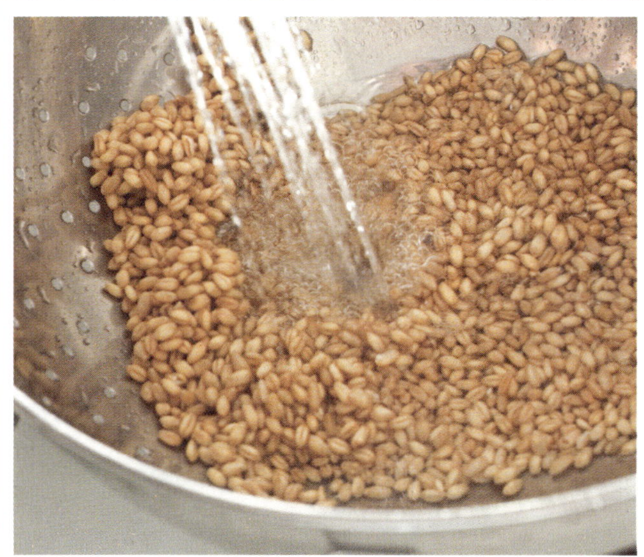

- It's important to rinse whole wheat grains because they have been harvested in a dirty field and may have a dirt crust on the outside.

- If you don't rinse the grains, the dirt will totally destroy the flavour of your meal.

- Or, you may find a nugget of dirt, which will dissolve under running water.

Whole-Wheat Grains Instead of Chips

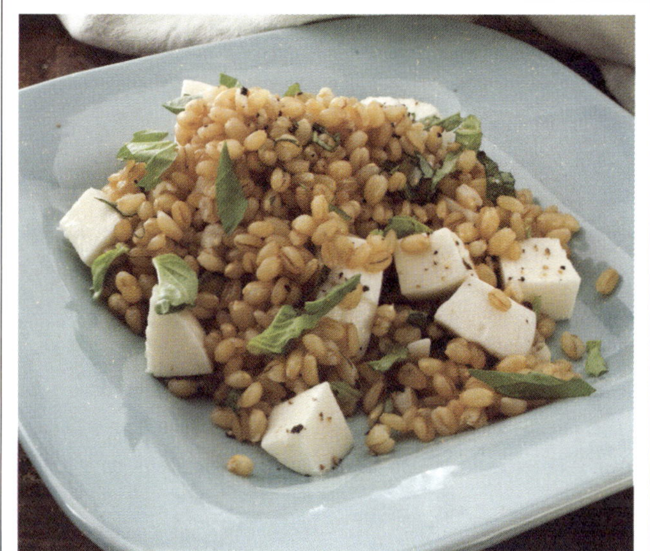

- What a treat! Set out a bowl of wheat drenched in vinaigrette with fresh basil and small chunks of low-fat mozzarella.

- For colour, add 150 g quartered cherry tomatoes and cubed green peppers.

- Scoop up the goodies by the spoonful on some thin slices of multigrain bread.

CHICKEN CURRY WITH RICE

You can make this curry in a hurry and please everyone's taste, from hot to mild

When you start to understand Indian cooking, you'll find that there is not just one spice blend that is the 'curry'. An experienced chef will mix his or her spices to suit the dish, the occasion and the personal tastes of family and guests.

For the purposes of this recipe, get a premium blend of Madras curry powder from your supermarket. You can always add some hot chillies or cayenne pepper to increase the heat if you want.

There are probably a thousand recipes for chicken curry. This one is quite easy and delicious. It's a wonderful party dish, as you can make a big batch in advance and keep it warm on a hot tray. Serve with rice and lots of garnishes.

Ingredients

Serves 8

1 tablespoon cooking oil, such as canola or groundnut

900 g chicken fillets cut into 2.5-cm pieces

2 onions, chopped

2 green chillies, cored and finely chopped (optional)

2 cloves garlic, peeled and chopped

1 tablespoon curry powder, or to taste

1 tablespoon fresh ginger, peeled and minced

120 ml canned low-fat condensed cream of chicken soup

120 ml unsweetened coconut milk

50 ml chicken stock

2 tablespoons ground cashews

400 g cooked brown rice

Calories 454, **Fat** 17 g, **Carbohydrates** 41 g, **Protein** 34 g, **Fibre** 4 g, **Saturated Fat** 7 g, **Cholesterol** 76 mg, **Sodium** 403 mg.

Chicken Curry with Rice

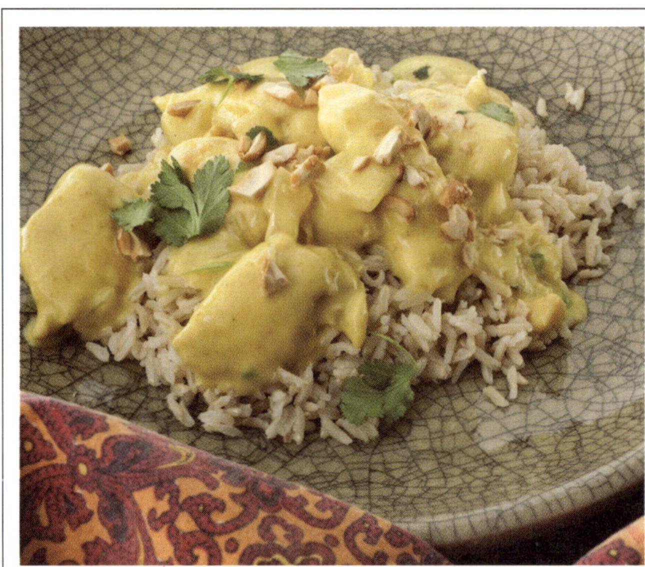

- Heat oil in a large pan. Sauté chicken pieces; when golden brown on both sides, remove from pan and set aside.

- Add onion, optional chillies and garlic; cook 5–7 minutes to soften. Stir in curry powder and blend well. Blend in ginger.

- Add remaining ingredients and stir, cooking over very low heat.

- Return chicken to pan; simmer for another 10 minutes. Serve with rice.

Garnishes for curry: Curry is enhanced by a number of garnishes. Bowls of cashews and peanuts are excellent. Cucumbers, chopped and marinated in lemony yogurt, make a refreshing accompaniment. A bowl of fresh pineapple chunks is cooling, as are orange slices.

• • • • RECIPE VARIATION • • • •

Fresh apple chutney: Use 2 cored, chopped apples (leave the skin on for colour), 1 small chopped onion, 1 teaspoon fresh ginger, 2 tablespoons cider vinegar, 1 teaspoon Splenda, $\frac{1}{8}$ teaspoon ground cloves, and $\frac{1}{8}$ teaspoon chilli powder, more or less to taste. Make it a day in advance; marinate the chicken, covered, in the refrigerator. Substitute peaches or mangos for apples.

Working with Chicken Fillets

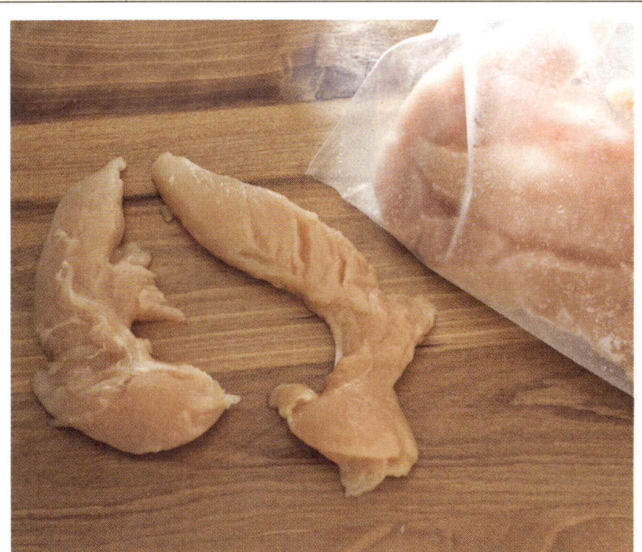

- Chicken fillets are a gift to any busy cook. They can go from freezer to pan with no fuss and in little time.

- They are excellent for people with diabetes and dieters, as they are skinless and lower in fat and calories.

- Cut them into strips for stir-frying, or into chunks for a quick addition to a pasta sauce.

- Or make a chicken pie with loads of vegetables and chicken fillets.

Adjusting Heat in Curry

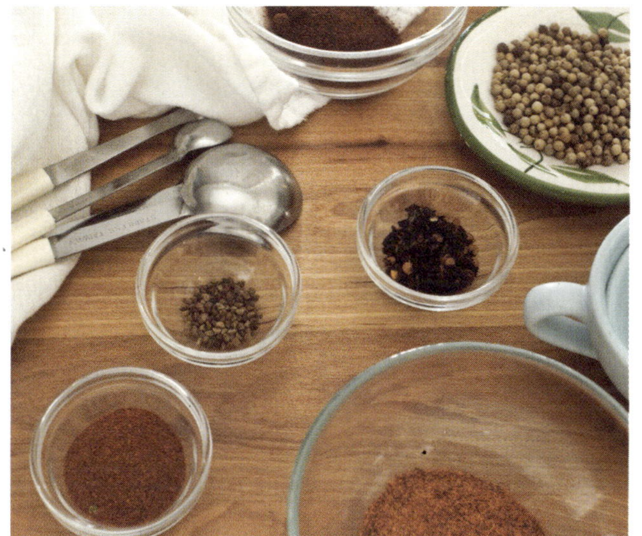

- Adjust the heat of a curry dish by adding or removing chilli.

- Lightly coloured curries often use white pepper.

- The heat in curry can come from a number of sources, including cayenne (ground chilli), red chilli flakes, chilli powder, black pepper, fresh chillies and hot paprika.

- Therefore, you can make your curry as hot or as mild as you wish. Remember, fresh chillies should be handled with care, as they can burn your skin.

SZECHUAN BEEF WITH VEGETABLES

Stir-fried beef with vegetables is a staple in many Chinese restaurants

This recipe features strips of fillet steak marinated briefly to add flavour. The fillet needs very little cooking.

Once you get into stir-frying and using a wok, you will absolutely depend on it for quick and diverse meals.

A good, stainless-steel wok is an excellent addition to any kitchen. If the bottom is copper clad, that's even better, and it should come with a stand to hold it steady on your stove.

You can use sugar snap or mangetout peas, bamboo shoots and/or any variety of bean sprouts. Frozen petits pois are also very good, and spring onions are an essential part of any stir-fry. Making a delicious marinade that's also used in cooking saves time, something we all appreciate.

Ingredients

Serves 6

For the marinade/sauce:

50 ml light soy sauce

2 teaspoons garlic powder

$1/2$ teaspoon Chinese five-spice powder

$1/2$ teaspoon ground coriander seeds

1 teaspoon ground black pepper

2 tablespoons sesame seed oil

450 g beef fillet, fat removed and cut into strips, 2.5 cm long and 12 mm wide

For the vegetables:

1 tablespoon canola oil

225 g sugar snap peas, ends trimmed

1 (175-g) can water chestnuts, drained, rinsed and halved

1 bunch spring onions, cut into 2.5 cm pieces

120 ml beef stock

Calories 358, **Fat** 19 g, **Carbohydrates** 18 g, **Protein** 29 g, **Fibre** 3 g, **Saturated Fat** 4 g, **Cholesterol** 82 mg, **Sodium** 744 mg.

Szechuan Beef with Vegetables

- Whisk sauce ingredients in a large bowl. Add beef; marinate for 20–30 minutes.

- Heat wok over medium-high heat and add oil. Add vegetables; cook for 2 minutes, stirring often. Push vegetables up the sides of the wok to slow the cooking process.

- Using a slotted spoon to drain marinade, add beef to the wok. Stir-fry beef in wok for 2 minutes.

- Stir in beef stock and remaining marinade. Reduce heat; cook, stirring (1 more minute for rare, 90 seconds for medium, or 3 minutes for well done).

Try this Asian-inspired variation: Start with the basic recipe, and just before serving add the following: 75 g chopped pineapple and 50 g red pepper, roasted, peeled and chopped (from a jar is fine). Roasted unsalted peanuts add crunch and flavour. A second variation is to add 1 tablespoon tangerine or clementine zest to the basic recipe, and sprinkle the chopped fruit of 2 tangerines or clementines on the dish just before serving. You can use coriander, a herb that adds a strong flavour spike. Try adding 2 tablespoons fresh, chopped coriander leaves. But remember, some people are allergic to coriander, while some just hate it.

Seasoning a Wok

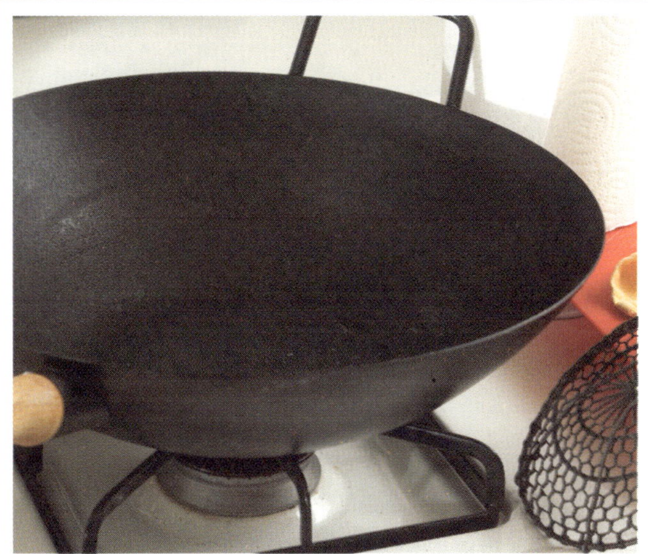

- Now that woks are made of stainless steel, seasoning them is not necessary. However, if you have a traditional steel wok, here's how to do it:

- Place cooking oil, preferably one with a high flash point such as grapeseed oil, in the wok and turn heat on low.

- Let it heat slowly. Then turn off heat, and leave the wok for 30–60 minutes.

- Wipe out the wok with a paper towel, and use it as often as possible. Cooking in it renews the seasoning.

Cutting Spring Onions

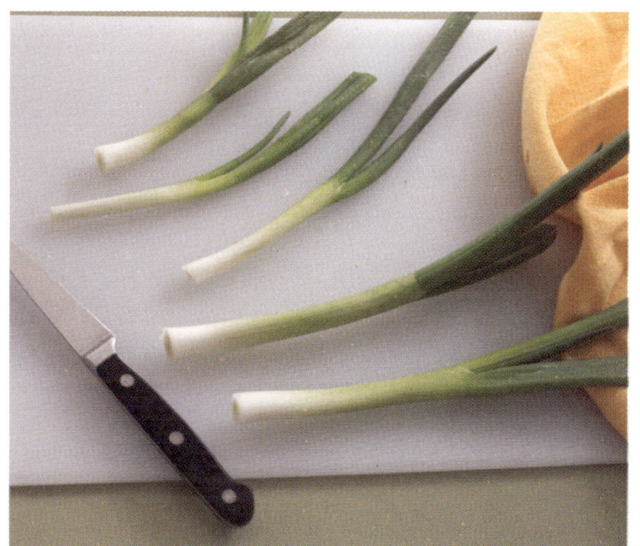

- When chopping a bunch of spring onions, first cut off the roots.

- Then, using a sharp paring knife, slit the papery skin remaining at the root end. Peel off the skin and discard.

- The white part of the onion is full of flavour and can be finely chopped.

- Use a pair of scissors to cut the green parts of the onions to desired lengths.

PORK SOUVLAKI

Marinated pork is grilled on skewers with onions and peppers

Souvlaki is the Greek word for 'skewer'. The dish consists of meat and vegetables threaded on to a skewer and barbecued or grilled until browned and juicy.

Kalamaki (or 'little reed') is made up of meat cut into small cubes and skewered on wooden skewers. Either way, the meat is marinated in a mixture of lemon, garlic, olive oil, wine and lots of herbs.

Lamb is traditionally used for this recipe, but you can use pork, chicken breasts or chicken thighs. The meat is always boneless and is marinated before grilling.

Serve souvlaki with tzatziki sauce, which is made from sour cream or yogurt and cucumber, a rice pilaf flavoured with oregano and mint and a cucumber and tomato salad. Follow with lemon meringue pie.

Ingredients

Serves 8

1 lemon

3 tablespoons olive oil

2 tablespoons balsamic vinegar

2 tablespoons red wine

1 teaspoon dill

¼ teaspoon dried mint

¼ teaspoon pepper

1 tablespoon fresh oregano

900 g pork tenderloin

2 red onions

3 green peppers

Calories 190, **Fat** 10 g, **Carbohydrates** 4 g, **Protein** 20 g, **Fibre** 1 g, **Saturated Fat** 3 g, **Cholesterol** 62 mg, **Sodium** 20 mg.

Pork Souvlaki

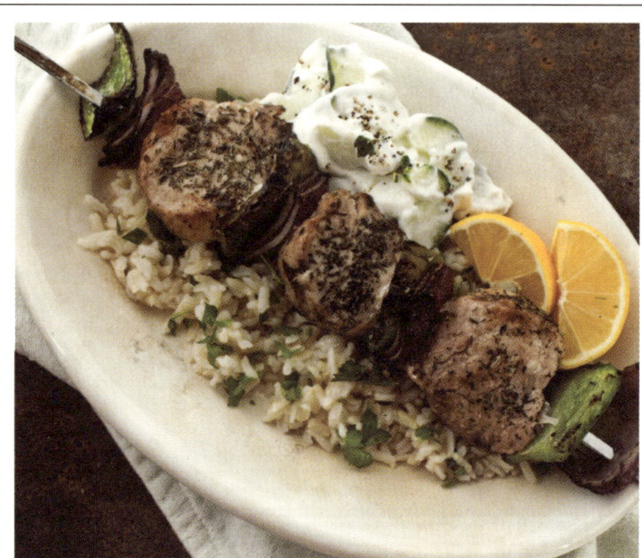

- Prepare grill. Zest lemon and squeeze juice. Combine juice, zest, olive oil, vinegar, wine, dill, mint, pepper and oregano in a bowl.

- Cut pork into 4-cm cubes and add to marinade. Cover and chill for 8–24 hours.

- Remove pork from marinade; reserve marinade. Cut each onion into 8 wedges; cut peppers into strips. Thread food on to skewers.

- Grill 15 cm from medium coals for 12–15 minutes, brushing with marinade, until pork is done. Discard remaining marinade. Serve with tzatziki sauce.

• • • • RECIPE VARIATION • • • •

Tzatziki sauce: Peel a cucumber and cut in half; remove seeds. Shred half the cucumber; drain on paper towels. Mix with 250 ml low-fat sour cream, 2 tablespoons lemon juice, 2 chopped garlic cloves, 1 tablespoon fresh dill, and ¼ teaspoon pepper. Serve with souvlaki.

Lamb souvlaki: Make recipe as directed, but use 900 g lean lamb shoulder instead of pork tenderloin. Omit dried mint; add 1 tablespoon chopped fresh mint leaves. Omit balsamic vinegar; add 2 tablespoons orange juice. Marinate and cook as directed.

Prepare Marinade

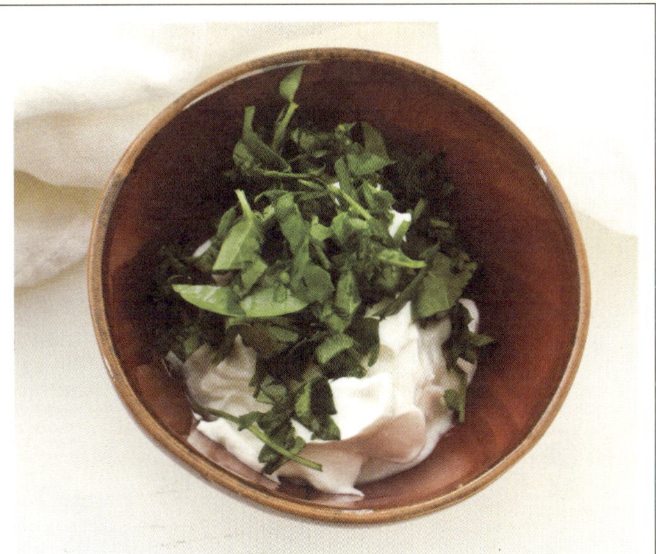

Thread on Skewers

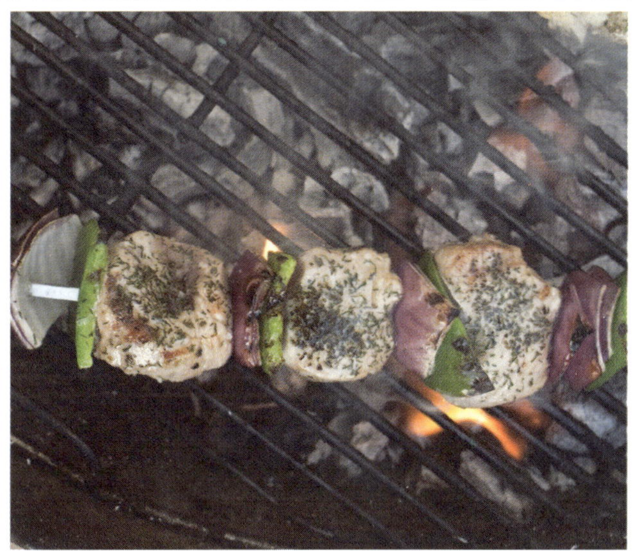

- This marinade recipe is quite variable and forgiving. You can use lime juice instead, add garlic or omit the mint.

- Use other fresh herbs, omit the balsamic vinegar, and add finely chopped chilli peppers.

- You can make the marinade ahead of time. Store it in the refrigerator for up to 2 days.

- If you change the marinade and love the results, remember to write down your formula. Soon, you'll have a notebook full of tried-and-true recipes.

- Metal skewers are the best choice for this type of recipe because the food grills longer than 7–8 minutes.

- The onions may be a bit difficult to push on the skewer. If so, use a sharp knife to start a hole.

- You can assemble the skewers ahead of time; cover and refrigerate for up to 8 hours.

- It's OK to marinate the pork longer than 24 hours; the meat will be very flavourful and tender.

VEAL STEW WITH CAPERS

Veal makes a most amiable stew, as it gets along happily with almost anything you add

Chunks of veal from the shoulder or flank are sold as stewing veal. Veal cut from the leg, and chops from the loin or rib, are a lot less expensive than veal cutlets.

Veal is tender and delicate meat with a light pink colour and a subtle flavour. Look for local veal raised in line with high welfare standards. Rosé veal, from pasture-fed calves, is also an excellent choice; it is slightly darker and fuller-flavoured.

Traditionally, veal and peppers in tomato sauce are the basic ingredients of an Italian stew. This recipe combines French and Italian influences. You can serve it with brown rice or mashed potatoes, with multigrain noodles or with some crusty French bread for mopping up the sauce.

Ingredients

Serves 6

25 g whole-wheat flour

$^1/_4$ teaspoon salt

Freshly ground black pepper to taste

1 teaspoon dried oregano

1 teaspoon dried basil

1 teaspoon dried rosemary

500 g stewing veal, cubed

1 tablespoon olive or canola oil

1 onion, peeled and chopped

1 carrot, peeled and chopped

2 cloves garlic, peeled and chopped

$^1/_2$ teaspoon Worcestershire sauce

120 ml dry white wine

120 ml chicken stock

2 tablespoons capers

Small bunch fresh parsley, rinsed and coarsely chopped

Calories 160, **Fat** 5 g, **Carbohydrates** 7 g, **Protein** 21 g, **Fibre** 1 g, **Saturated Fat** 1 g, **Cholesterol** 79 mg, **Sodium** 414 mg.

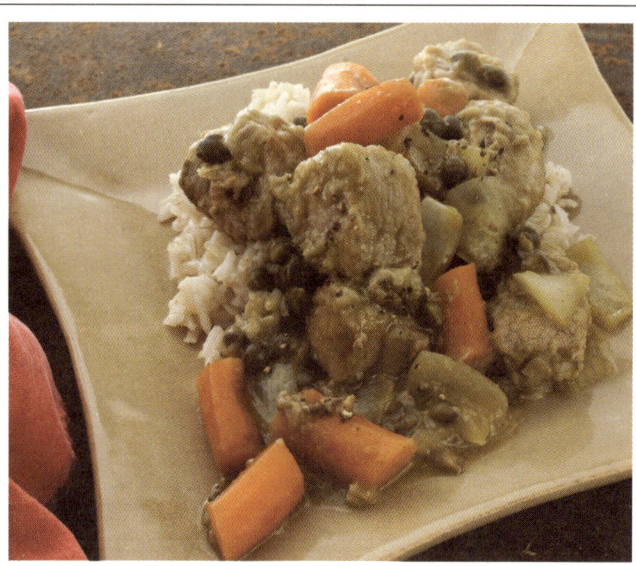

Veal Stew with Capers

- On a piece of greaseproof paper, mix flour, salt, pepper and herbs. Roll meat in the flour mixture.

- Heat oil in a large pan over medium heat. Add veal and brown on all sides. Push to one side of the pan, and add onion, carrot and garlic.

- Sauté for 4 minutes, stirring occasionally. Slowly blend in Worcestershire sauce, wine, stock and capers. Reduce heat and cover.

- Simmer for 1 hour or until very tender. Sprinkle with parsley. Serve with brown rice or whole-grain noodles (optional).

French veal stew: Veal stew cooks more quickly than beef or lamb stew. White wine will tenderize the meat, especially if you marinate it for a couple of hours. You can turn this into a French Provençal-style stew with 2 cans drained and rinsed haricot beans and lots of herbes de Provence. Sauté 2 cleaned and chopped red peppers with 1 chopped onion along with the veal, then add 500 ml of a garlicky tomato sauce to the pan; cover and simmer for 1–2 hours. Since the stew needs to cook for at least an hour, it's sensible to make a double quantity and freeze half. When you defrost it, you can add 75 g sliced, sautéed mushrooms. Brown mushrooms have more flavour than white ones.

Thickening Stews and Soups

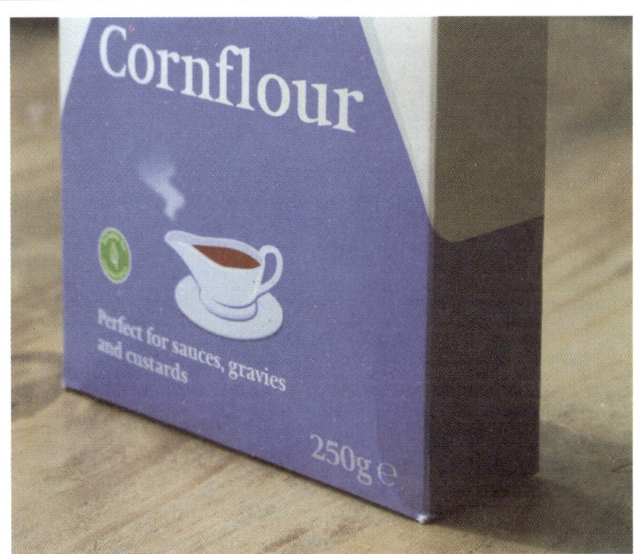

- Tossing meat in flour before sautéing helps to give body to a sauce, but you may want to thicken it more at the end of cooking.

- Make a paste with equal amounts soft butter or low-fat margarine and flour. Drop in a little at a time, stirring constantly.

- Or combine 1 tablespoon cornflour with 120 ml cold water. Whisk with a fork until smoothly blended. Slowly stir in some of the hot liquid, then add to stew.

- Don't add ordinary raw flour to hot liquid: you will end up with an unpleasantly lumpy stew or soup.

Turning Stew into Soup

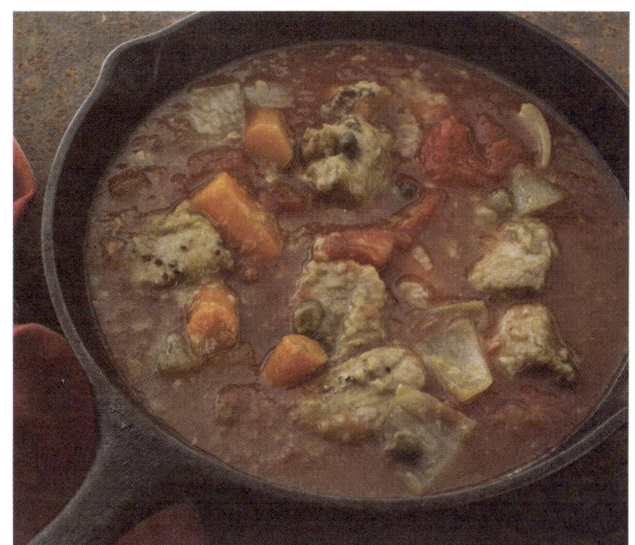

- Turn your stew into soup by adding liquids.

- A can of chopped tomatoes, with their juice, will transform your veal stew into soup.

- Chicken stock, wine or water will also thin the stew and stretch it.

- Stews and soups can also be stretched by the addition of stock, fresh or frozen vegetables such as pearl onions, baby carrots or courgettes, or a can of aduki or haricot beans.

NONA'S MEATBALLS WITH RICOTTA

Adding ricotta cheese to meatballs improves the flavour and texture

This recipe came from chef Nick Martshenko's grandmother. His *Nona* ('grandmother' in Italian) started him on a career that went from the Culinary Institute of America to executive chef at a prestigious restaurant.

  Martshenko delights customers at Match Restaurant in Stamford, Connecticut, serving Nona's recipe as an appetizer with tomato sauce and crusty bread. With spaghetti, it's a great meal. Adding ricotta gives meatballs a rich flavour and a nice consistency. Nick's grandmother used lean minced sirloin, which made the meatballs top-of-the-line. Either skirt or chuck steak would also be fine, though chuck is typically a little more fatty. Traditionally cooks fry their meatballs, adding a lot of calories from oil. Health-conscious cooks prefer to bake them.

Ingredients

Serves 8

450 g lean minced beef (sirloin, skirt, or chuck)

225 g low-fat ricotta

1 egg

40 g grated Parmesan cheese

50 g fresh soft breadcrumbs

¼ teaspoon cinnamon

2 teaspoons dried basil

2 teaspoons dried oregano

Salt and freshly ground black pepper to taste

½ teaspoon flax seed or ¼ teaspoon aniseed (optional)

50 g dry breadcrumbs

Calories 247, **Fat** 12 g, **Carbohydrates** 12 g, **Protein** 21 g, **Fibre** 1 g, **Saturated Fat** 5 g, **Cholesterol** 62 mg, **Sodium** 266 mg.

Nona's Meatballs with Ricotta

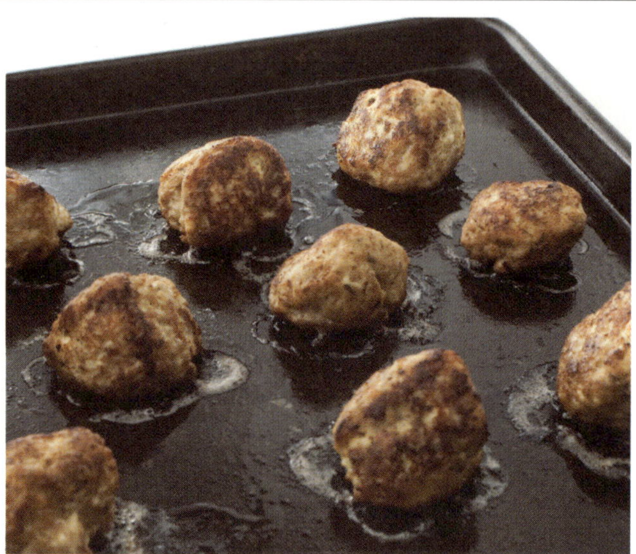

- Preheat oven to 180°C. Combine beef, ricotta, egg, Parmesan and soft breadcrumbs in a large bowl.

- Sprinkle cinnamon, basil, oregano, salt, pepper and flax seed or aniseed over meat mixture. Work mixture until well blended.

- Oil a baking sheet or line it with baking parchment. Make meatballs, rolling them between your palms. Roll them in dry breadcrumbs; place on sheet.

- Bake for 35–40 minutes or until well done and nicely browned.

Spicy and sweet suggestions: Combining beef, pork and veal is one way to vary this recipe. Substitute minced turkey to reduce calories. With turkey, add 50 g dried cranberries or raisins. A few dried apricots, chopped and soaked for 30 minutes until plump, along with ½ teaspoon cinnamon give meatballs a Moroccan touch.

Fun variations: The addition of 65 g pine nuts changes the texture considerably, amd 50 g chopped fennel bulb gives meatballs a bit of crunch. Use fine crumbs from a multigrain French-style baguette. Serve meatballs with raw or lightly sautéed baby spinach to enhance the nutritional value.

Frying Meatballs

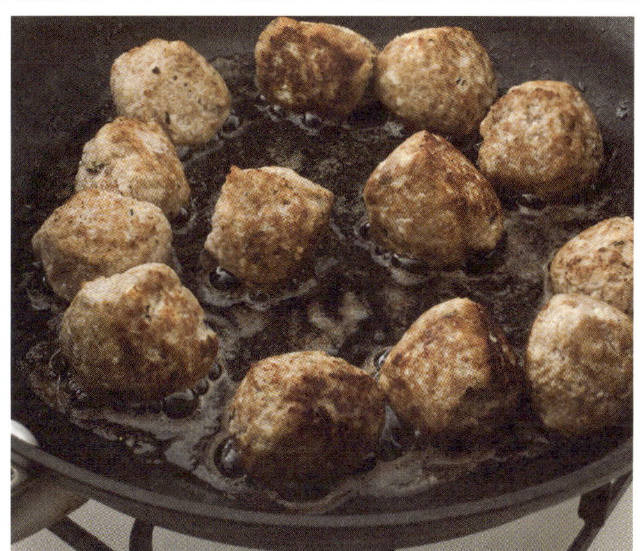

- To fry meatballs, pour 2.5 cm of oil, such as canola, grapeseed or groundnut, into a frying pan.

- If you use a deep-fat fryer with a basket, you will need more oil. But don't fill it too full; the oil bubbles up and expands when hot.

- Bring oil temperature to 180°C. Don't add meatballs all at once; start with two, bring oil back to temperature, turn meatballs over, and add two more.

- When completely browned, drain meatballs on paper towels, turning so that oil drains off.

Storing Meatballs

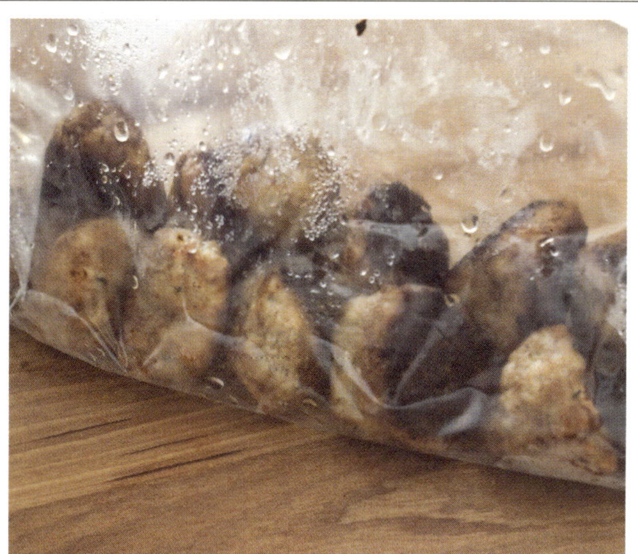

- If you are going to store unsauced meatballs, whether baked or fried, first let them cool down.

- Place them on a foil-covered baking sheet, making sure they are not touching.

- Freeze meatballs solid.

- Put them in a resealable plastic bag and store in the freezer, using them as needed.

MEDITERRANEAN CASSEROLE

This is a healthy take on paella, the famous Spanish dish made with rice and seafood

For this recipe, you can certainly use frozen prawns as opposed to fresh. A few pieces of chicken are also a very good addition, and you can substitute fresh or frozen scallops for the prawns. All the seafood, chicken and chorizo add flavour to the rice as it absorbs the cooking juices. Herbs and saffron will make your baked rice dish very special. Although saffron is the most expensive spice in the world, it's worth it for a special-occasion dinner.

A garnish of chopped green olives, capers or green peppercorns will enhance the dish.

Ingredients

Serves 8

50 ml olive oil

1 small chicken, cut into 8 pieces

Freshly ground black pepper

A little plain flour

1 medium onion, peeled and chopped

2 cloves garlic, peeled and chopped

1 sweet green or red pepper, cored, seeded and diced

115 g chorizo sausage, cut into 6-mm slices

350 mg short-grain rice

500 ml chicken stock

250 ml dry white wine

250 seafood stock or water

$^1/_2$ teaspoon turmeric

$^1/_2$ teaspoon cumin

1 tablespoon oregano

$^1/_2$ teaspoon saffron

32 clams

32 cleaned mussels

32 raw jumbo prawns, peeled and deveined

Calories 442, **Fat** 14 g, **Carbohydrates** 46 g, **Protein** 30 g, **Fibre** 0, **Saturated Fat** 3 g, **Cholesterol** 97 mg, **Sodium** 366 mg.

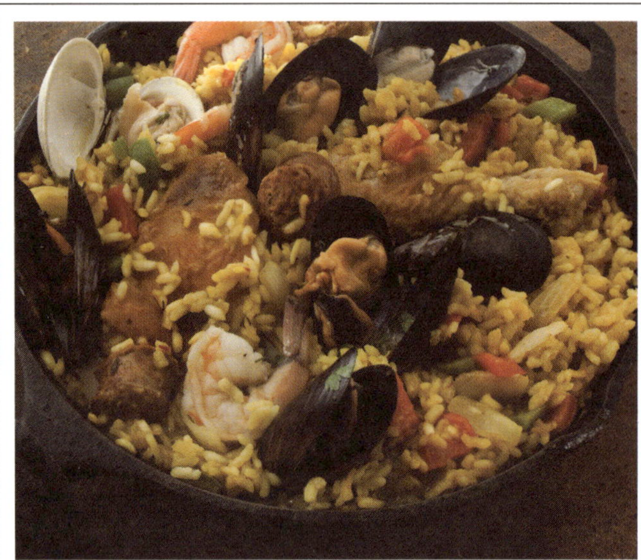

Mediterranean Casserole

- Preheat oven to 180°C. Heat oil over medium-high heat in a large flameproof dish.

- Sprinkle chicken with pepper and flour. Sauté for 5 minutes, turning, to brown both sides. Add onion, garlic and peppers. Sauté, stirring occasionally, for 8 minutes. Mix in chorizo.

- Blend in rice and cook, stirring, for 5–6 minutes. Pour in liquids, a little at a time, stirring. Add seasonings. Bake for 15 minutes. Press clams and mussels into rice. Return to oven. When rice blooms, add prawns, pressing into rice mixture. Cook until all shellfish are open and prawns are pink.

About rice: Rice has been cultivated in Asia for 5,000 years. A staple of Chinese, Indian, Japanese and Southeast Asian cooking, it sustains huge populations. Rice migrated to Japan, India and the Middle East from China. Then it made a short trip across the Mediterranean to Europe. In the 1800s, slave owners transported skilled Africans from Angola and settled them on islands off the coast of the Carolinas to grow rice, introducing the crop to America. Brown rice is unpolished and less processed than white rice. It has more fibre, texture, vitamins and minerals as well. Quick-cooking rice is highly processed. Although it takes only a minute to make, you lose some flavour, nutrition and texture.

Know When the Rice Is Done

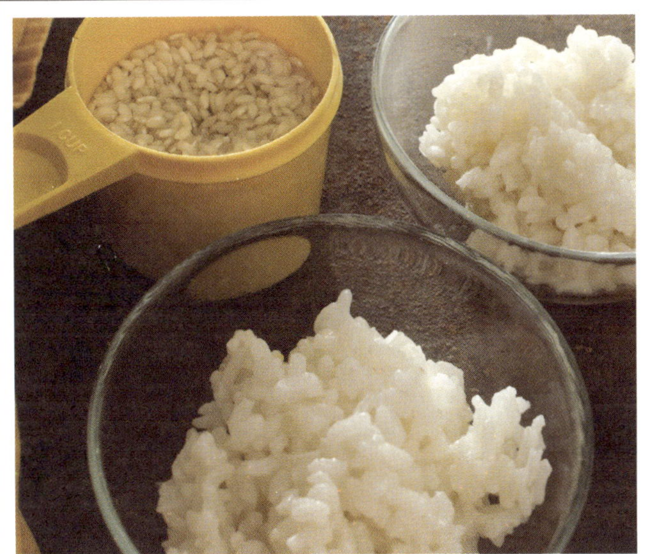

- Rice should not be al dente; you don't want anyone to crack a tooth. You don't want mushy or burned rice, either.

- The easiest way to check that rice is cooked is to take a teaspoonful and taste it.

- Rice actually 'blooms', which means that it expands, absorbing the flavours in the stock and seasonings.

- If the rice is not done but is drying out, pour in a bit more liquid and continue cooking.

The Order of Addition

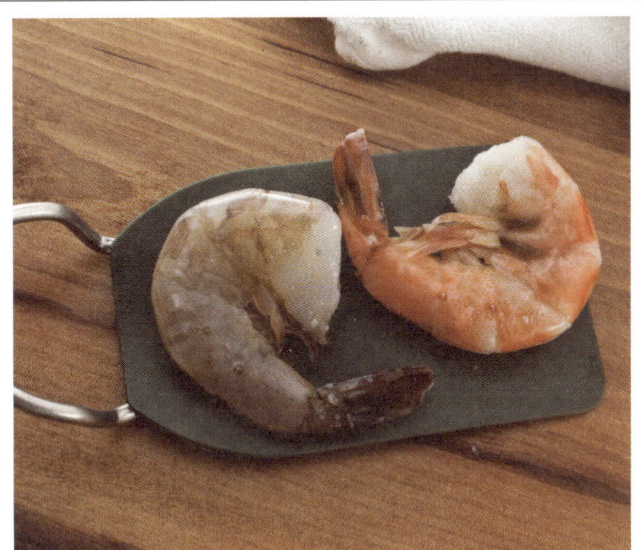

- When adding seafood to a dish, you don't want to overcook or undercook it.

- Seafood must always be carefully watched. It's too easy to ruin and too expensive to waste.

- Overcooked prawns have the texture of rubber. The same goes for scallops, which need very little cooking.

- An underdone clam or mussel is not opened. Give it more heat; discard any shellfish that does not open. If a prawn is pink on one side and grey on the other, turn it over.

187

TINY TURKEY MEATBALLS

These are excellent for an afterschool snack or for adults in a hurry

There is so much more to turkey than Christmas dinner. It's low in fat, high in protein, and can be the base for everything from meatballs to chilli.

This is a simple recipe. It is easy to make and very nutritious, and baking the meatballs keeps them low in fat.

People should eat a small amount of food frequently; eating a little bit helps to keep blood sugar steady, avoiding metabolic highs and lows. For dieters, snacks keep energy levels high and prevent the body from going into 'starvation mode'. Neither situation is good for any human being.

Don't skip a meal; eat a little, eat often, and eat healthily.

Ingredients

Makes 32 small meatballs

For the meatballs:

1 egg

1/2 teaspoon ground black pepper, or to taste

1/2 teaspoon hot pepper sauce, or to taste

1 teaspoon salt

1 teaspoon cumin

1 teaspoon garlic powder, or to taste

1/4 teaspoon cinnamon

1 tablespoon tomato purée

450 g minced turkey

40 g seasoned breadcrumbs

40 g raisins

1 tablespoon ground walnuts

For the coating:

1 egg

1/2 teaspoon Tabasco sauce

1 teaspoon chilli sauce

150 g multigrain cereal, ground in food processor

Calories 127, **Fat** 5 g, **Carbohydrates** 12 g, **Protein** 9 g, **Fibre** 1 g, **Saturated Fat** 2 g, **Cholesterol** 54 mg, **Sodium** 414 mg.

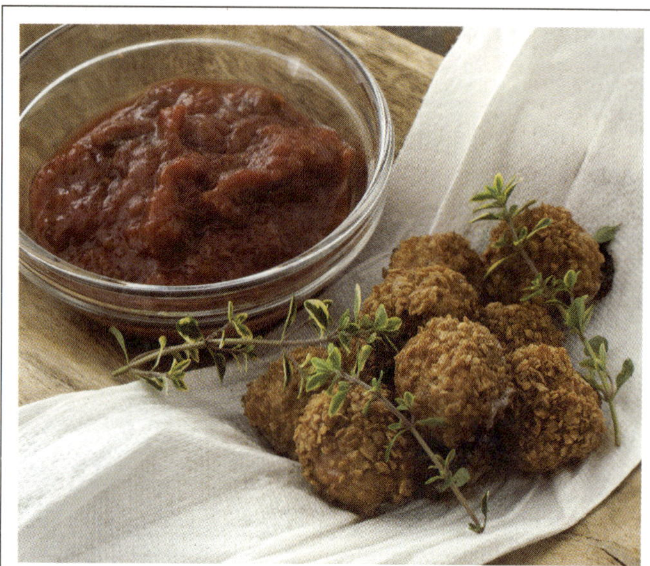

Tiny Turkey Meatballs

- Preheat oven to 180°C. Lightly oil a large baking tray.

- Whisk together the first eight ingredients. Work in the minced turkey and breadcrumbs. Mix in raisins and nuts. Form 32 small meatballs, about 2.5-cm in diameter.

- Whisk egg, Tabasco and chilli sauce together. Roll meatballs in egg mixture, then in crushed cereal.

- Place meatballs on prepared baking tray. Bake for 35 minutes, or until well browned. Cool.

Turkey meatballs are high in protein, yet have additional nutritive qualities from nuts, onions and garlic to make them a great choice. Transform your meatballs with Mexican seasonings. With a salsa dip and some corn chips (eaten in moderation) turkey meatballs make a wonderful party snack, and are very good to take on a picnic.

Enriching the meatballs: Meat from the drumstick and thigh of turkey is richer, moister and somewhat higher in calories than white breast meat. Enrich the basic turkey meatball recipe with 25 g finely chopped toasted walnuts, raisins, currants or pine nuts. Throw in an extra egg white, 50 ml milk and 25 g grated Parmesan cheese.

Coating Meatballs

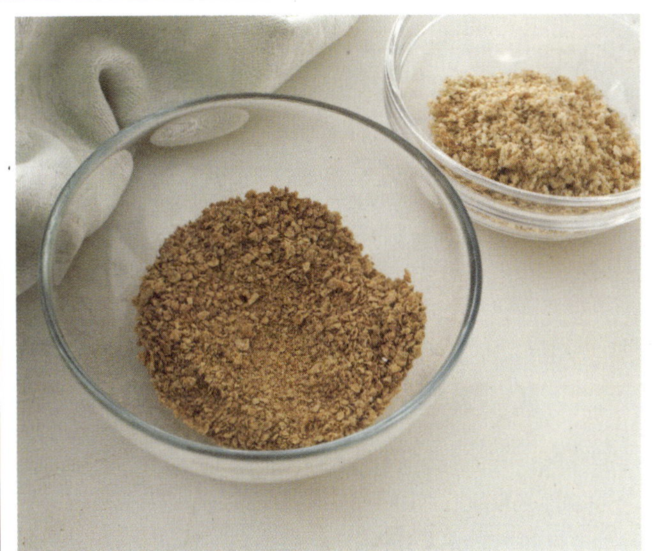

- There are many good coatings for meatballs, which should have a nice, crisp crust. Making your own crumbs from multigrain bread is ideal.

- Commercial crumbs are fine, but read labels for seasonings and salt.

- Ground crackers are usually too salty to be good for people with diabetes. Many cereals are too sweet.

- Crumbled homemade corn bread produces an excellent coating, but you have to retoast the bread after you've made crumbs.

Shaping Meatballs

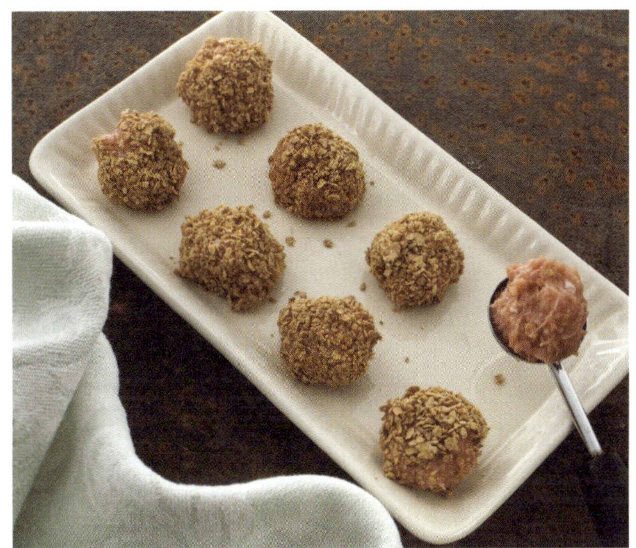

- Toss the meat, crumbs and other ingredients with two forks.

- If you pat the meat and roll it too tightly, it will be denser than desired.

- Try using a melon ball scoop to make meatballs of equal size, which is important for uniform baking.

APPLE & WALNUT CHEESE SPREAD

This low-fat treat is perfect for kids as well as adults with a sweet tooth

It's important for children and adults alike to snack on foods that will nourish and provide energy without adding sugar or fat to their diets. Obesity in children is linked to early-onset type 2 diabetes.

You can provide great school and workplace snacks for the family with little effort. Low-fat cottage cheese is an excellent base for many flavourful spreads. The spark of a tart apple, the crunch of nuts and a touch of Splenda, cinnamon or nutmeg will give you a spread that goes on mini waffles or crackers. Cheese adds calcium, and fruit and nuts add fibre and other nutrients. Keep one pot of this spread at work and another at home for snacking.

Ingredients

Makes 350 ml (nutritional analysis based on 25-g serving)

225 g low-fat cottage cheese

3 tablespoons chopped, toasted walnuts

1 small tart apple, cored and chopped, skin on

Juice of 1/2 lemon

1 teaspoon Splenda

1/2 teaspoon cinnamon

Pinch of nutmeg

Apple and Walnut Cheese Spread

- Mix cottage cheese and nuts in a bowl.

- In a separate bowl, sprinkle chopped apple with lemon juice to prevent the apple from browning.

- Work Splenda and spices into the cheese; mix in apple pieces. Store in an airtight container, and refrigerate leftover spread.

- Serve on small waffles, toast or crackers.

Calories 20, **Fat** 0, **Carbohydrates** 2 g, **Protein** 2 g, **Fibre** 0, **Saturated Fat** 0, **Cholesterol** 1 mg, **Sodium** 111 mg.

Fruits and nuts: Vary the types of fruits and nuts you add to the low-fat cottage cheese. Chopped toasted almonds, pecans or peanuts are all fine. Just make sure that they are not salted. Any fruit you like can be substituted for apples. Try using chopped fresh figs for a terrific treat.

From sweet to savoury: Transform this sweet treat into a savoury one by omitting the sugar and adding 1 tablespoon grated Parmesan or Gorgonzola cheese. Finely chopped radishes, carrots, celeriac, fennel or celery are also wonderful additions, all with negligible calories. Dried or fresh herbs to add for a savoury combination include basil, oregano, rosemary or thyme. Lots of black pepper is another good addition.

How to Mix Successfully

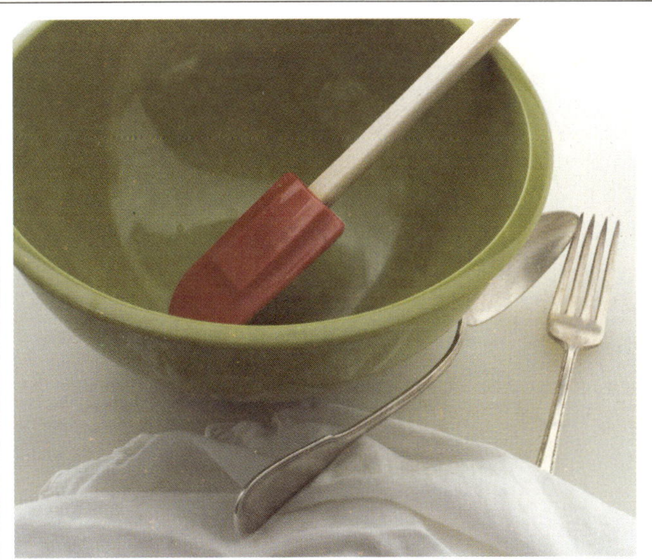

- The last thing you want is to bite into a concentrated lump of Splenda or find that all of the cinnamon has landed in one place.

- The best way to blend the cheese with the sugar and spice is to pre-mix them in a bowl with a fork.

- Using a rubber scraper, mix from the outside in.

- Repeat the process until well blended, then add the apple.

Roasting and Toasting Nuts

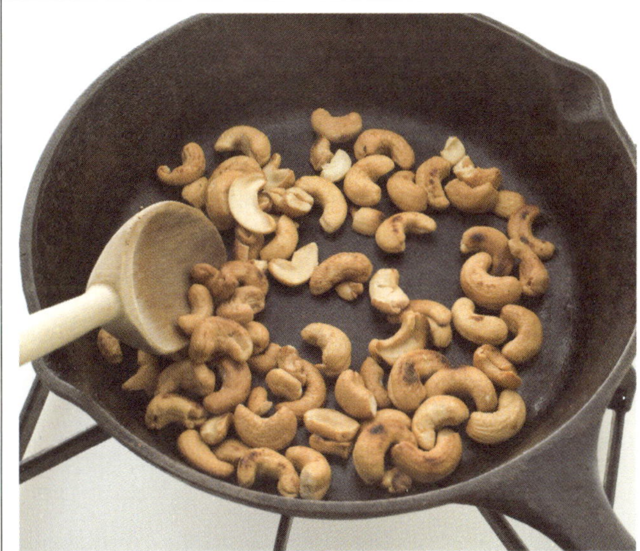

- There are basically two ways to roast or toast nuts.

- One is to do it in a hot frying pan, preferably a heavy-bottomed, cast-iron pan. As soon as the pan is hot, add the nuts; keep them moving and turn often.

- Another method is to bake them in the oven at 170°C for 10–15 minutes.

- Running them under the grill is risky – it's all too easy to burn the nuts, even if you only look away for a second.

COURGETTE CREAM CHEESE PIZZA

You can't go wrong with a healthy, delicious pizza, topped with courgettes and low-fat cheese

Making a truly healthy, low-fat pizza is not all that hard. For this recipe, use low-fat cream cheese in place of mozzarella or mascarpone, a rich and very creamy cheese that's loaded with calories.

Low-fat cream cheese is fat reduced, and lots of flavour is gained with the addition of a little grated Parmesan. Oregano, chilli flakes and a bit of extra-virgin olive oil will give your pizza a lot of zing.

You can put as many different vegetables on a 'white' pizza (one made without tomato sauce) as you would on a 'red' pizza. Use a ready-made pizza base or your favourite multigrain or whole-wheat pizza dough recipe.

Ingredients

Serves 12 as a snack

Large pizza base or 450 g fresh pizza dough, preferably multigrain or whole wheat

Extra-virgin olive oil, in a spray bottle or mister

115 g low-fat cream cheese, at room temperature

1 teaspoon dried oregano

1 teaspoon red chilli flakes, or to taste

25 g finely grated Parmesan cheese

1 large or 2 medium-size courgettes, sliced very thinly

Calories 192, **Fat** 10 g, **Carbohydrates** 20 g, **Protein** 6 g, **Fibre** 3 g, **Saturated Fat** 1 g, **Cholesterol** 6 mg, **Sodium** 293 mg.

Courgette Cream Cheese Pizza

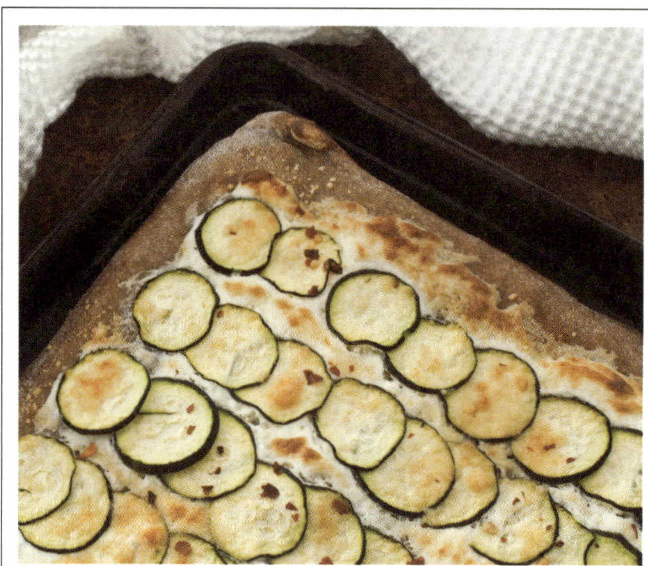

- Preheat oven to 220°C and lightly oil a baking sheet.

- Arrange pizza base on sheet or roll dough into a 22 x 30-cm rectangle, and lay it on the baking sheet. Spray it lightly with olive oil.

- Spread dough with cream cheese; sprinkle with oregano, red chilli flakes and half the Parmesan.

- Arrange courgette slices over top. Sprinkle with the remaining cheese, and give it another misting of olive oil. Bake for 14–16 minutes, or until crust is golden brown.

Lots and lots of vegetables: Vary this basic pizza with other vegetables. Try substituting 175 g chopped, cooked turnip tops for the courgettes. Cooked, chopped broccoli also makes a wonderful topping. Or try 30 g fresh baby spinach leaves spread on the pizza, but be sure to give it a good spritz of olive oil.

Cheese variations: There's no reason why you can't make pizzas with different cheeses. Try using 175 g grated Manchego cheese from Spain as an alternative. Gorgonzola is wonderful with broccoli or courgettes. Stay away from the heavy, creamy cheeses, such as Brie and Camembert. And remember, pizza is a treat, not part of your daily diet.

Arranging Pizza Toppings

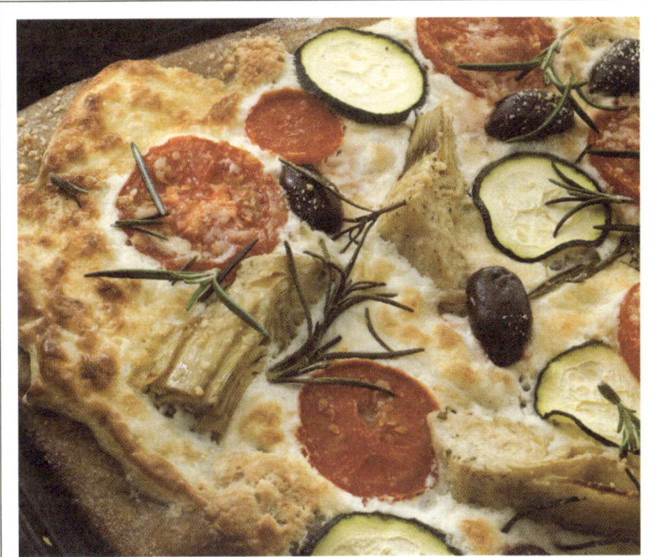

- The top of a pizza can be a work of art or a mess.

- Arranging the toppings artfully takes a bit more time than just throwing stuff on the dough. Make a geometric design with courgettes, pepperoni, and/or pepper strips.

- Don't let the cheese clump in one place; sprinkle or spread it evenly.

- If your oven heats unevenly, turn the pizza around halfway through the cooking time so that it will brown evenly.

Grating Cheese

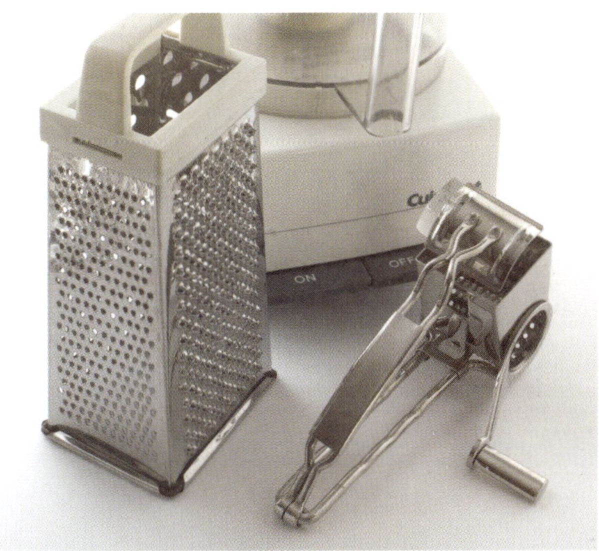

- An old-fashioned box grater does a fine job with semi-soft and even some hard cheeses. You get a coarse grate, which is fine for some dishes.

- For a large quantity, it's worth using the grater attachment on your food processor.

- When you attempt to grate soft cheeses, such as mozzarella or Brie, they clump.

- For pizza, a finer grind of Parmesan is better than a coarse one.

CROSTINI WITH MUSHROOMS

Yet another Italian creation, crostini are so much better than ordinary crackers

Crostini can be made large with Italian bread, or small with a baguette. Either way, use a multigrain loaf if possible. The combination of grains results in extra crunch and gives the bread a wonderful nutty flavour.

Crostini can be classically topped with garlic, tomato and basil. Or you can go wild with toppings. Sautéed mushrooms are lovely when dressed with vinaigrette and spread on the crostini while still warm. Follow your taste preferences.

Very low in salt, crostini have almost no sugar, and multigrain varieties have an added value with fibre. The health benefits of crostini far outweigh those of any commercial cracker.

Ingredients

Makes 32 (nutritional analysis based on serving of 4 crostini)

For the topping:

1 tablespoon olive oil

2 shallots, peeled and finely chopped

75 g cleaned, chopped mushrooms (shiitake, porcini, or white)

2 tablespoons red wine vinegar

1 teaspoon dried thyme

1 tablespoon low-fat mayonnaise

25 g finely grated Parmesan cheese

For the crostini:

1 multigrain baguette, about 30 cm long

Olive oil, in a spray bottle or mister

1 tablespoon garlic powder

1 tablespoon dried oregano

Calories 137, **Fat** 5 g, **Carbohydrates** 17 g, **Protein** 6 g, **Fibre** 1 g, **Saturated Fat** 2 g, **Cholesterol** 6 mg, **Sodium** 283 mg.

Crostini with Mushrooms

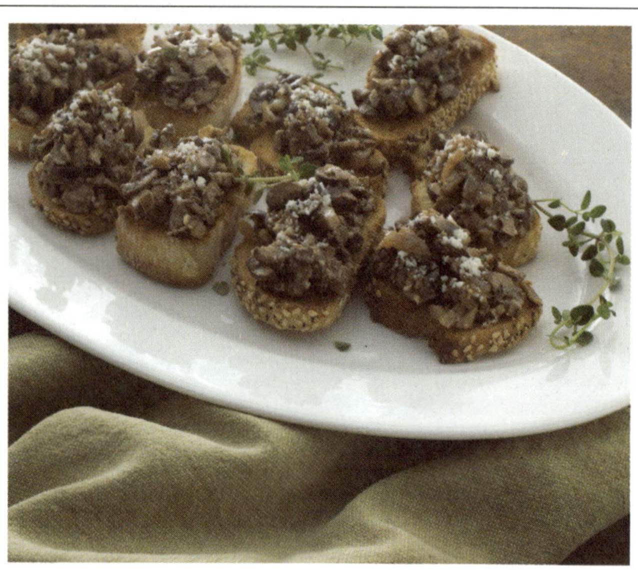

- Heat oil in a frying pan over medium-high heat. Sauté shallots and mushrooms until softened, about 10 minutes. Add vinegar, thyme and mayonnaise; cool. Sprinkle with cheese.

- Preheat oven to 200°C. Lightly oil a baking sheet.

- Cut baguette diagonally into 6 mm slices. Arrange on baking sheet; bake until lightly brown. Turn over. Spray with oil; sprinkle with garlic powder and oregano. Bake until crisp and brown.

- Spread each crostini with 1 tablespoon of the spread.

• • • • RECIPE VARIATION • • • •

Diversity in toppings: After you've toasted one side of the crostini, you can put a topping on the other side and bake it a bit longer for a melted treat. Various cheeses are excellent; try 225 g crumbled Gorgonzola or low-fat Emmental mixed with 175 g chopped, low-salt ham, 150 g chopped fresh figs or, as in this recipe, 75 g mushrooms. Or you can simply spray the untoasted side of the crostini with olive oil; sprinkle with 1 tablespoon each of oregano, garlic powder and pepper; and toast some more. Crostini are fine plain or served with a dip. A mixture of fresh chopped tomatoes with fresh basil and diced mozzarella is very good and can be served hot or cold – if you heat this on the crostini, the cheese melts. Experiment with goats' cheese, olives, figs and apples as toppings.

Chopping

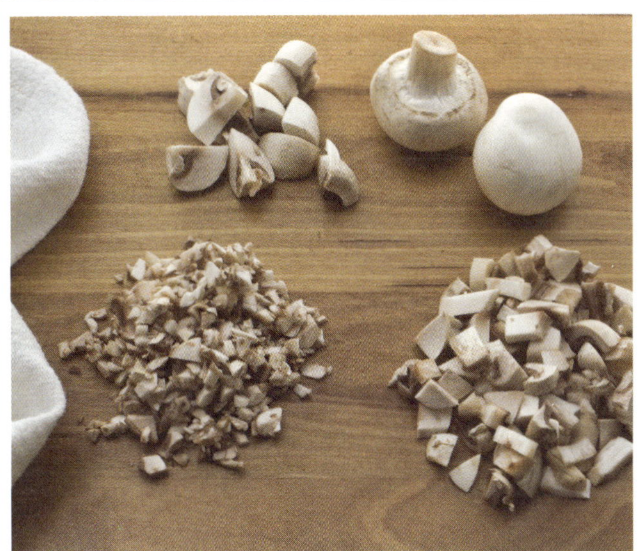

- To chop really finely, you need a chef's knife or a Chinese cleaver.

- The Chinese call this work 'march chop' because it makes the sound of a very fast march. When you've chopped all the food in one direction, revolve the chopping board, or move ingredients around and chop them the other way.

- If you use a food processor, keep pulsing it until you reach the desired size.

- Dicing means cutting vegetables into squares, which can vary in size.

Bake or Grill?

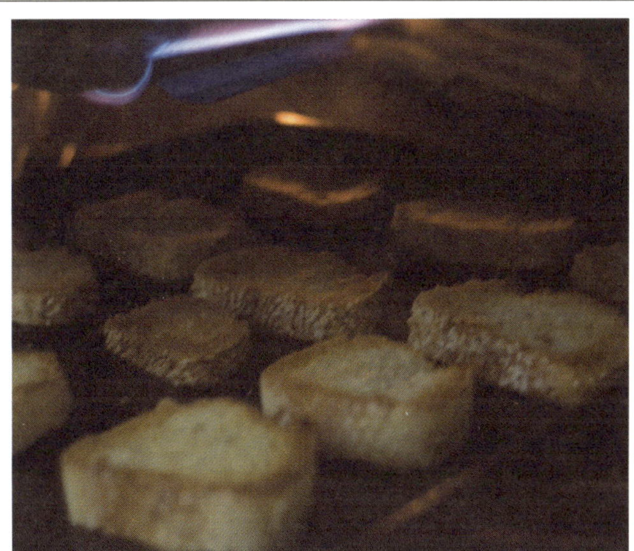

- Under a very hot grill, one side will be done in about 30 seconds, and the other side in 8–10 seconds.

- Baking at 230°C takes slightly more time; the crostini will be a bit crisper if you grill them.

- No matter what you do, watch the crostini – they burn very easily.

- Whichever way you toast them, don't char the crostini.

DEVILLED EGGS WITH PRAWNS

A popular snack for decades, here is a healthier version of devilled eggs

Dill and baby prawns turn devilled eggs into a gourmet treat. Buy the smallest eggs you can find for snacking. You may have to settle for medium eggs, but don't get large or extra large eggs, or you risk having your snack turn into a meal.

The 'devil' in the eggs can be extremely hot or just a bit spicy. Mustard is essential, as is mayonnaise, which gives the egg yolks their silky texture. After that, you can mix in all kinds of other ingredients.

Most people love devilled eggs. On most cocktail buffets, they are among the first items to disappear. Reduce the calories in devilled eggs by using low-fat mayonnaise.

Ingredients

Serves 6

For the devilled eggs:

6 hard-boiled eggs, cooled and peeled

2 tablespoons low-fat mayonnaise

2 teaspoons prepared yellow mustard or Dijon-style mustard

Salt to taste

Tabasco sauce to taste

For the topping:

1 tablespoon olive oil

Juice of $^1/_2$ lemon

Salt to taste

Freshly ground black pepper to taste

1 teaspoon dried dill

12 small cooked prawns, peeled

Calories 136, **Fat** 10 g, **Carbohydrates** 2 g, **Protein** 12 g, **Fibre** 0, **Saturated Fat** 3 g, **Cholesterol** 279 mg, **Sodium** 324 mg.

Devilled Eggs with Prawns

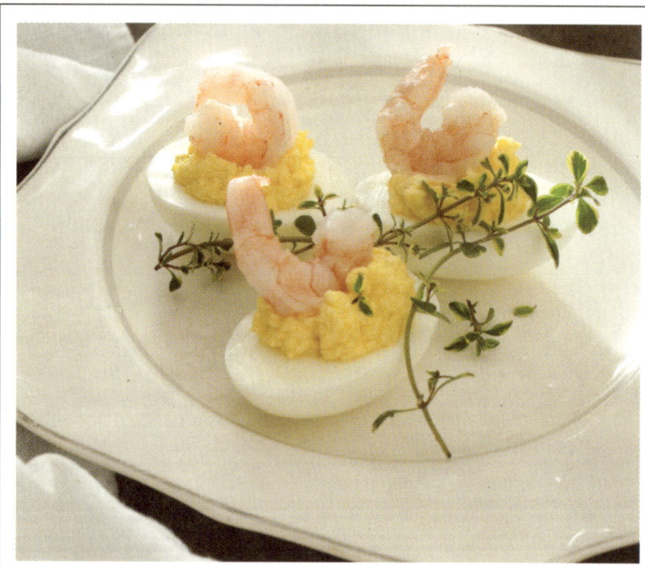

- Cut eggs in half and arrange the whites on a plate.

- Place three of the yolks with the next four ingredients in food processor and pulse until very smooth. Pause every 10 seconds to scrape sides of bowl.

- Taste for seasoning, then spoon into whites.

- Make topping by whisking all but prawns in bowl. Add prawns; toss gently to coat.

- Gently press a prawn into the whipped yolks in each half egg.

Endless versatility: When you start with a basic recipe for devilled eggs, there is no limit to what you can add. By mixing 3 tablespoons chopped smoked salmon into the yolks, you will have a whole different egg. Or you can simply place snips of salmon on top. A sprinkling of red or black caviar is classic and great with champagne for a special party.

Flavouring eggs: Four green peppercorns on top of each egg make them really come alive, as do 4 capers. A teaspoon of crabmeat salad pressed down into each of the whipped yolks is also very good. Two tablespoons of finely chopped spring onions added to the yolk mixture is also nice, as are snipped fresh chives on top.

How to Hard-Boil Eggs

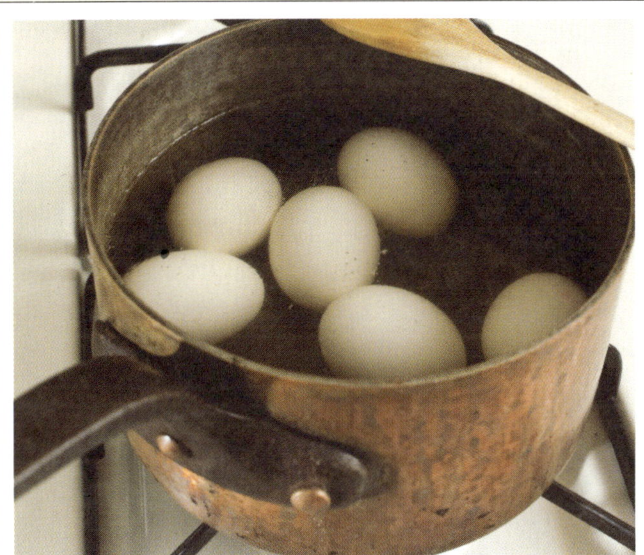

- Place eggs in saucepan of cold water on stove. Turn the heat on high.

- When the water is scalding hot (small bubbles showing at the edges of the pan), turn the heat to simmer and cover eggs. If you are using a very heavy pan, remove it from the stove.

- Let eggs sit for 10–12 minutes in the hot water.

- Place pan of eggs under cold running water. As soon as you can touch them, crack each egg and return it to the pan of cold water. When all are cracked, peel the eggs.

How to Peel Eggs Easily

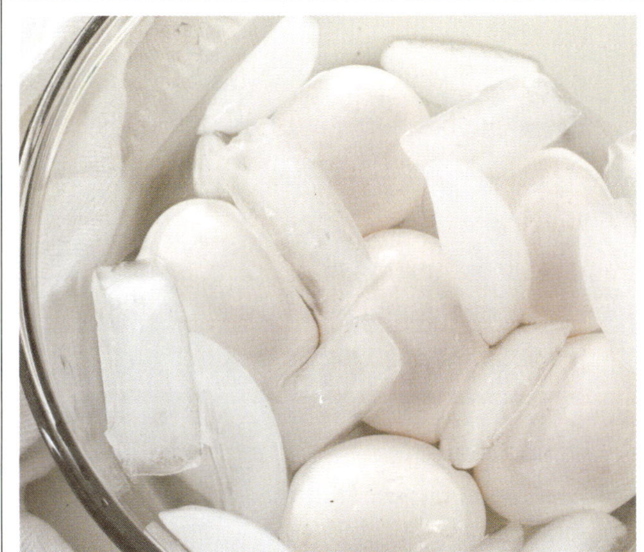

- Sometimes an egg is hard to peel because it's almost too fresh.

- Return it to the boiling water, then plunge it in iced water to shrink the egg.

- If your eggs turn into an irretrievable mess, looking moth-eaten and rough, simply make egg salad, placing the mixture in a bowl, with crackers or crostini on the side. Then add your prawn garnish for a new 'egg-sperience.'

CHICKEN WITH PEANUT SAUCE

These tender chunks of chicken can be served hot, cold or at room temperature

Barbecued or grilled, the results are pretty much the same with chicken fillets. When they are marinated and either charcoal-grilled or run under the grill, they are an excellent and flavourful source of protein.

The fillet is the strip across the very top of the chicken breast, and its size reflects the size of the chicken. A bag of frozen chicken fillets is wonderful to have on hand – it covers you in almost any food emergency. Whether it's the soccer team showing up ravenous after practice, or the bridge club playing at your house, you can make an instant snack that will please everyone.

Ingredients

Serves 8

For the chicken:

120 ml light soy sauce

50 ml fresh orange juice

1 tablespoon sesame seed oil

1 tablespoon finely chopped fresh ginger

675 g chicken fillets, cut into bite-size pieces

For the sauce:

50 ml reduced-fat peanut butter

Juice of ½ fresh lime

1 teaspoon finely chopped fresh ginger

3 tablespoons low-sodium soy sauce

Dash of Tabasco or other hot pepper sauce

Calories 155, **Fat** 7 g, **Carbohydrates** 4 g, **Protein** 12 g, **Fibre** 1 g, **Saturated Fat** 1 g, **Cholesterol** 43 mg, **Sodium** 465 mg.

Chicken with Peanut Sauce

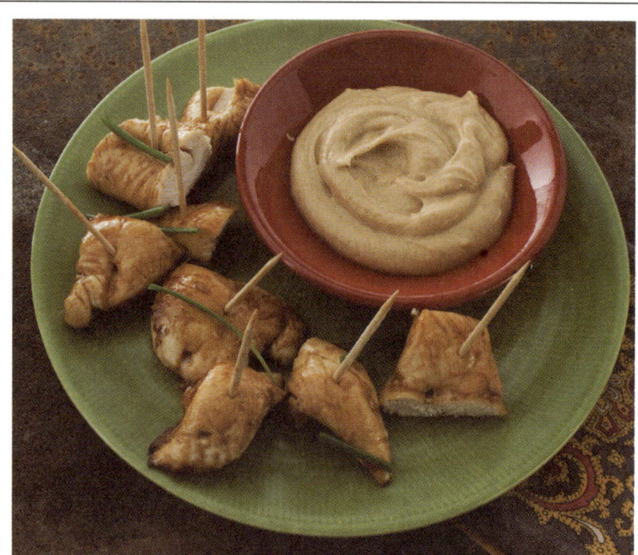

- Whisk the first four ingredients in a bowl; add chicken. Marinate for 30 minutes; drain marinade.

- Preheat barbecue or grill to 200°C. For barbecue, thread chicken on 8 long skewers. If grilling, arrange chicken on a lightly oiled grill pan.

- Barbecue or grill chicken until well browned, about 4 minutes per side.

- Whisk sauce ingredients in a bowl. Serve chicken on cocktail sticks with the sauce handy for dipping.

Chicken fillets can be barbecued on skewers over hot coals or run under the grill. If you are using wooden skewers, you'll need to soak them to stop them burning. Using metal skewers saves having to do this. If you are cooking the chicken under the grill there's no need to skewer the pieces, simply spread them out in the grill pan. Then, pierce them with cocktail sticks for easy dipping and eating. You can add a bit of sugar-free barbecue sauce to the cooked chicken pieces to make a snack children will love. Or make an easy curry sauce for lunch. Chopped cooked chicken fillets served in wraps are easy to hold and not messy.

Picking Cocktail Sticks and Skewers

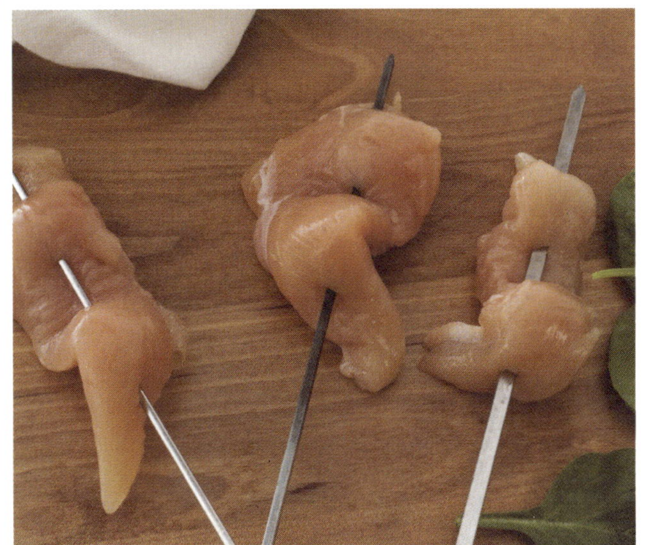

- Never insert plastic cocktail sticks until after food has been cooked. Otherwise, the heated plastic will melt into the food.

- If you use wooden skewers, soak them prior to cooking, or they will catch fire. If you are charcoal-grilling the chicken pieces, use metal skewers.

- If you are grilling them in the oven, don't bother with skewers; spear them with cocktail sticks when done.

Switching Up Sizes

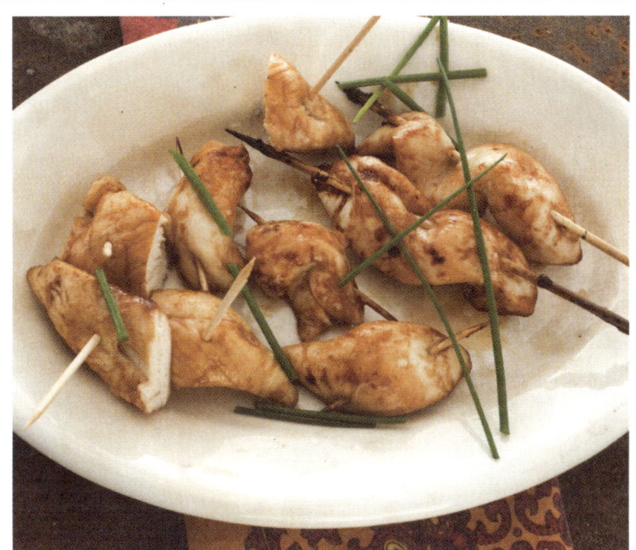

- If you are cooking the chicken to 'grab and go,' you should probably make the pieces bite-size.

- When preparing them for a crowd who will be sitting around and eating, you can make them larger.

- If you are feeding them to little children as a snack, you may prefer not to use cocktail sticks or wooden skewers, but just serve them as finger food with plenty of paper napkins.

HOMEMADE TOMATO KETCHUP

Better restaurants make their own tomato ketchup, and you can too

Commercial tomato ketchup is usually quite sweet and salty. No one needs all that sugar and sodium. When you make your own, you are in control.

You can also add your own personal touch when you spice up ketchup with sharp vinegar, various types of citrus juice and/or zest, cardamom and extra cloves, cinnamon and cumin. Salt and sugar substitutes also work very well.

Turn the ketchup into an American-style seafood cocktail sauce by adding horseradish and lemon juice to the basic recipe. If you are going to eat the ketchup with burgers, add some beef extract to give it a beefy flavour. Extra Worcestershire sauce is another ingredient that works well when you make your own ketchup.

Ingredients

Makes 1 litre (nutritional analysis based on 2-tablespoon serving)

4 (400-g) cans chopped tomatoes or 40 fresh tomatoes, blanched, skinned and seeded

120 ml cider vinegar

50 g Splenda

2 teaspoons cinnamon

6 whole cloves

1 teaspoon garlic powder

1 teaspoon onion powder

1 teaspoon chilli powder

1 teaspoon cumin

Salt to taste

1 teaspoon cayenne pepper, or to taste

Calories 22, **Fat** 0, **Carbohydrates** 5 g, **Protein** 1 g, **Fibre** 1 g, **Saturated Fat** 0, **Cholesterol** 0, **Sodium** 21 mg.

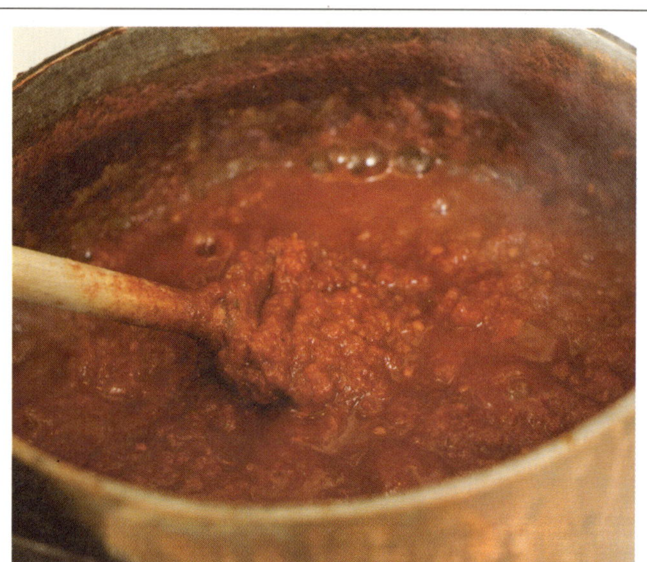

Homemade Tomato Ketchup

- Mix all the ingredients together in a large saucepan; bring to the boil over medium-high heat.

- Reduce heat to a simmer; cover partially, with enough venting to let the steam escape, as you want the sauce to cook down.

- Simmer for 3–4 hours, or until the ketchup is thick, rich and smooth.

Chilli sauce: It's easy to transform homemade ketchup into low-salt and low-sugar chilli sauce or barbecue sauce. To make chilli sauce, start with the basic ketchup recipe. Add 115 g tomato purée to the mixture, and cook the mixture down to 750 ml. Add ¼ teaspoon ground cloves and 1 tablespoon Splenda.

Barbecue sauce: Add 1 tablespoon mustard, extra hot sauce to taste and 1 tablespoon molasses. One teaspoon liquid smoke will give your barbecue sauce an outdoor flavour, even when you are cooking in the oven. If your menu features chicken, try adding 50 ml raspberry vinegar and 25 ml orange juice to the sauce.

Blanching Tomatoes

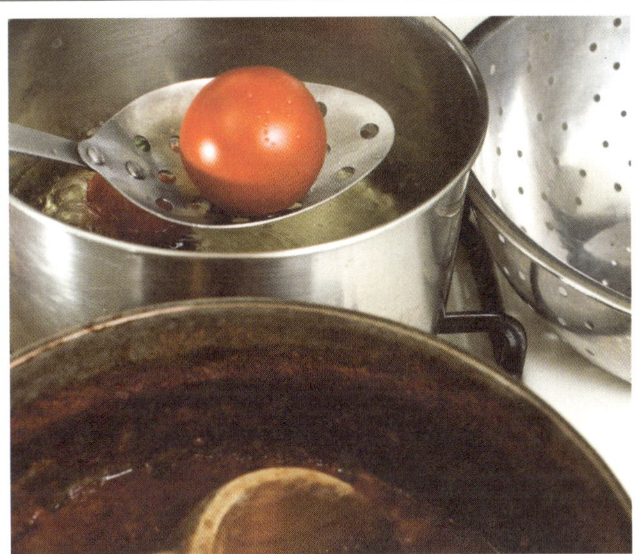

- If you are using fresh tomatoes, you will need to blanch them to remove the skins.

- Prepare a large pan of boiling water, and have a slotted spoon and colander ready.

- Slowly add the tomatoes to the boiling water, keeping track of the order in which you have immersed them. It takes 2–3 minutes of cooking to loosen the skins.

- Remove tomatoes to the colander. Allow them to cool, then slip the skins off. Remove the cores and seeds, and chop the tomatoes in a food processor.

Using Plum Tomatoes

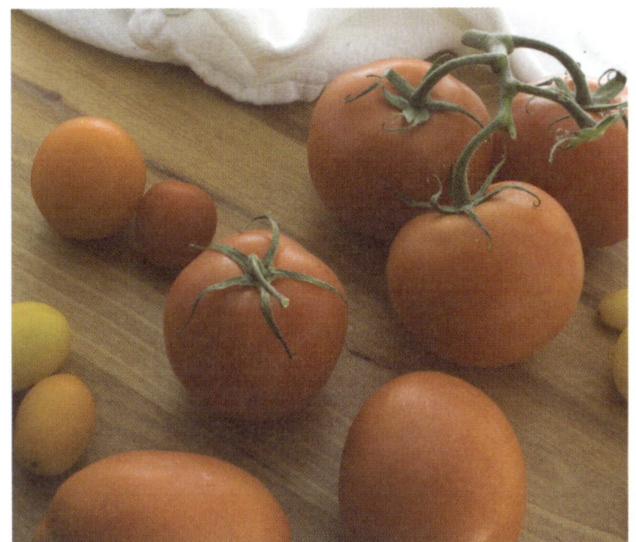

- Although most tomatoes are available year-round, you will find plum tomatoes in abundance starting in August in most places.

- Plum tomatoes have almost no core, are not very juicy, and have very few seeds. They are dense and meaty.

- They are also called sauce tomatoes or Roma tomatoes.

HOMEMADE VINAIGRETTE

A basic vinaigrette is always useful and should be on hand at all times

The most basic vinaigrette recipe is elegantly simple: it's a mixture of vinegar and olive oil. The proportion of vinegar to oil varies. It can be $1/3$ vinegar to $2/3$ oil, or ¼ vinegar to ¾ oil.

The fun part is adding such goodies as chopped shallots, basil oil, hot pepper oil and varying amounts of garlic and herbs. Citrus and fruit vinaigrettes are wonderful with fish and chicken. Fruity ones made with raspberry vinegar are enticing when blended with a fresh peach. Mango and curry vinaigrettes are also excellent options for the creative cook.

Lots of garlic and basil will make a delectable pesto vinaigrette. Add some mint, and use the vinaigrette to dress cold roast lamb for a summer treat.

Ingredients

Makes 250 ml (nutritional analysis based on 2-tablespoon serving)

50 ml red wine vinegar

2 tablespoons fresh lemon juice

1 teaspoon dry mustard or Dijon-style prepared mustard

$1/2$ teaspoon Worcestershire sauce

1 clove garlic, peeled and mashed

1 shallot, peeled and mashed

1 teaspoon dried oregano, basil or rosemary (or all three)

Salt and freshly ground black pepper to taste

$1/2$ teaspoon Splenda

50 ml water

120 ml extra-virgin olive or canola oil

Calories 83, **Fat** 9 g, **Carbohydrates** 1 g, **Protein** 9 g, **Fibre** 0, **Saturated Fat** 1 g, **Cholesterol** 0, **Sodium** 0.

Homemade Vinaigrette

- Place all the ingredients except the water and oil in a food processor.

- Process until well mixed.

- Slowly pour the water and oil into the mixture, pausing to let the oil 'digest' the mixture.

- Scrape down the sides of the processor, and give it another whirl. Pour into a glass bottle for serving or short-term storage.

Vinegar variations: Try to find different vinegars whenever you shop. Substitute sherry vinegar from Spain for red wine vinegar. Spanish cuisine is replete with aromatic and delightful sherry vinegar. You can also find Pinot Grigio and champagne vinegars. Raspberry vinegar is amazing with fruit, as is balsamic vinegar. Simply use as substitutes in the standard recipe.

Oil variations: For Asian flavouring, mix 2 tablespoons sesame seed oil into olive or canola oil. Walnut oil is marvellous as a flavouring added to olive or canola oil. Use half canola and half olive oil for a light flavour. White truffle oil is delicious. Deduct 25 ml oil from the basic recipe, and whisk in truffle oil. You can also substitute low-fat mayonnaise for oil to make a creamy dressing.

Whisking vs. Blending

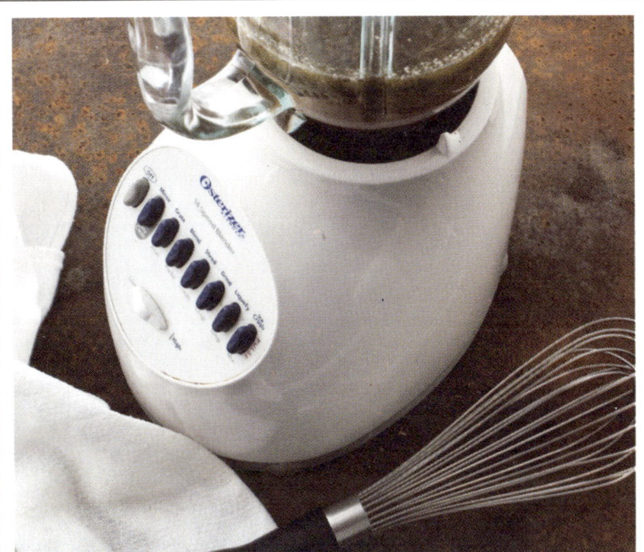

- A wire whisk is the traditional tool for making dressings. Whisking will take longer than using the blender. You will have an entirely unique consistency, as the dressing will separate more easily.

- Blending purées the herbs, fresh or dry, and the aromatic vegetables.

- Use a blender to assure a fully emulsified dressing. And always use a blender for large batches of dressing.

Caesar Salad Dressing

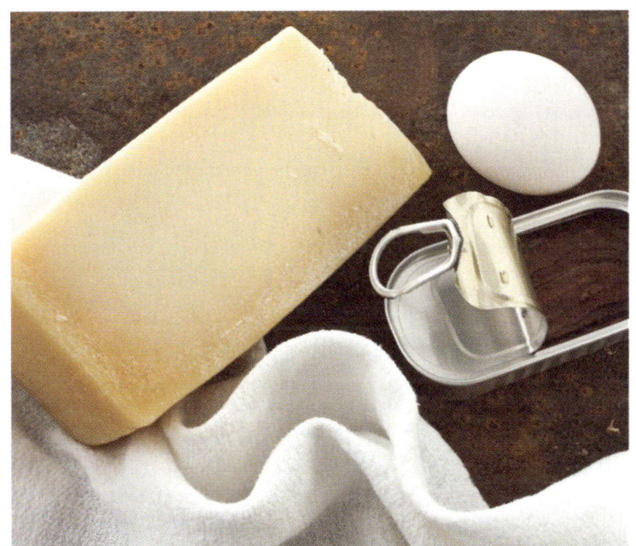

- To create Caesar salad dressing, add 1 anchovy or 1 cm anchovy paste to the basic vinaigrette recipe and blend well.

- Add 1 egg and blend well.

- Pour over 4 servings of prepared romaine lettuce leaves sprinkled with 25 g grated Parmesan cheese.

- Garnish with 2–3 low-fat croutons, if desired.

HOMEMADE MUSTARD

This spread can be adjusted to your preference for heat and spice

Jeremiah Colman began processing mustard in 1814, and in 1866 his product was given Queen Victoria's seal of approval. Colman's English Mustard is still around and is available in most supermarkets. In its powdered form, mustard is easy to mix into sauces and pastes.

Mustard grows just about everywhere, and the leaves, flowers and seeds are all edible. The three most popular mustard varieties are black, brown and white. English mustard is a blend of brown and white mustard. French mustard is blended with vinegar, giving a milder flavour, and American mustard, coloured with turmeric, is very mild.

The ancient Greeks and Romans used mustard for medicinal purposes in poultices and dressings. Today, mustard is second only to black pepper in popularity as a seasoning.

Ingredients

Makes 120 ml (nutritional analysis based on 1-teaspoon serving)

25 g English mustard powder

50 ml cold water

3 tablespoons olive oil

75 ml white wine or champagne vinegar

$1/2$ teaspoon salt

$1/2$ teaspoon Splenda

$1/2$ teaspoon Tabasco sauce

Optional: $1/2$ teaspoon celery salt, 1 teaspoon Worcestershire sauce

Homemade Mustard

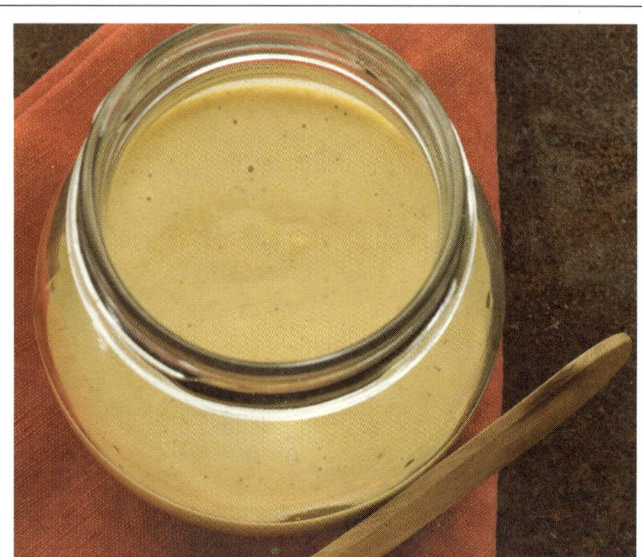

- Using a fork, blend the powdered mustard and cold water until smooth and free of lumps.

- Pour the mustard and remaining ingredients into a blender, and mix until smooth.

- Taste for seasonings and add more Tabasco, Splenda, salt, vinegar or optional ingredients as desired.

- Place in a glass jar and store in the refrigerator. It will keep for months.

Calories 49, **Fat** 5 g, **Carbohydrates** 1 g, **Protein** 1 g, **Fibre** 1 g, **Saturated Fat** 0, **Cholesterol** 0, **Sodium** 99 mg.

More on mustard: Most mustard contains some honey or sugar. When you are making mustard at home, sweeten it with Splenda. Using a mortar and pestle, it's easy to grind brown, black or white mustard seeds to as coarse a consistency as you want. Mixing mustard powder with various types of vinegar, juice and wine also creates delightful variations. Mustard is an essential ingredient in many barbecue sauces, pickle relishes and salad dressings. It is a subtle ingredient in Hollandaise sauce, and essential in mayonnaise and white sauce for fish and chicken. Mustard makes an excellent sauce for beef when mixed with soy sauce, and it's the 'devil' in devilled eggs. And what would a hot dog be without mustard?

Grainy Mustard

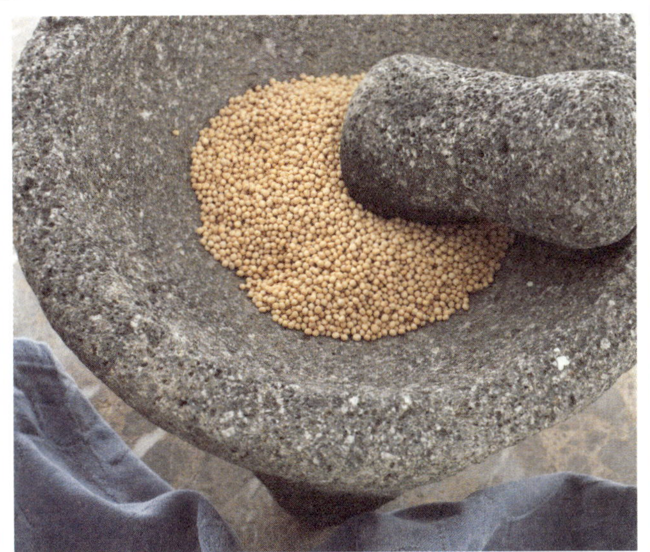

- Mustard seeds are available in many health food and gourmet shops. Buy 50 g at a time.

- Grind the seeds a tablespoon at a time to the desired consistency using a mortar and pestle.

- Follow the above recipe, substituting the freshly ground mustard.

- Store in a jar or crock, and refrigerate.

Changing the Flavour

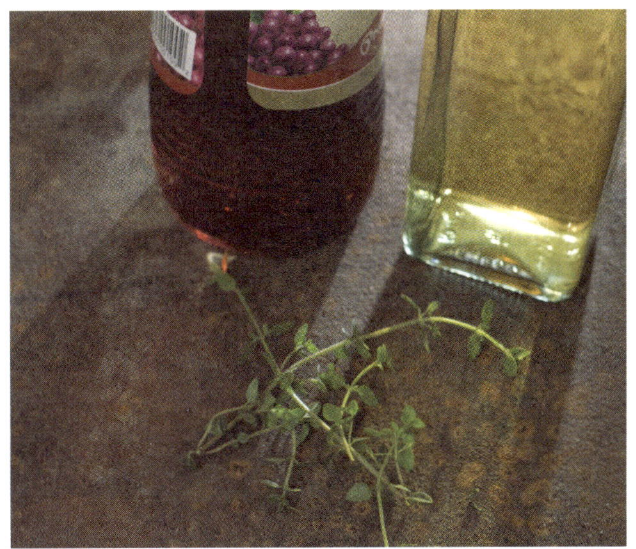

- Vinegar comes in a variety of flavours that you can use to change the flavour of your mustard at will.

- Try substituting 50 ml sherry or raspberry vinegar for the white wine vinegar. Or, substitute 50 ml orange juice for the water.

- Another way to change the flavour is to mix lemon zest into your mustard.

- You can add various herbs at will – just keep experimenting with flavours to develop a combination that is very much your own.

FRUIT COULIS

Liven up meat dishes with the addition of a seasonal fruit coulis

Making coulis requires the use of a blender. Historically, chefs put the fruit through a fine sieve or chinoise to make a perfectly smooth purée, and you might want to do that today to remove the seeds of raspberries or blackberries if you use them. If someone in your circle has digestive issues, he or she may not be able to handle the seeds even after they've been puréed in the blender.

Fresh fruit is best. Frozen berries are never quite as good as fresh, and canned fruit is too soft for a coulis. Use any fruit that is in season. Mangos with a bit of lime juice are excellent. Strawberries, blueberries and blackberries are also possibilities. Peaches are very good and can be used as a sauce on pork or duck.

Ingredients

Makes 250 ml, serves 4

250 g fresh raspberries, rinsed

1 tablespoon Splenda

$1/_2$ teaspoon salt

Optional: $1/_2$ teaspoon hot pepper sauce, 1 tablespoon fresh rosemary leaves, or 4 fresh mint leaves

Fruit Coulis

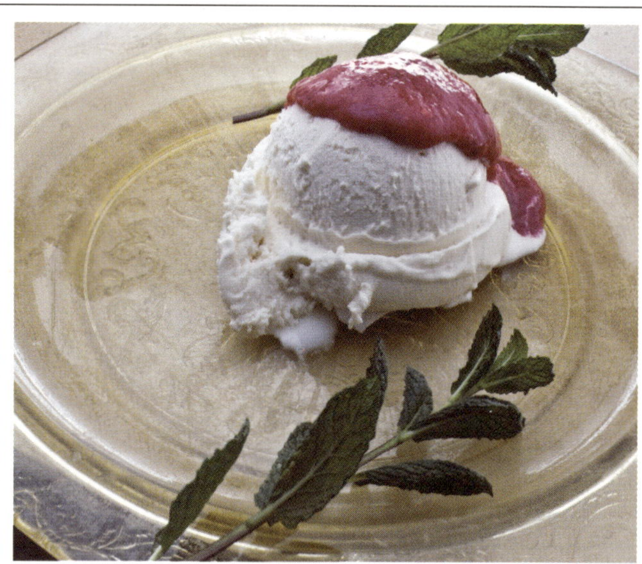

- Pick over the raspberries to make sure there are no stems or bad berries.

- Place all the ingredients in a blender and mix until puréed.

- Add optional ingredients, if desired.

- Store the coulis in a glass jar with a tight-fitting lid in the refrigerator. It will keep for about 1 week.

Calories 24, **Fat** 0, **Carbohydrates** 6 g, **Protein** 1 g, **Fibre** 3 g, **Saturated Fat** 0, **Cholesterol** 0, **Sodium** 1 mg.

Savoury coulis: By adding spices and/or herbs to the fruit, you will discover a number of creative and wonderful variations. Mixing, as in the recipe below, 250 g fresh raspberries with 1 tablespoon fresh rosemary and 1 teaspoon hot sauce or curry powder results in a terrific sauce for duck or chicken. Two ripe pears (skins on), cut up and blended with 1 tablespoon lemon juice and 1 cinnamon stick produce a fresh sauce that's delightful on chicken or turkey. Mixing fruit is also an option. Try 3 blanched, peeled and stoned ripe peaches and 125 g raspberries for a melba-type sauce that's as good for dessert as it is with pork or poultry. If you are making a coulis for use with meat or chicken, use less Splenda; a bit is fine, but you don't want the result to be too sweet.

Straining Coulis

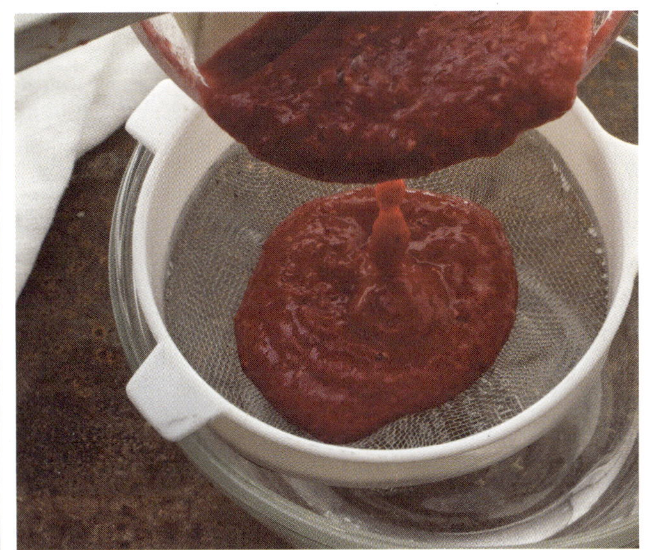

- If you are feeding a person who has denture trouble or certain digestive problems, you may want to strain even the ground-up seeds out of the coulis.

- Simply put the sauce through a fine sieve, stirring with a spoon.

- You may need to add 1 tablespoon hot water to make it easier to get the pulp through the sieve.

- Discard remaining seeds.

Using Hot Coulis as a Sauce

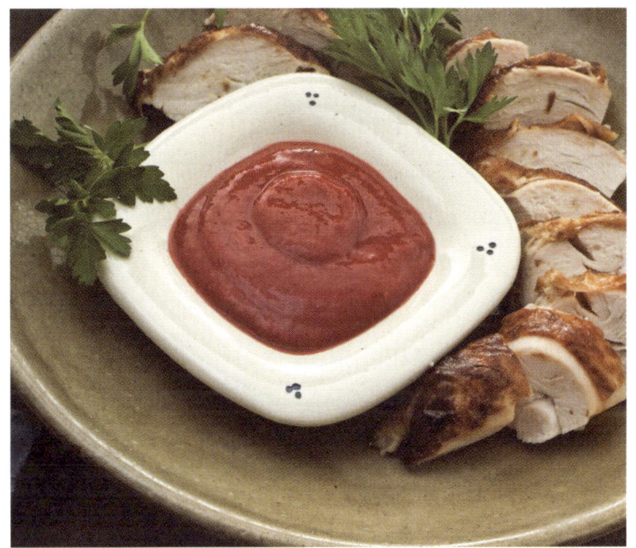

- By heating your coulis, you will transform it from a dessert sauce to one that is very good with meat.

- This technique is adaptable to various flavours of fruit coulis to go with different poultry, meat or seafood dishes.

- Do not boil it; coulis can burn easily.

- Pour the coulis into the top of a double boiler and heat, keeping the water in the base 1 cm away from the top pot to warm it without burning.

BASIC WHITE SAUCE

There's no limit to what a good cook can do with a basic white sauce

Everyone who cooks needs to know the basics of sauce making. If you can whip up a sauce, you can turn everyday dishes into amazing creations. This version of the basic recipe keeps the calories and sodium down to a minimum.

This white sauce is perfect for vegetables, and it can be spiced up for chicken, seafood or anything else you are cooking. It is also the base of many creamy soups with the addition of more milk and/or stock. The addition of sautéed mushrooms produces an excellent sauce for chicken. Adding chopped pieces of cooked chicken gives you chicken á la king. Two tablespoons of Parmesan cheese will also transform this sauce, giving it extra flavour.

Ingredients

Makes 250 ml, serves 4

2 tablespoons low-fat margarine

2 shallots, peeled and finely chopped

2 tablespoons plain flour

1 cup warm low-fat milk

$^{1}/_{2}$ teaspoon salt

$^{1}/_{4}$ teaspoon Worcestershire sauce

$^{1}/_{2}$ teaspoon ground white pepper

Optional: $^{1}/_{8}$ teaspoon ground nutmeg; 1 teaspoon chopped chives; 1 teaspoon sweet paprika; 1 hard-boiled egg, chopped; 1 teaspoon curry powder; 1 teaspoon prepared Dijon-style mustard

Calories 85, **Fat** 5 g, **Carbohydrates** 8 g, **Protein** 3 g, **Fibre** 0, **Saturated Fat** 1 g, **Cholesterol** 3 mg, **Sodium** 3 mg.

Basic White Sauce

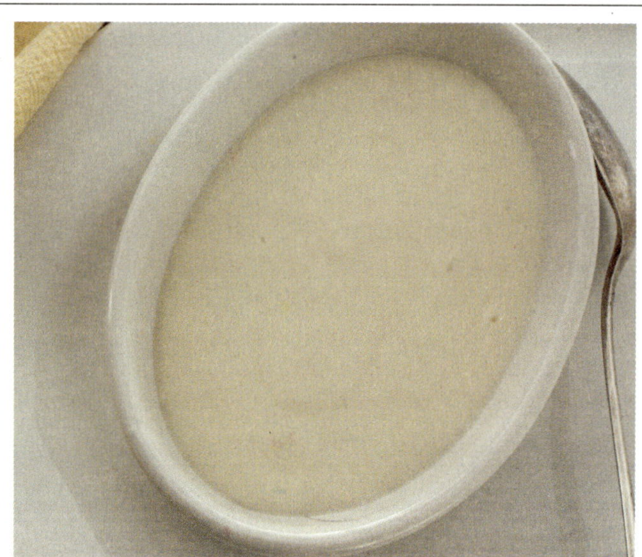

- Heat margarine in a saucepan over medium heat. Stir in chopped shallot and cook until softened.

- Whisk in flour and cook, stirring, until well blended with the margarine, about 3 minutes.

- Stir in warm milk, adding it slowly and making sure it blends, or you will have lumps in your sauce.

- Mix in salt, Worcestershire sauce and pepper. Reduce heat to low, and stir until very smooth and creamy. Add any of the optional ingredients you desire; serve.

Turning white sauce brown: You can completely change this sauce by substituting 250 ml beef stock for the milk. Brown sauce is superb with all sorts of meats, especially if you mix it into the pan juices from roasting or grilling a piece of beef. Sautéing 75 g mushrooms with the shallots is also a nice addition to the sauce.

Varying the flavour: Vary the flavour by adding 1 tablespoon dry red wine to the brown sauce. Adding 75 g roasted, peeled and chopped chestnuts will make the brown sauce perfect for roast beef or venison. To make a spicy, hot sauce, simply sauté 1 chopped jalapeño pepper along with the shallots.

Making a Smooth Sauce

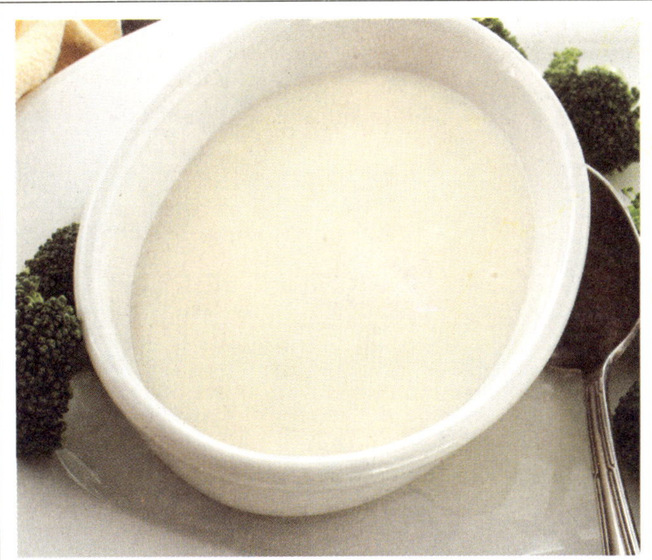

- If you don't sauté the flour prior to adding the milk, you will end up with a lumpy sauce and a raw flavour.

- If you add cold as opposed to warm milk to the sauce, you will get lumps.

- When adding lemon juice, do so just before serving, or the sauce will curdle or separate.

- Curdled sauce is lumpy, with an undesirable separation between the whey of the milk and the fats.

Turning a White Sauce into a Brown Sauce

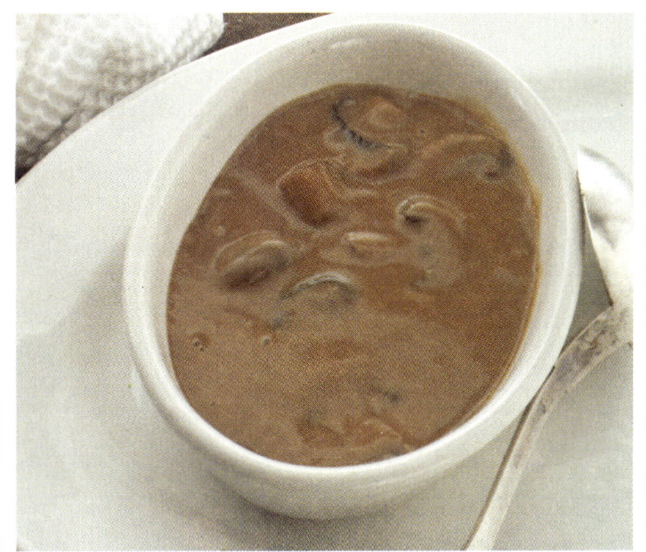

- When you are sautéing the shallots in the melted margarine, add 40 g chopped mushrooms to turn this into a brown sauce.

- Substitute warm beef stock for the warm milk. Follow the recipe as directed.

- Serve with roast beef or steak, or add to stew.

- You can also flavour the sauce with 50 ml red wine.

MANGO SALSA

The perfect recipe for the cook who wants easy and elegant results

Mangos have been cultivated for 6,000 years in Southeast Asia and India. They are in the same family as cashew nuts, pistachios and poison ivy.

There are 40 varieties of mangos, varying in skin colour from red to yellow to purple. Mexico is the world's largest exporter of mangos. They are the most eaten fruit in the world, growing generously in warm climates.

Mangos are an excellent source of vitamins A and C. Because they are, like most fruit, high in sugar, a little bit of salsa goes a long way. So serve it by the tablespoon or as a dip. A little bit mixed with low-fat mayonnaise is wonderfully tasty.

Ingredients

Makes about 250 ml, serves 24

1 tablespoon olive oil

1 small onion, finely chopped

2 serrano (for extra hot) or jalapeño (for just plain hot) chilli peppers, seeded and finely chopped, more or less to taste

1 clove garlic, peeled and chopped

1 teaspoon ground cumin

2.5 cm fresh ginger, finely chopped

Salt to taste

Pinch of Splenda

2 large or 3 medium mangos, peeled and chopped

Juice of 1 lime

2 tablespoons fresh coriander, finely chopped

Calories 111, **Fat** 4 g, **Carbohydrates** 21 g, **Protein** 1 g, **Fibre** 2 g, **Saturated Fat** 1 g, **Cholesterol** 0, **Sodium** 4 mg.

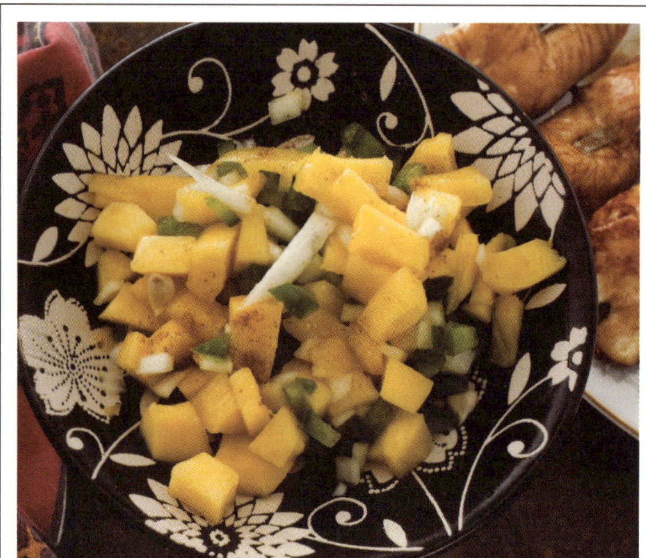

Mango Salsa

- Heat oil in a sauté pan over medium-high heat. Stir in onion, chillies, garlic, cumin and ginger.

- Cook, stirring often, until vegetables soften. Place in a large bowl, and add the remaining ingredients.

- Cover and refrigerate for 30–60 minutes before serving.

Serving mango salsa: When you serve mango salsa as a dip for cold cooked prawns, your guests will ask you for the recipe, and you may have to make a second batch. Mango salsa is also great spooned over cold chicken, lamb or lobster. The lobster can be served hot or cold, and the mango salsa can replace butter or mayonnaise as a dipping sauce. Mix it with mayonnaise and add it to turkey salad. Fruit goes amazingly well with seafood, poultry and meat. Most people serve cranberry relish with turkey and apple sauce with pork, but fruit salsas are much spicier. Serve mango salsa on the side.

Removing a Stone from a Mango

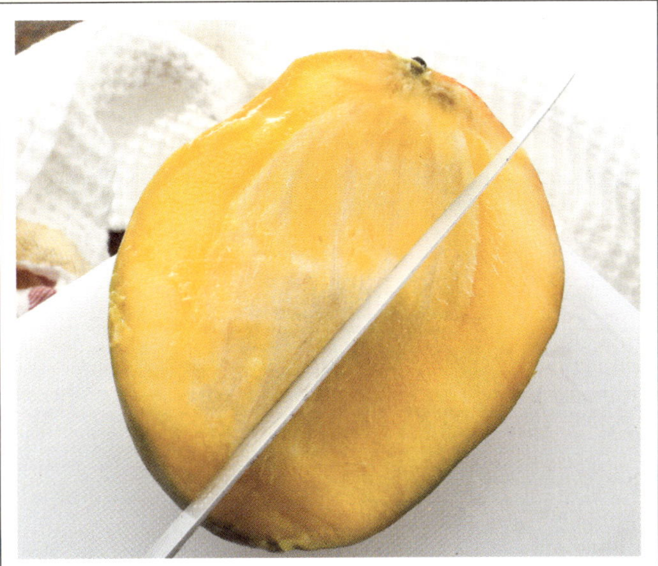

- To remove a stone from a mango, first cut the mango in half and twist it to release one side.

- Bang the side of the knife with the sharp edge down into the pit.

- Pull the pit out of the mango by retracting the knife from the fruit.

- Do not peel the mango. If you aren't going to use it immediately, sprinkle the fruit with lime juice to keep it fresh.

Dicing the Mango

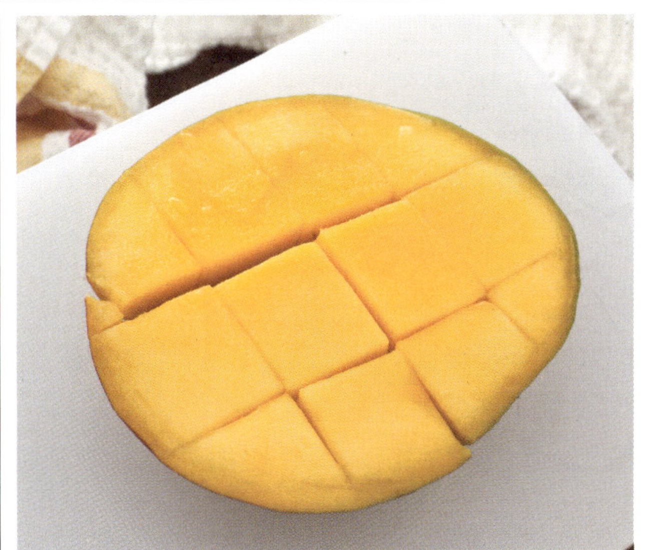

- Make cuts crosswise through the unpeeled mango. Do not pierce the skin.

- Make cuts lengthwise without piercing the skin. You will see the mango has been divided into dice.

- Using a spoon, scrape the fruit from the skin and into a bowl.

- Be sure to use the mango soon after slicing to ensure freshness.

BAKED PEARS WITH CLOVES

A classic dessert is lightened up with low-fat vanilla yogurt

Baked pears are a natural in autumn, served warm and well spiced; you will find everyone loves them.

You can use almost any kind of pear for this recipe; 240 varieties are grown worldwide. If they are thin skinned, such as Williams, you don't even have to peel them; however, they will absorb more wine if you do.

The pears are served with vanilla-flavoured frozen yogurt.

You could add a scattering of toasted walnuts or pecans for a wonderful contrast of textures and flavours.

Although traditional recipes for cooked pears often call for a sweet wine, this one does not. The sweetness comes from the pears and a bit of Splenda. The pears can be baked for just a little while and eaten al dente, or for long enough for the wine to become syrupy.

Ingredients

Serves 4

4 ripe pears, peeled, halved and cored

24 whole cloves

120 ml dry red wine

50 ml water

2 teaspoons Splenda

1 teaspoon orange zest

Topping: sugar-free vanilla frozen yogurt

Calories 143, **Fat** 2 g, **Carbohydrates** 31 g, **Protein** 1 g, **Fibre** 8 g, **Saturated Fat** 0, **Cholesterol** 0, **Sodium** 19 mg.

Baked Pears with Cloves

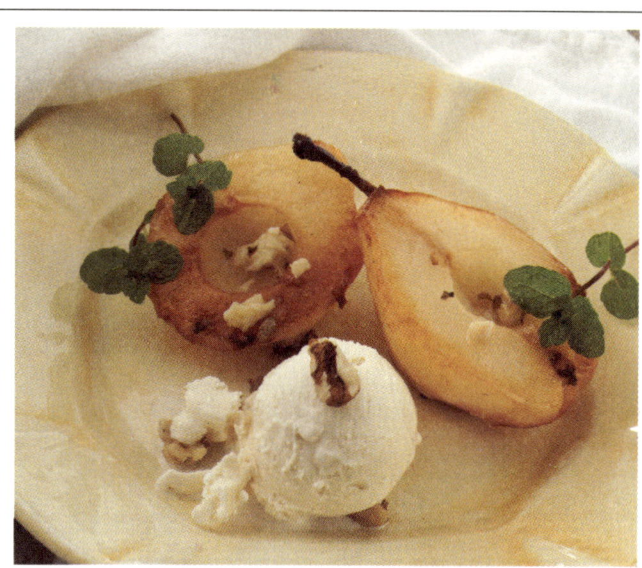

- Preheat oven to 180°C. Lightly oil a baking dish that will hold the pears without overlapping.

- Arrange pears cut side down in the dish. Stud each pear half with 3 whole cloves. Add the liquids. Sprinkle pears with Splenda and orange zest.

- Bake until pears are soft, about 20 minutes, basting from time to time.

- Turn pears, cut side up, on to serving dishes. Add spoonfuls of frozen yogurt. Drizzle sauce over the tops of the pears.

Simple and sensational: You can whip up this appetizer in no time. It's especially refreshing in late summer, when pears are first available. Cut 2 small ripe pears in half and remove the cores. In a small bowl, combine 4 tablespoons ricotta cheese with 1 tablespoon chopped pistachio nuts. Spread this mixture on to the cut sides of the pears and garnish with a few extra whole pistachio nuts.

Quick pear sauce: Serve this with chops. Core 2 firm but ripe pears; cut into 12-mm slices. Add pears to pan in which you cooked chops. Sprinkle pear slices with 1 tablespoon Splenda and ½ teaspoon crushed dried rosemary. Cook over medium-low heat for 3 minutes, stirring often. Pour 120 ml apple juice into pan; return pork to pan; simmer for 5 minutes.

How to Core a Pear

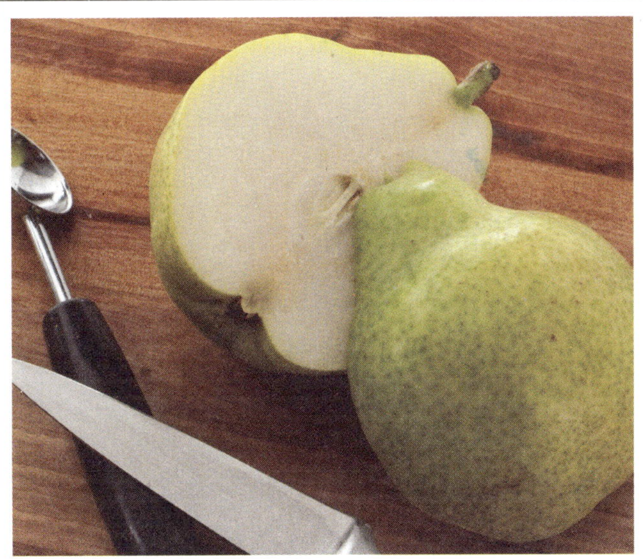

- Peel the pear, and cut it in half lengthwise.

- Using a paring knife, remove the stem and cut around the core.

- With a melon ball scoop, twist a circle around the core, and gently remove it.

- If your melon ball scoop doesn't go all the way around the core, the pear is likely to break.

Know When a Pear Is Ripe

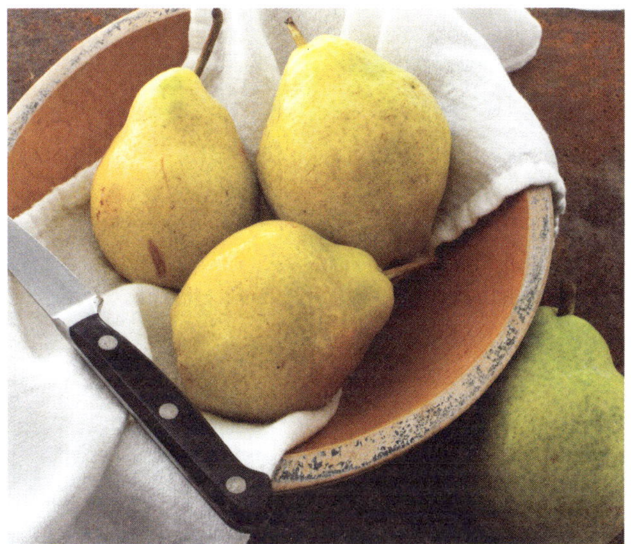

- To find out whether a pear is ripe, first sniff it. The pear should have a rich, fruity aroma.

- Then, using a paring knife, snip off a tiny bit of the fruit, right next to the stem.

- If it's hard and difficult to get the knife in, the pear is not ripe.

- If the knife slides into the stem end easily and the pear drips juice, it's ripe and ready to eat.

WATERMELON SORBET

Picture-pretty berries add to the high nutritional value of this dessert

Watermelon is an extremely low-calorie food: a serving of 150 g contains only 46 calories, and is packed with phytochemicals that are thought to boost your resistance to certain types of cancer.

The rule of thumb for 'power' fruits and vegetables is that the deeper and more intense their colour, the more nutritious and valuable they are for cancer prevention.

Watermelon not only boosts your 'health esteem', it is also practically a multivitamin in itself, containing excellent levels of vitamin A (important for optimal eye health), vitamin B6 (used to manufacture brain chemicals that help us cope with anxiety), and vitamin C (which helps bolster the immune system). The addition of the lemon juice and zest adds tang to this sorbet.

Ingredients

Serves 4

275 g watermelon, seeds removed, no white or green part

Juice and zest of 1/2 lemon

3 teaspoons Splenda, or to taste

Pinch of salt

Dash of Tabasco sauce (optional)

1 cup fresh blueberries, washed and picked over

4 fresh mint leaves

Watermelon Sorbet

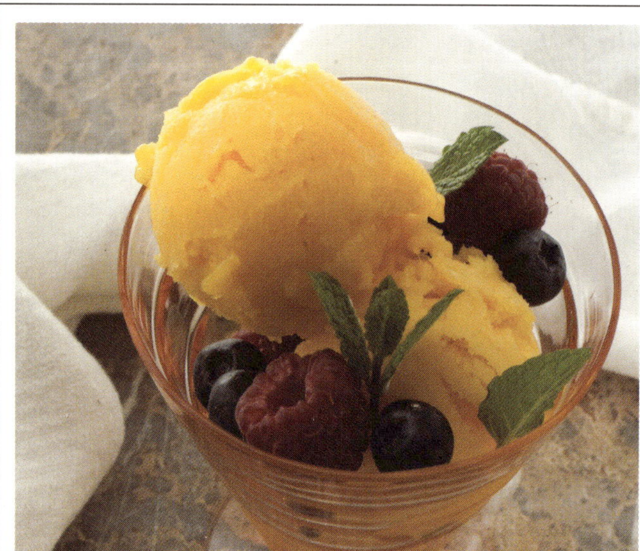

- Place the first four ingredients and the Tabasco sauce, if using, in a blender.

- Whirl until puréed; the mixture will expand a bit when blended. Stop the blender from time to time to scrape down the sides.

- Place in an ice cream maker and freeze according to the manufacturer's directions.

- Serve garnished with fresh berries and a mint leaf.

Calories 45, **Fat** 0, **Carbohydrates** 12 g, **Protein** 1 g, **Fibre** 1 g, **Saturated Fat** 0, **Cholesterol** 0, **Sodium** 79 mg.

Watermelon sorbet: The sorbet can take on a whole new flavour with the addition of 2 blanched peaches. Simply add the peeled, stoned peaches to the watermelon while you are blending it. Make dessert smoothies with watermelon sorbet: just add 250 ml plain yogurt and blend. Fresh raspberries also make a good addition to the sorbet: add 175 g to the purée as you freeze it. The whole berries freeze into icy nuggets that are very tasty and do not require any added sugar. Your sorbet will be a different colour if you use yellow or golden watermelon instead of the red/rosy variety. For a complete change of pace, make sorbet using honeydew or cantaloupe melon. The same quantities of melon and the same directions work perfectly well.

No Ice Cream Maker?

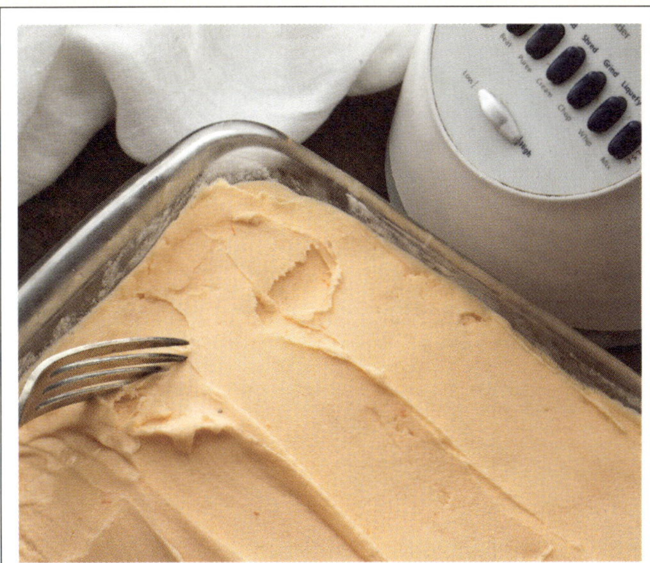

- Place the sorbet in a freezer container or a square baking dish.

- Place in the freezer. When the mixture begins to freeze, whisk it with a fork.

- When the sorbet is quite stiff, break it up and put it back into the blender.

- Return to the freezer. When stiff, place in a plastic container and keep frozen until ready to serve.

Sorbet and Ice Cream

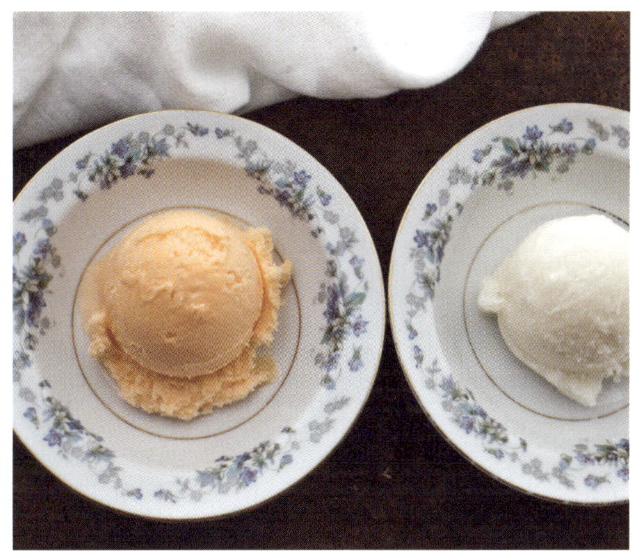

- Sorbet is basically a water ice made with fruit purée and syrup.

- If you make your own sorbet, it will contain fewer calories, and you can control the amount of sugar and the type of fruit in it.

- Ice cream is a frozen dessert made from dairy products, and sometimes based on an egg custard mixture.

- Some fruit ice creams are made using a sorbet base with the addition of double cream.

PEACH FLAN

The naturally sweet taste of summer is now available year-round

Flan is an incredibly simple dessert. It is equally good in the summer as it is in the winter. Very popular in France, Spain and Italy, this dish uses various seasonal fruits.

Flan can also be made as a very rich custard, when it is usually known as crème caramel. This classic and super-rich dessert is made with lots of whole eggs and cream. Sugar is caramelized on the bottom of a soufflé dish or ring-form mould. When the custard has cooked, it's turned out and the caramel forms the topping and flows over the custard to make a sauce.

This recipe has just fruit and more egg whites than yolks. The creamy, satiny effect is achieved with very few calories, and the sweetness from the peaches and Splenda is quite enough to make it delicious.

Ingredients

Serves 6

6 large ripe peaches, blanched to remove skin, stoned and sliced

Juice of $1/2$ lemon

250 ml semi-skimmed milk

25 g granulated Splenda

40 g plain flour

40 g whole-wheat flour

3 egg whites

2 whole eggs

2 teaspoons pure vanilla extract

$1/2$ teaspoon salt

Calories 167, **Fat** 3 g, **Carbohydrates** 28 g, **Protein** 9 g, **Fibre** 3 g, **Saturated Fat** 1 g, **Cholesterol** 72 mg, **Sodium** 75 mg.

Peach Flan

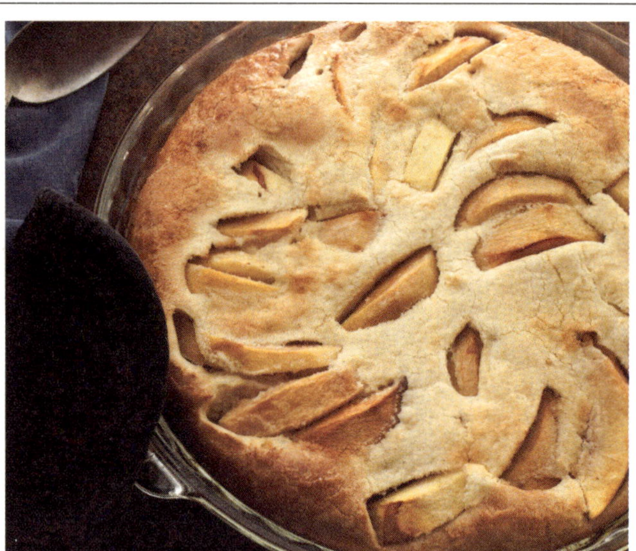

- Preheat oven to 180°C. Sprinkle sliced peaches with lemon juice. Toss.

- Place remaining ingredients in a blender, pulsing after each addition.

- Lightly oil a flameproof pie dish and add enough batter to thinly coat the bottom.

- Place dish over medium heat on the hob for 2–3 minutes to set batter.

- Remove from heat; place peaches on top of set batter. Pour in remaining batter; bake for 1 hour.

Peach substitutions: Flan can be made with apples, pears berries – just about any fruit you like and whatever's in season. For apple flan, peel, core and slice 4 large apples. Sprinkle with ½ teaspoon cinnamon, and proceed as you would with peaches. Have fun by mixing fruit when you make flan. Try adding 50 g dried cranberries to the apple flan, and 100 g fresh or frozen blueberries to the peach flan. You can also try plums and nectarines in the flan. If you leave the skins on thin-skinned fruit, you will add to the fibre content of the dish. This is especially true of plums and nectarines, as well as certain varieties of pears. Make use of whatever is in season.

Blanching Peaches

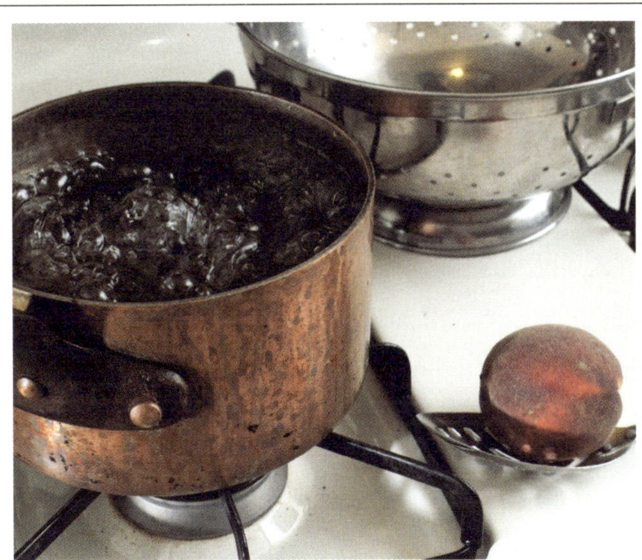

- Many fruits require blanching to remove their skins. Blanching is far more efficient than peeling, which removes a great deal of fruit along with the skin.

- To blanch, start with a pan of boiling water. Ease one piece of fruit at a time into the pan; return the water to the boil before adding more fruit.

- After a minute or so, remove the fruit with a slotted spoon, and leave in a colander to cool.

- Using a paring knife, slip the skin from the fruit.

Acid and Oxidization

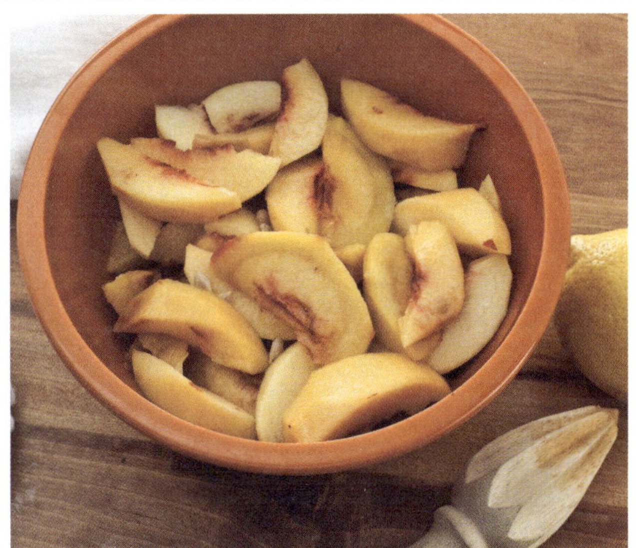

- Apples, bananas, potatoes, peaches and pears are some of the foods that will turn brown when exposed to oxygen.

- The brown is not harmful but can be unsightly.

- To prevent this, add vinegar or citrus juice to the item that will brown.

- In the case of peaches, apples or bananas, simply toss them with some lemon, orange or lime juice. Vinegar is better for potatoes.

MERINGUE NESTS WITH FRUIT

A classic dessert that just about everyone adores

The irresistible fruit-filled meringue dessert known as a Pavlova was created for, and named after, the famous Russian ballerina Anna Pavlova in the 1920s. There is controversy over the exact origin of the recipe. Some food historians say it was created in Australia; others claim it came from Europe.

Meringue nests are rather spectacular, whether you make one large one or, as here, individual servings. However, there is one warning: if the weather is damp or humid, make the meringue at the last minute. Humidity in the air or in the kitchen will soak into it and make it gluey. It should have a crisp shell and a soft interior.

To make the crust even more interesting, fold 25 g ground nuts into the stiffly whipped egg whites. Another good addition is fresh lemon or orange zest.

Ingredients

Serves 8

For the meringue nests:

5 egg whites

1 tablespoon plain flour

$1/2$ teaspoon white vinegar

2 tablespoons Splenda (for baking)

For the filling:

1 banana, peeled and sliced

120 ml whipping cream, whipped, or low-calorie whipped topping

225 g strawberries, hulled and sliced

1 tablespoon Splenda

Calories 85, **Fat** 3 g, **Carbohydrates** 11 g, **Protein** 4 g, **Fibre** 2 g, **Saturated Fat** 2 g, **Cholesterol** 11 mg, **Sodium** 50 mg.

Meringue Nests with Fruit

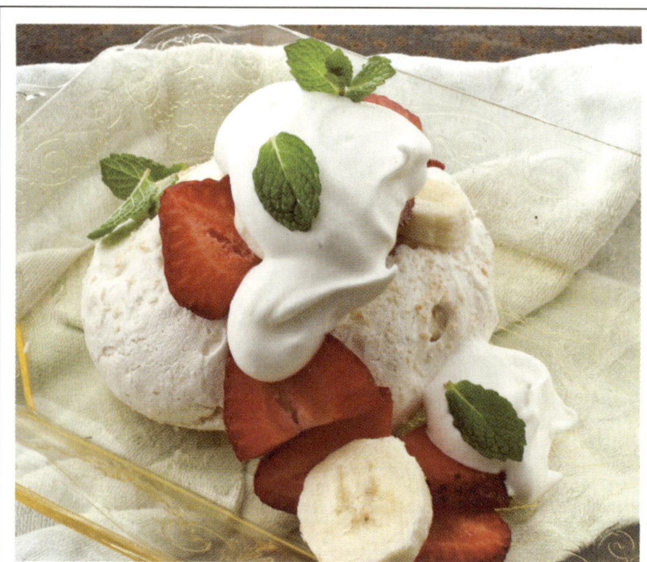

- Preheat oven to 120°C. Whip egg whites until foamy; add flour and keep beating. Add vinegar and Splenda; whip until high, stiff peaks form.

- Using a piping bag, pipe 8 meringue shells of equal size on a baking sheet. Bake for 60–90 minutes, or until shells dry out. Turn oven off; open the door slightly. Leave shells in oven.

- When dry, place slices of banana in the bottom of each nest. Cover with whipped cream and strawberries. Sprinkle with Splenda and decorate with reserved berries.

Fillings for meringues: Low-calorie fillings are delicious in a meringue nest. Try using vanilla, chocolate or butterscotch instant pudding. Place a layer, as in the recipe, of bananas on the bottom, and then add a layer of pudding. Decorate the top with fresh mint leaves.

The healthiest way to make this recipe is with all the fresh fruit you can find. Prepare all the fruit in advance and refrigerate it. Then, use low-calorie whipped topping between the layers. Don't fill the meringue in advance or it will get soggy. Have all your fillings at the ready, and then fill just before serving.

Separating Egg Whites

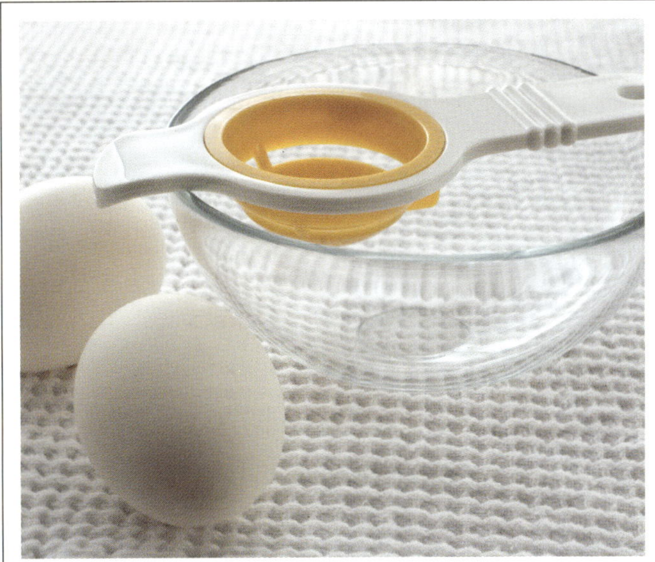

- There is a tool for separating yolks and whites. Place it over a cup or bowl, and break the egg over it. The yolk remains in the separator while the white slips through slits at the sides.

- Alternatively, break the egg and tip it so that the yolk sits in the small end of the shell. Pour the egg white into a bowl. Slide the yolk into the other shell.

- Add the rest of the white to the bowl. Pour the yolk into another bowl.

- Examine the egg white carefully to make sure there is no yolk in it.

No Yolks, Grease or Fat

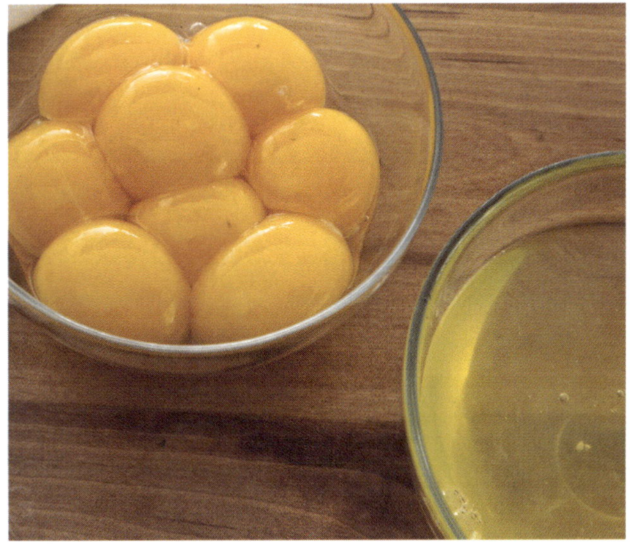

- In order to whip egg whites into stiff peaks, there must not be even a tiny speck of yolk in the whites.

- The beaters must be grease-free and immaculately clean, or the eggs will not whip into peaks.

- The bowl in which you whip the eggs must also be totally clean and free of grease.

- If there is even a bit of yolk, grease, or fat on any part of the equipment, the eggs will foam slightly but not get stiff.

WALNUT-STUFFED BAKED APPLES

Old-fashioned baked apples are as delicious as apple pie and less fattening

Almost every variety of apple is suitable for baking. Eating apples such as Russets will keep their shape, while cooking varieties such as Bramley tend to explode into a light apple foam when cooked.

Some apples are higher in sugar than others. All apples – especially when they are eaten with the skin on, as in this recipe – are high in fibre. They are also high in phytochemicals, which are cancer preventatives, and they promote regularity, as any high-fibre food does. Hence the old saying, 'An apple a day keeps the doctor away.'

This recipes provides a healthy alternative to a traditional apple pie dessert.

Ingredients

Serves 4

4 teaspoons finely chopped walnuts

4 teaspoons Splenda

1 teaspoon cinnamon

4 large apples

2 teaspoons low-fat margarine

250 ml cloudy apple juice

4 tablespoons sugar-free vanilla frozen yogurt or sugar-free ice cream

Calories 199, **Fat** 5 g, **Carbohydrates** 41 g, **Protein** 3 g, **Fibre** 6 g, **Saturated Fat** 1 g, **Cholesterol** 1 mg, **Sodium** 30 mg.

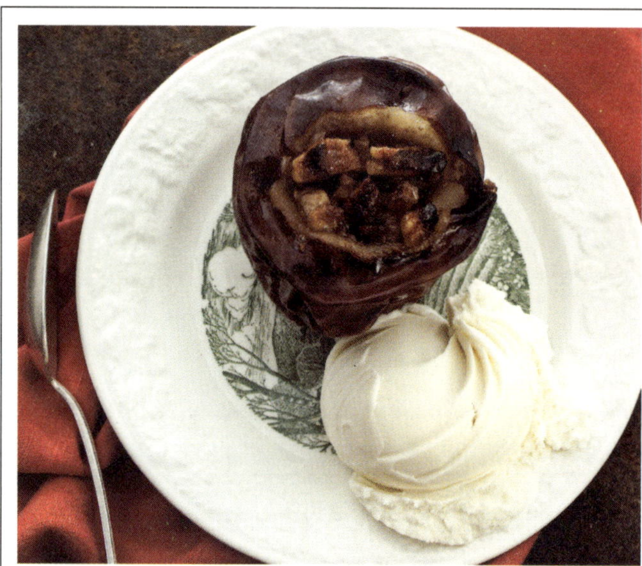

Walnut-Stuffed Baked Apples

- Preheat oven to 180°C and lightly oil a baking dish.

- Mix walnuts, Splenda, and cinnamon in bowl.

- Core apples. Stuff nut mixture into apples and arrange in dish close together so that they hold each other up.

- Dot tops of apples with low-fat margarine and pour apple juice over the top.

- Bake for 25 minutes. Don't let them dry out: add more juice or water if necessary.

- Serve with 1 tablespoon frozen yogurt or ice cream.

Baked stuffed apples cut in half: Baked stuffed apples don't always have to be cored with a vertical hole going down the centre. Try simply cutting the apple in half from top to bottom, and scooping the core out with a grapefruit spoon or melon ball scoop. Place apple skin-side down in a baking dish. Mound the entire half with 1 heaped table-spoon mixed chopped nuts, raisins, Splenda and the spices in the recipe. Sprinkle with 1 tablespoonful breadcrumbs. Moisten each apple with 1 tablespoon apple juice and 1 teaspoon low-calorie margarine. Bake until apple halves are softened and topping is golden brown. Alternatively, mound chopped nuts, pecans, almonds or walnuts on apples. Sprinkle chopped nuts with fresh orange zest and moisten with orange juice.

Barbecued Fruit

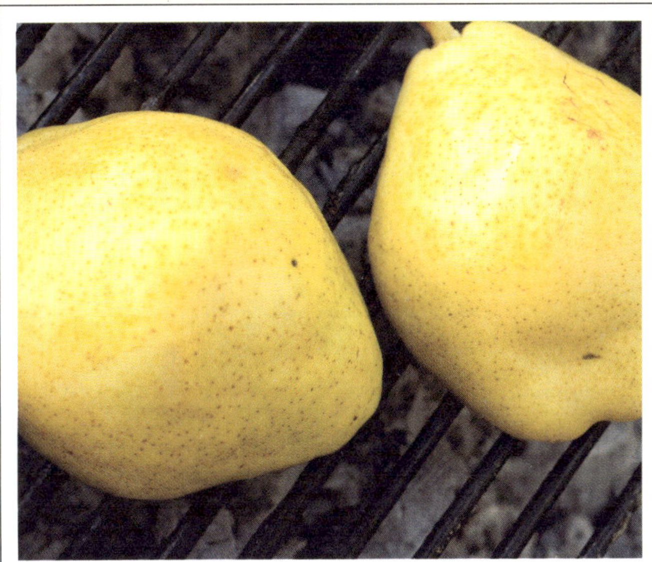

- Many types of fruit are excellent when cooked on a charcoal or gas barbecue as opposed to being baked in the oven.

- When you barbecue a pear or peach, don't skin the fruit. Brush it with lemon juice. You don't have to barbecue the fruit for a long time, just until it's very hot.

- Because it's drier than baked fruit, barbecued fruit needs to be dressed with a sauce, a bit of low-fat margarine or a sweetened cheese, such as low-calorie cream cheese mixed with Splenda.

Macerated Fruit

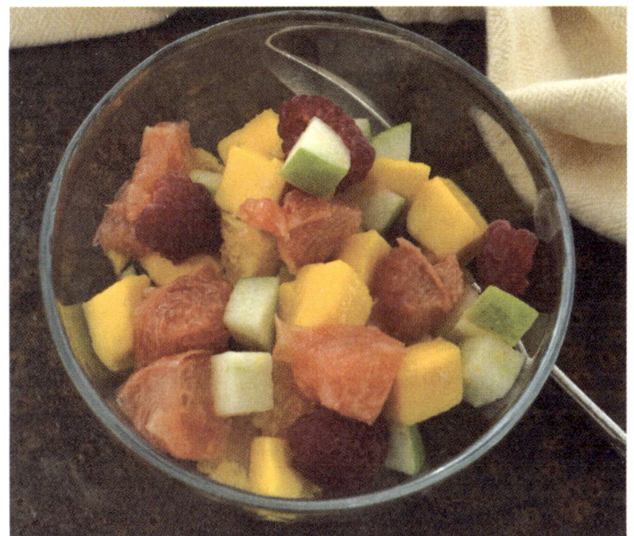

- Macerated fruit is basically fruit that's been 'cooked' in citrus juice. This is an easy way to prepare a mixture of fruit.

- Fill a 1-litre bowl with a mix-ture of seasonal fruits, such as bananas and pineapples, that have been peeled, stoned and cut into pieces.

- Add 120 ml orange juice, 1 teaspoon curry powder and Splenda to taste. You can also use a liqueur, but this will add sugar and calories.

- Toss to coat well. Leave to 'cook' in the refrigerator for 1–2 hours, then serve.

GLOSSARY
The language of cooking

Baste: To brush food with a liquid during cooking to keep it moist as it roasts or bakes.

Beat: To manipulate food with a spoon, mixer or whisk to amalgamate ingredients and incorporate air.

Blanch: To briefly cook food, primarily vegetables or fruits, to remove skin or fix colour.

Brown: To cook food so that the surface caramelizes, adding colour and flavour.

Caramelize: To cook until the sugars and proteins in a food combine to form complex compounds, browning the food and creating appetizing flavours.

Charcoal: Real charcoal is made by burning solid wood in a controlled atmosphere without carbon; it becomes almost pure carbon.

Chill: To refrigerate a food or place it in an ice-water bath to cool rapidly.

Chop: To cut food into small pieces using a chef's knife or a food processor.

Coat: To cover food in another ingredient to provide a protective flavoured or textured surface, such as coating chicken breasts with breadcrumbs.

Deglaze: To add liquid to a pan that has been used to sauté meat, fish or vegetables, to release caramelized residue stuck to the pan, which flavours the sauce.

Dice: To cut food into small, even cubes, usually about 6 mm square.

Flake: To encourage cooked fish to break into small pieces; also to cut food into thin slivers.

Fold: To combine two soft or liquid mixtures together, using a gentle over-and-under action with a large spoon, to avoid beating out previously incorporated air.

Grate: To remove small pieces or shreds of food such as cheese, chocolate or citrus fruit zest, using a box grater, rotary grater or microplane.

Grill: To cook food quickly close to the heat source, as under an overhead grill or on a griddle or barbecue.

Marinade: A mixture of an acid, such as citrus, oil and seasonings used to flavour meat, fruits and vegetables before cooking.

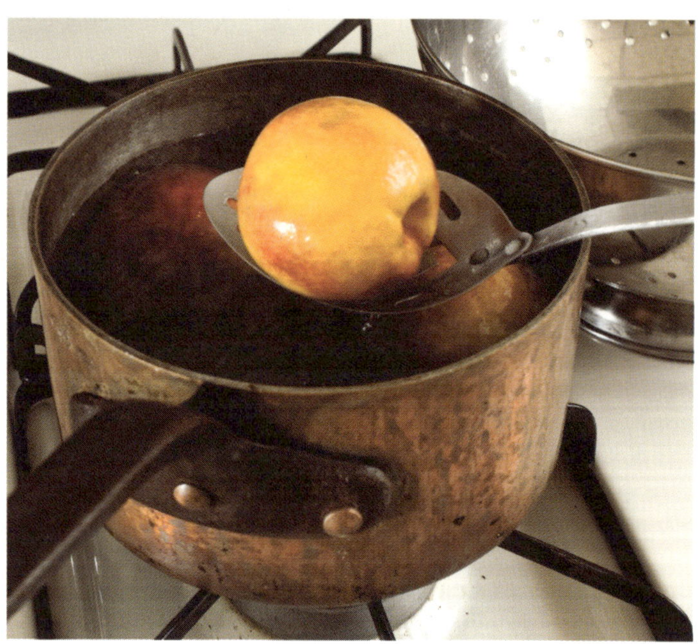

Marinate: To steep meat, fish or vegetables in a mixture of an acid and oil, to tenderize and add flavour and succulence.

Melt: To turn a solid into a liquid, by the addition of heat.

Pan-fry: To cook quickly in a shallow pan, in a small amount of fat over relatively high heat.

Shred: To use a coarse grater to create small strips of food, or to pull meat such as chicken apart into small pieces.

Simmer: A state of liquid cooking over very gentle heat, where the liquid stays just below boiling point.

Skewer: As a noun, a sharp metal or wooden stick threaded with food. As a verb, to place food on a skewer to make kebabs.

Slow cooker: A thermostatically controlled appliance that cooks food by surrounding it with low, steady heat.

Soup: A mixture of solids and liquids served hot or cold, as a main dish or part of a multicourse meal.

Steam: To cook food by immersing it in steam. Food is set in a perforated container over boiling liquid.

Stock: Flavoured liquid obtained by cooking meat, bones, vegetables or fish in water, used as the basis for soups and sauces.

Toss: To combine food using two spoons or a spoon and a fork until mixed.

Whisk: Both a mixing tool, which is made of loops of steel, and a method, which combines food until smooth while incorporating air in the mixture.

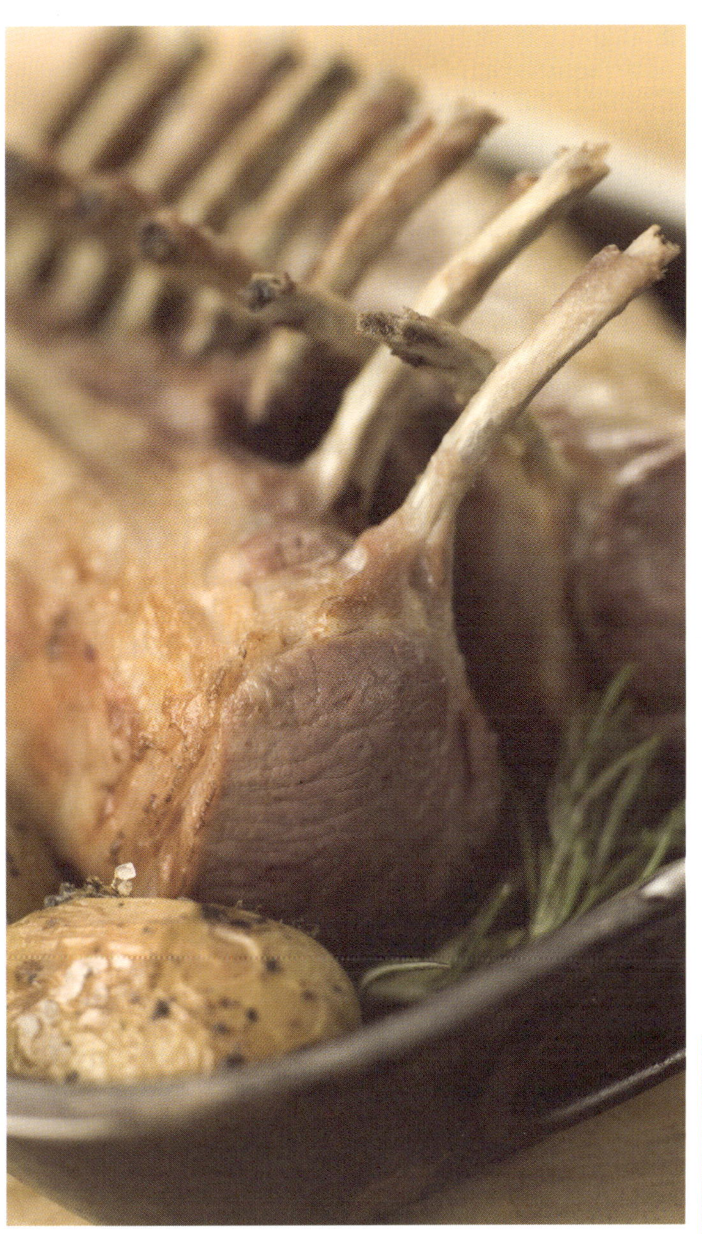

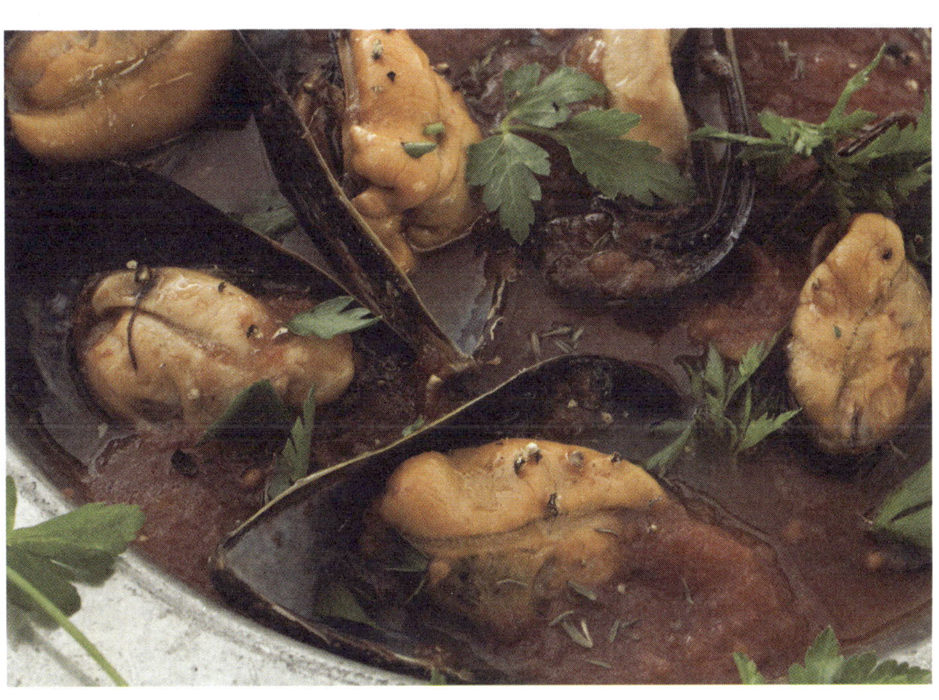

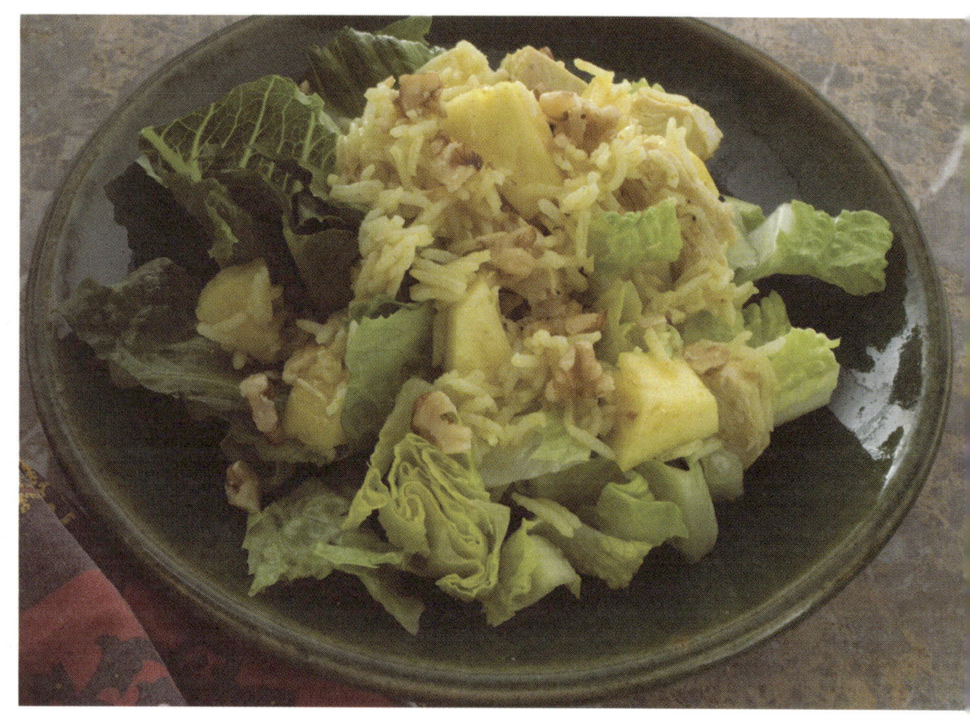

226